MAY 0 3 2010

W9-AOA-069

Medical Uses
of Statistics

3rd Edition

Medical Uses
of Statistics

3rd Edition

 The NEW ENGLAND
JOURNAL of MEDICINE

EDITED BY

JOHN C. BAILAR III
DAVID C. HOAGLIN

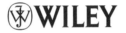

A JOHN WILEY & SONS, INC., PUBLICATION

RA
409
.M43
2009
science
Library

Copyright © 2009 by Massachusetts Medical Society. All rights reserved.

Published by John Wiley & Sons, Inc., Hoboken, New Jersey.
Published simultaneously in Canada

No part of this publication may be reproduced, stored in a retrieval system, or transmitted in any form or by any means, electronic, mechanical, photocopying, recording, scanning, or otherwise, except as permitted under Section 107 or 108 of the 1976 United States Copyright Act, without either the prior written permission of the Publisher, or authorization through payment of the appropriate per-copy fee to the Copyright Clearance Center, Inc., 222 Rosewood Drive, Danvers, MA 01923, 978-750-8400, fax 978-750-4470, or on the web at www.copyright.com. Requests to the Publisher for permission should be addressed to the Permissions Department, Massachusetts Medical Society, 860 Winter Street, Waltham, MA 02451.

Limit of Liability/Disclaimer of Warranty: While the publisher and author have used their best efforts in preparing this book, they make no representation or warranties with respect to the accuracy or completeness of the contents of this book and specifically disclaim any implied warranties of merchantability or fitness for a particular purpose. No warranty may be created or extended by sales representatives or written sales materials. The advice and strategies contained herein may not be suitable for your situation. You should consult with a professional where appropriate. Neither the publisher nor the author shall be liable for any loss of profit or any other commercial damages, including but not limited to special, incidental, consequential, or other damages.

For general information on our other products and services or for technical support, please contact our Customer Care Department within the United States at 877-762-2974, outside the United States at 317-572-3993 or fax 317-572-4002.

Wiley also published its books in a variety of electronic formats. Some content that appears in print may not be available in electronic formats. For more information about Wiley products, visit our web site at www.wiley.com.

Library of Congress Cataloging in Publication Data:
Medical uses of statistics / edited by John C. Bailar III, David C. Hoaglin. — 3rd ed.
    p. ; cm.
  Includes articles originally published in the New England journal of medicine.
  Includes bibliographical references and index.
  ISBN 978-0-470-43952-4 (cloth) — ISBN 978-0-470-43953-1 (pbk.)
1. Medical statistics. 2. Clinical medicine — Research — Statistical methods. I. Bailar III, John C. (John Christian), 1932- II. Hoaglin, David C. (David Caster), 1944- III. New England Journal of Medicine.
  [DNLM: 1. Statistics as Topic — Collected Works. 2. Research — methods — Collected Works. WA 950 M489 2009]
RA409.M43 2009
610.72—dc22
                                                              2009017256

Printed in the United States of America
10 9 8 7 6 5 4 3 2 1

262427444

To

Frederick Mosteller (1916–2006)

superb teacher

supportive friend

and wise collaborator

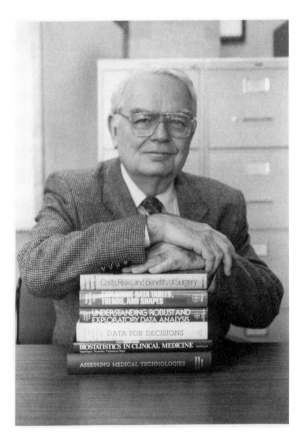

Contents

Contributors

Shilpi Agarwal, M.B.B.S.
Department of Epidemiology; Harvard School of Public Health

Paul S. Albert, Ph.D.
Biometric Research Branch, National Cancer Institute

John C. Bailar III, M.D., Ph.D.
Professor Emeritus, University of Chicago; Scholar in Residence, National Academies

A. John Bailer, Ph.D.
Department of Mathematics & Statistics, Miami University

Graham A. Colditz, M.D., Dr.P.H.
Department of Surgery, Washington University School of Medicine

Fernando Delgado, M.S.
Colombia, South America

Christl Donnelly, D.Sc.
Department of Biostatistics, School of Public Health, Harvard University

Jeffrey M. Drazen, M.D.
Editor-in-Chief, New England Journal of Medicine

John D. Emerson, Ph.D.
Department of Mathematics, Middlebury College

Mark S. Goldberg, Ph.D.
Department of Medicine, McGill University

David C. Hoaglin, Ph.D.
Abt Bio-Pharma Solutions, Inc.

Hossein Hosseini, Ph.D.
Digital Equipment Corporation, Irvine, California

David J. Hunter, M.B.B.S.
Department of Medicine, Brigham & Women's Hospital; Harvard School of Public Health

xi

Joseph A. Ingelfinger, M.D.
Bowdoin Street Health Center, Harvard Medical School

Thorsten Kurz, Ph.D.
Core Facility Genomics, University Hospital Freiburg, Germany

Stephen W. Lagakos, Ph.D.
Department of Biostatistics, School of Public Health, Harvard University

Philip W. Lavori, Ph.D.
Department of Psychiatry and Human Behavior, Brown University

Thomas A. Louis, Ph.D.
Department of Biostatistics, Johns Hopkins Bloomberg School of Public Health

Nancy E. Mayo, Ph.D.
Division of Clinical Epidemiology, Department of Medicine, McGill University

Stephen Morrissey, Ph.D.
New England Journal of Medicine

Lincoln E. Moses, Ph.D. (1921–2006)
Department of Statistics, Stanford University

Frederick Mosteller, Ph.D. (1916–2006)
Department of Statistics, Harvard University

Dan L. Nicolae, Ph.D.
Department of Medicine and Department of Statistics, University of Chicago

Carole Ober, Ph.D.
Department of Human Genetics, University of Chicago

Margaret Perkins, M.A.
New England Journal of Medicine

Marcia Polansky, D.Sc.,
Department of Biometrics and Computing, Drexel University

Amita Rastogi, M.D., M.H.A.
Ingenix, Inc.

Paul J. Rathouz, Ph.D.
  Department of Health Studies, University of Chicago

Michael A. Stoto, Ph.D.
  School of Nursing & Health Studies, Georgetown University

Rui Wang, Ph.D.
  Biostatistics Center, Massachusetts General Hospital; Department of Biostatistics, Harvard School of Public Health

James H. Ware, Ph.D.
  Department of Biostatistics, School of Public Health, Harvard University

Preface

The practice of medicine combines science and art. The science part of medicine derives largely from inferences drawn from experiments, often performed with the invaluable assistance of patients who put themselves at risk to become research participants. These brave and altruistic people have all or part of their medical care driven by the requirements of research participation rather than by their specific clinical needs. Investigators measure various outcomes and assemble the results of their observations in research reports, which medical journals review and publish to help guide the community's thinking about how best to approach the biology, prevention, diagnosis, and treatment of the condition under study.

It comes as no surprise that the clinical and laboratory observations involve many sources of variation, including measurement errors, intrinsic patient biological variability, and differences among patients in adherence to treatment protocols. These multiple sources of variation lead to uncertainty in assessments of outcome and in the clinical inferences drawn from them. Medical researchers apply statistical methods to these inherently noisy data and derive reasonably precise conclusions from them, taking into account not only the uncertainty but also other limitations of the data. Their experience with this process and its results also guides them in designing new studies. The conclusions drawn from these inferences drive clinical practice.

This third edition of *Medical Uses of Statistics* provides a broad first course in understanding the key ideas of quantitative methods that guide this process. Because we are interested in helping people understand the approaches used to study and solve problems rather than in providing a detailed manual for the investigator, concepts are explained with minimal use of mathematics. The approach maintains the emphasis in the first two editions, but this edition has been updated to include new methods and new disciplines. In the 17 years since publication of the second edition, new methods such as those used in genome-wide association studies or in multiple imputation for missing data have come into common use in medical journals. Because medicine is taught by example, the authors include multiple examples drawn from published articles, particularly from the *New England Journal of Medicine*, to illustrate each of the approaches and keep the presentation on firm practical ground. For the novice the book outlines the major statistical approaches used in medical analysis; for the expert the examples can provide hints about optimal study design and improvements in reporting results.

Regardless of your prior experience and expertise, it is highly likely, $p<0.001$, that this book will be a useful companion in the search for better information to guide clinical thinking. You can bet on it—keep reading, and you will see.

Jeffrey M. Drazen, M.D.
Editor-in-Chief, *New England Journal of Medicine*

Preface to the Second Edition (1992)

The first edition of this book, published over five years ago, found favor with a gratifyingly large number of readers and was widely praised as a unique contribution to its field. The Preface to the first edition, reprinted in almost its entirety, describes the book's origins and purposes. This second edition builds on the strengths of the first, extending its scope to new topics, while revising and updating treatment of many of the old ones and replacing a few of the original chapters with entirely new material.

The result is a slightly longer book, but I believe it is even better and more useful than its predecessor. The general philosophy and organization remain the same, but the range of subjects is broader and the overall treatment more comprehensive. Every effort has been made to achieve a readable and interesting text that explains the important ideas behind current medical uses of statistics without burdening the reader with the technical details of mathematical manipulations.

I found this new edition more interesting and accessible than the first. I trust readers will enjoy it as much as I did.

Arnold S. Relman, M.D.
Editor-in-Chief Emeritus, *New England Journal of Medicine*

Preface to the First Edition (1986)*

No one who reads the current medical literature, and certainly no one who performs clinical studies these days, can be unaware of the growing importance of statistics. Sound clinical research, as well as the ability to understand published results of research, increasingly depends on a clear comprehension of the fundamental concepts of statistical design and analysis.

This book is the fruit of an idea that originated in 1977, in conversations with John Bailar and Frederick Mosteller of the Department of Biostatistics of the Harvard School of Public Health. Convinced that the readers of the *New England Journal of Medicine* needed a clearer idea of how statistical techniques were being applied in current clinical studies, my editorial colleagues and I (including most prominently our former Deputy Editor, Dr. Drummond Rennie) suggested to Bailar and Mosteller that they organize a study of the research papers published in recent volumes of the *Journal* (and some other important medical journals), to determine what statistical methods were actually being used. We also asked them to tell us whether the methods were appropriately applied and how their use might be improved, and we asked them to do so in simple language that would be understood even by readers who had no education in biostatistics.

With the aid of a generous grant from the Rockefeller Foundation, Bailar and Mosteller, assisted by a host of colleagues at Harvard and elsewhere, set out to do just that. Their work was greatly helped by encouragement from Dr. Kenneth Warren, Director of the Division of Health Sciences, and Dr. Kerr White, Special Projects Officer at the Rockefeller Foundation.

The result, in my view, has been spectacular. First of all, they carried out a survey of statistical practice in the *New England Journal* and a few other journals, demonstrating the frequency with which different types of statistical methods were applied and identifying the need for improvement in the selection and use of these methods. In addition, the group produced a series of articles on a wide range of statistical subjects, drawn from the insights gained during their survey of actual practice.

All together, more than 30 papers have come from this project so far. Some have appeared in the *Journal* as part of our "Statistics in Practice" series. A dozen or so have been published in other journals or as book chapters. Still others have been reserved for first publication in this book.

---

*Text appears as published in the second edition.

There are many books on biostatistics, but there are two unique and important characteristics of this one that I believe set it apart. First of all, as already noted, it is based on current usage, and it is concerned with improving that usage. Unlike most standard textbooks, this book takes an empirical, practical approach. It does not simply use examples from the literature to illustrate didactic points; it carefully surveys what clinical investigators are actually doing with statistical methods, as revealed mostly in the pages of the *Journal*. It tells readers what they need to know to understand those methods, and it points out ways in which medical writers can make their reporting of methods and results more informative and their analyses of data more useful.

Secondly, the orientation of this book is toward an understanding of ideas—when and why to use certain statistical techniques. There are many textbooks that explain statistical calculations but few or none that attempt, as this one does, to get behind the calculations and tell what they are all about. This book does not concern itself with the mechanics of statistical computation. There are no instructions on how to perform calculations, and there are few mathematical formulas. The emphasis here is on explaining the purpose of the statistical methods, so that the general reader will have a better understanding of the strategy to be employed and the alternatives that need to be considered. Most chapters, however, cite other "how-to" textbooks of statistics, to which readers may refer for detailed explanations of the mathematical calculations.

The authors have striven to write in a straightforward style, as unencumbered by biostatistical jargon as possible. Their object has been to make this book understandable to almost anyone who has a nodding acquaintance with biomedical research and an elementary grasp of numerical concepts. How well they have succeeded only the reader can judge, but, as an amateur myself, I have found their writing lucid and readable. I should think that most medical students and physicians—even those with no formal statistical education—would agree.

I should note here that this book constitutes one of the *Journal*'s first ventures in book publishing. We hope it meets the standards of quality we have always tried to maintain for the *Journal*, and that it will find favor with a broad cross-section of physicians and students.

Arnold S. Relman, M.D.
Editor, *New England Journal of Medicine*

Acknowledgments

M any people have contributed to the completion of this third edition of *Medical Uses of Statistics*. First is Fred Mosteller, who developed the vision for the first edition and extended it in the second edition. Fred worked on the present update as long as he could, and then suggested that Dave Hoaglin take his place. He was, as usual, exactly right in his assessment of who could work well with whom. We are pleased to dedicate this edition to Fred.

Jeff Drazen first suggested that Fred Mosteller and John Bailar prepare a third edition, and Jeff has been a constant source of encouragement and support through the entire process, including reading and commenting on each chapter as it reached its final stages.

Doris Peter also had a critical role; as facilitator in the later years of writing, she kept us moving ahead even when moving was difficult. Doris had an invaluable role in managing the many versions of each manuscript chapter, and in seeing those manuscripts turned into print. Without Fred, Jeff, and Doris this book would not exist.

Joe Elia provided important support and advice as this edition was being blocked out. Elizabeth Platt copy-edited the entire book. Kent Anderson, at the *New England Journal of Medicine*, and Steve Quigley, at John Wiley & Sons, worked out the details of what was necessarily a difficult and complicated sharing of responsibilities for the completion and publication of the product.

We thank John D. Emerson and Kay Larholt for timely advice.

We are grateful to all of the contributors for their hard work, dedication, and patience in writing with a level and style that were unfamiliar to almost all of them. And we are grateful to readers of the first and second editions who told us about additions and other changes that they would like to see in a future edition. We hope that readers of the present volume will follow their example.

Origins of Chapters

Chapter 1.   Substantially revised, expanded, and updated for the second edition from an article originally published in the *New England Journal of Medicine* (1985; 312:890–7); slightly revised for the third edition.

Chapter 2.   Based on an original publication in the Carolina Environmental Essay Series (1988; No. 9), Institute for Environmental Studies, University of North Carolina at Chapel Hill, with some new examples for this edition. Printed with permission of the publisher.

Chapter 3.   Updated from the original article published in the *New England Journal of Medicine* (1983; 309:709–13) and from the second edition.*

Chapter 4.   This article was written for this edition of this book. It replaces an article in the second edition.*

Chapter 5.   Updated from the original article published in the *New England Journal of Medicine* (1984; 310:24–31) and from the second edition.

Chapter 6.   Updated from the original article published in the *New England Journal of Medicine* (1984; 311:705–10).

Chapter 7.   This article was written for this edition of this book.*

Chapter 8.   This article was written for the second edition of this book and updated for this edition. The version prepared for the first edition was based heavily on material in Ingelfinger JA, Mosteller F, Thibodeau LA, Ware JH. What are P values? In: *Biostatistics in Clinical Medicine.* New York: Macmillan Publishing Co., Inc. 1983:160–76. Printed with permission of the publisher.

Chapter 9.   This article was written for this edition of this book.*

Chapter 10.   This article was written for this edition of this book. It replaces an article in the second edition.*

Chapter 11.   This article was written for the second edition of this book and updated and extended for this edition.

Chapter 12.   This article was written for this edition of this book. It replaces an article in the second edition.*

Chapter 13.   Updated and shortened from the original article published in the *New England Journal of Medicine* (1984; 311:442–8).

Chapter 14.   This article is substantially revised and updated from the second edition. The original article, slightly modified for the second edition, appeared in the *Annals of Internal Medicine* (1988; 108:266–73). Printed with permission of the publisher.*

Chapter 15.   Slightly revised from the original published in the *New England Journal of Medicine* (2007; 357:2189–94).

Chapter 16.   This article was written for the first edition of this book, updated for the second edition, and substantially revised and updated for this edition.

Chapter 17.   This article was written for this edition of this book. It replaces an article in the second edition.*

Chapter 18.   This article was written for this edition of this book.*

Chapter 19.   This article was written for this edition of this book.*

Chapter 20.   This article was written for this edition of this book.*

Chapter 21.   This article was written for this edition of this book.*

**Indicates a chapter new to this edition or completely rewritten for this edition.*

Introduction

S tatistics is increasingly important to practitioners of medicine an
other medical sciences, including biomedical research investigators, bi
changes are so rapid that their knowledge of statistical concepts, meth
ods, and techniques may be out of date within a few years. As in the first tw
editions, we focus on the critical ideas, not on the mechanics. This is largely
book for the readers, not the doers, of statistics, though the latter might pro
from knowing more about the nature of the procedures they use. No prior s
tistical knowledge is assumed. Accordingly, there are few formulas of any kii
and fewer computing formulas. Our hope is that practitioners and students
medicine and other health fields will find here the resources they need to unc
stand the statistical methods that they encounter in the *Journal* and elsewher
the medical literature.

Changes in the medical uses of statistics are indeed marked. Agarwal, C
itz, and Emerson show how the use of statistical methods and concepts ir
Journal has changed from 1978–1979, to 1989, and now to 2004. They re
(in Chapter 3) that a reader with no statistical knowledge beyond such si
descriptive measures as means, percentages, and variances could fully ur
stand 27% of *Journal* articles in 1978–1979, but only 12% in 2004. Furthe:
kinds of statistical knowledge needed have changed markedly. Now, 66
Journal papers require some knowledge of survival analysis, compared to
in 1978–1979. Similarly, the proportion requiring some knowledge of (
miologic methods has increased to 53%, from only 9%. Uses of contir
tables and statistical power calculations have also seen major increases.
methods have decreased in frequency of use, *t*-tests and Pearson corre
coefficients among them. A substantially larger proportion of papers us
than one statistical method.

Thus, the needs of readers have changed with time. The 1989 survey
some changes in the content of the second edition of this book (1992),
shift in *Journal* content since then requires much more substantial changes
erage. We have replaced a chapter on clinical trials and added a second (
added two on statistical methods in epidemiology, and added two on stat
genetics. Other new or replacement chapters discuss linear regression, (
cal data analysis, meta-analysis, subgroup analysis, and risk analysis. '
kept a few chapters from the first and second editions because their mes:
current, but the chapters on statistical thinking, statistical content of th
cross-over designs, survival analysis, guidelines for reporting research re:

writing about numbers have been extensively updated, and a chapter on ordered categories also has been updated and shortened. Overall, more than two-thirds of the content is new; only three chapters are substantially unchanged.

This book is meant to provide self-instruction in basic aspects of statistics as used in medicine and other health-related fields, as well as to serve as a textbook for readers who are full-time students or taking continuing education courses. With few exceptions, we stress the concepts underlying statistics rather than its more technical how-to-do-it aspects. Most of our examples come from the pages of the *New England Journal of Medicine*. We deal with both the results of investigation and the presentation of results.

Although readers can find review and didactic papers on specific statistical methods in textbooks or journals, they may not always know when or how their knowledge is incomplete or out of date, and they may have nowhere to turn for overviews of the field. This book surveys statistical applications now used in clinical research and illustrates good and poor uses of methods.

Although each chapter stands alone and can be read as a separate work, they make up five broad sections. Section I opens with a chapter (Statistical Concepts Fundamental to Investigations) on the larger concepts of statistics. That chapter surveys some of the ideas that are central to statistical methods and techniques—ideas that guide all statistical work. These broad concepts are important even when no numbers appear in a research article: Users of statistical methods should not think of numerical techniques (such as estimation or special methods of testing hypotheses) as the main ideas in statistics, while leaving the big ideas unrecognized and neglected. Chapter 2 (Some Uses of Statistical Thinking) extends the concepts in the first chapter, and illustrates with four examples how the practicalities of real life often make the uncertainty associated with statistical inferences much larger than the usual formulas for confidence limits would indicate. Such challenges arise from the need for sound data in statistical analysis, errors in critical assumptions, and uncertainty about generalizing results in complicated situations, such as moving from data acquired from animal experiments to future human experience. The chapter includes an illustration of how a complex problem can be attacked as a sequence of somewhat simpler problems. The next chapter (Use of Statistical Analysis in the *Journal*), the third in a series, tells how often various statistical procedures were used in one volume of the *Journal* and what a reader should know to understand journal reports; this chapter on frequency of use offers practical guidance to persons planning a program of study, whether they are instructors developing courses or interested readers pursuing their own education.

Section II deals with a major statistical area—the design of investigations in the medical sciences. Chapter 4 focuses on randomized trials, which have come to dominate much medical research; it discusses issues of specifying

the question, choosing the method for assigning subjects to groups, appraising the choice of outcomes, weighing the statistical power of the study, and recognizing a need to end a study early. An understanding of these matters is important to readers whether the topic is treatment, prevention, or earlier and more accurate diagnosis. Chapter 5, on crossover and self-controlled designs, deals with two related, powerful, and often under-used tools of investigation. More-detailed comment on simple reporting of experience with a series of cases is then offered in Chapter 6 (The Series of Consecutive Cases), including some discussion of the difficulties in interpreting series of cases and of precautions that can be taken to improve their strength. Chapter 7 first illustrates the extent to which the concepts and methods of epidemiology have penetrated a broad range of areas of clinical interest, then presents and discusses some questions that the reader as well as the author should consider in any medical study of human subjects. No reader can really understand the current medical literature without a good grasp of these matters.

Although an investigation must start with a study design, analysis becomes the focus after the data are in. Section III describes some central topics in data analysis. Chapter 8 (p-values) discusses the meaning of p-values, the usual way of stating the results of tests of significance, which are widely used but often misunderstood. The chapter explains the assumptions that underlie p-values, which have a straightforward meaning only in the presence of likely alternative hypotheses. It is most important to understand the strengths of p-values in terms of achieving objectivity, as well as their weaknesses for decisions or policy. Therefore, this chapter deals with both uses and misuses. Section III then turns to five specific categories of methods. Four of these deal with major types of statistical analysis in the medical sciences—linear regression (Chapter 10), survival analysis (Chapter 11), categorical data (Chapter 12), and ordered categories (Chapter 13). This section also includes further discussion of some issues in the analysis and interpretation of randomized trials (Chapter 9, which extends the discussion in Chapter 4).

The increased use of survival analysis in the clinical literature has caused us to extend the discussion of failure-time data in Chapter 11. Survival analyses must ordinarily account for the fact that not all subjects in an investigation will have experienced some key event, such as death or stroke, by the time the analysis must be made. Competing risks are explained, as are the widely used Kaplan-Meier method of estimating survival distributions and the Cox proportional-hazards model.

Contingency tables are widely used to describe patients under study and to analyze the consequences of treatment. Thus, Chapter 12 (Categorical Data) explains notions related to the 2×2 contingency table, including odds ratios, Fisher's exact test, and the paradoxes that arise when tables are collapsed. One common generalization brings together 2×2 tables from several strata. The much-used technique of logistic regression extends the ideas of regression to situations where the outcome variable is dichotomous (0 or 1).

The chapters in this section make clear that investigators must have in mind specific questions about a set of data before they can make a rational choice of analytic methods, and that readers need to know what the investigators were after and how their goal shaped the design and analysis of a study—and what can or cannot be learned from it.

Once an investigation has been executed, the results must be conveyed. Readers and investigators may find the help they need in Chapters 14, 15, and 16 in Section IV on communicating results. When faced with the masses of numbers produced by any large quantitative study, one must consider what parts of the background and results to present. Chapter 14 (Guidelines for Statistical Reporting) gives the investigator some general ideas about what to offer readers and what to keep in one's notebooks. The chapter expands on the brief statistical guidelines given as the Uniform Requirements for Manuscripts Submitted to Biomedical Journals, published and periodically updated by the International Committee of Medical Journal Editors, and comments on some other guidelines. It gives advice about 17 specific issues that frequently arise in preparing a clinical paper containing numerical data. Chapter 15 discusses the interpretation of results seen for subgroups of a study population, which raises a vexing issue commonly known as "multiple comparisons," a matter that arises in several other chapters. The apparently simple act of writing about numbers (Chapter 16) can be much improved by understanding how to simplify, condense, and present quantitative data in text, tables, or figures. This chapter describes some common but easily avoided perils to those whose experience is primarily in working with words rather than numbers. It offers some conventions and rules about reporting numerical data.

Section V deals with five more-specialized topics. Reviewers of the literature assemble information about a particular topic from many papers. This assembly often goes beyond narrative review of the literature to a more-formal integration of quantitative information from different reports, often called meta-analysis. Chapter 17 (Combining Results) describes the various features of the research synthesis carried out by meta-analysts, illustrates the variety of methods used, and explains what a reader should be looking for in appraising a meta-analysis. Chapter 18 extends the discussion in Chapter 7 with diverse examples of regression methods applied to epidemiologic data. Chapters 19 and 20 take up a new topic, the statistical analysis of genetic data, including the investigation of hypotheses about genetic influences on human health and identifying specific genes that contribute to disease risk by genetic association studies. Chapter 21 surveys a field important to clinicians, assessing risks of various kinds to their patients.

Whereas the writing team for the first two editions was heavily concentrated at Harvard University, the authors of this edition are scattered over North America. Thus, we have given special attention to gaps and overlaps in coverage and to cross-references within the book.

John C. Bailar III
David C. Hoaglin

Broad Concepts and Analytic Techniques

CHAPTER 1

Statistical Concepts Fundamental to Investigations

LINCOLN E. MOSES, PH.D.

ABSTRACT   Statistics is a body of methods for learning from experience. Clinical research often draws on statistical methods, and an accurate understanding of their rationale is therefore important for clinicians as well as research investigators. This chapter examines the underlying logic of statistical methods as applied to clinical research. The discussion focuses on four key concepts: operational definition, the precise specification of terms and procedures; the infinite-data case, a way of considering what conclusions might be reached if the study were so large that statistical variation was negligible; probabilistic thinking, which focuses on the resemblance to be expected between the study's outcome and the results of an infinitely large study; and induction, the process of reaching conclusions about future cases on the basis of the data in the present study. The design of an investigation needs to take these concepts into account. The publication reporting the study should disclose fully and clearly how the study was done, what analyses were used, and how the authors interpret the results.

S tatistics may be defined as a body of methods for learning from experience—usually in the form of data from many separate measurements showing individual variations. Because many qualitative matters of clinical interest, such as alive or dead, improved or worse, and male or female, can be presented as counts, rates, or proportions, the scope of statistical reasoning and methods is surprisingly broad. Nearly all scientific investigators find that their work sometimes presents statistical problems that demand solutions; similarly, nearly all readers of research reports find that understanding a study's reported results often requires an understanding of statistical issues and of the way in which the investigators have addressed those issues.

Even more striking than the range of clinical studies where statistical issues arise is the importance of a few statistical concepts that apply to many different types of studies. This chapter presents and discusses four of these broad concepts.

The first key concept is *operational definition*. To learn from experience, we must first be able to state what that experience is. Labels are insufficient for this purpose. "Stage II disease" can have different meanings in different clinical settings. "Suicide" rates are likely to be very different in jurisdictions that do and do not require the presence of a suicide note before applying the term. A statistic reports the outcome of some measurement process; unless we specify that process, we cannot know the meaning of the statistic. It is this kind of specification that is meant by the term "operational definition."

Before they consider finite sets of data, statisticians usually find it valuable to consider what conclusions might be reached if the data set were infinitely large, so that statistical variation was negligible. In thinking about this *infinite-data case*, they pose these questions: If we had a very large quantity of data of the kind under consideration, would the data answer our questions? How would we analyze that infinite data set to explore and reveal its meaning? Could we change some feature of the data-gathering process to make that body of data more useful or informative?

Any actual study produces only a finite body of data, which can be regarded as approximating the infinite data set. *Probabilistic thinking*, which focuses on the closeness of that approximation, takes account of the number of observations and makes use of such statistical concepts as bias and variability. Its premise is that when the laws of probability are known to have governed the acquisition of data, then statistical inferences have the force of logical consequences of these laws.

Statistical inference, or *induction*, is ordinarily—perhaps always—a two-stage process. First, we must ask how well the data reflect what we would learn from an infinite body of data collected in the same way. We hope to discover how chance may have distorted the resemblance of our finite-data set to its corresponding infinite-data set. The issue raised by this question is sometimes labeled *internal validity*. A second question follows: If the data had been collected instead in a somewhat different way (e.g., by including patients younger than 55, by considering patients from community hospitals as well as teaching hospitals, or without excluding patients with diabetes), how closely might the data from our sample resemble the infinite-data case corresponding to such a modification? This question raises the issue sometimes labeled *external validity*. Internal validity is primarily a statistical issue; external validity can be evaluated only with the help of expertise and judgment in areas outside statistics.

The next four sections of this chapter discuss these four key concepts in detail and provide examples of their importance in clinical research. Two sections follow, examining the effects of all four concepts on study design and statistical reporting.

OPERATIONAL DEFINITION

Many medical investigations follow a characteristic pattern: the investigator imposes one or more treatments on certain kinds of subjects under controlled conditions, observes and perhaps compares outcomes, and then tries to reach conclusions about the effects of the treatments. The specific meaning of such a study grows out of the answers to a host of questions about the patients, the treatments as actually applied, the outcomes, and how the outcomes were assessed. For these answers to be accurate, they must faithfully take into account the actual procedures used in the study, and they must be precise and specific.

Description of Terms

Reports of laboratory investigations typically include specific accounts of equipment, procedures, and materials. An operational account of a clinical investigation is equally necessary, but often more demanding. A statement that patients have "disease A, Stages II and III" sounds definite enough, but the diagnosis of disease A may be somewhat tricky. We need to know how that diagnosis was made. What criteria were applied? How were the patients assessed? Were all cases assigned stages by the same person, team, or committee? If not, then how were disease stages determined? How reproducible is the staging? For instance, were any cases staged twice and blindly? If laboratory or microscopic confirmation was required, what is the effect of leaving out subjects with disease A who did not have that confirmation?

Measured characteristics present analogous demands. "Cardiac output" may be one thing if measured by angiography, another if assessed from blood gases. Blood pressure can vary greatly, depending on the state of the subject, the person who measures, and the device used. It is important to know how a measurement was made and whether the same method was used for all subjects. An often useful way to dispel ambiguity about the measurement of some elusive yet important variable is to employ a standard well-known instrument for the purpose; examples include the New York Heart Association Index of Cardiac Function, the Karnofsky Scale for disability in cancer patients, and the Mini Mental State Examination for cognitive function in the elderly.

Treatments are often not what investigators believe and intend them to be, and careful operational definition can require subtle distinctions. Drug A administered by mouth in a syrup also includes the syrup. (A series of deaths in the early days of sulfanilamide treatment attests tragically to this fact.[1]) A medicine prescribed is not necessarily a medication actually used. The analgesic pill has both its active ingredient and its function as a placebo to relieve the patient's pain. An office procedure comprises both the procedure and the visit, with whatever effects on well-being each may entail. Here we see highlighted the need for carefully devising (and operationally defining) any control treatment.

Phases in a Study

A comparative trial of treatments typically comprises several sequential phases: determination of a patient's eligibility for the study, the patient's entry into the study, assignment of treatment, the care itself (using the assigned treatment and any adjuvant treatments), evaluation of the patient's outcome (perhaps after a follow-up interval), statistical analysis of the data (including the information on this patient and others), and reporting. Fair comparison of treatments can be difficult if at any of these phases knowledge of the treatment assigned to the patient influences other aspects of the process. Thus, if the decision to enroll each patient in the trial can involve knowledge of the treatment the next patient will receive, then ample opportunity exists for constructing noncomparable treatment groups. If evaluation of subjective endpoints is made by observers who know which treatment the patient received, then another potential source of bias exists (hence the value of double-blind studies). Different follow-up periods for different treatment groups may conceal some mortality (or longevity), to the advantage of one treatment or the other. Careful planning of the processes at each phase can reduce the risk that knowledge of treatment assignment or results may lead to contamination of the conclusions.

Integrity of Operational Definition

When we move from studies where the investigators impose treatments to those where they simply observe different groups or similar groups in different epochs, the problems are likely to be markedly more difficult to solve. For example, the record may not always contain sufficient information for the operational definition of crucial matters. In such a situation, the conclusions of the study rest heavily on assumptions about the undefined terms and procedures, along with data about those that are adequately defined.

Concern for the integrity of operational definitions leads investigators to take important precautions in well-conducted studies. Identification of disease stages and laboratory analysis may be checked by introducing, blindly, occasional standard specimens. Samples of study records may be checked against clinical records. Visits and audits by personnel from a center that is charged with responsibility for quality control may be routinely conducted in multicenter studies. All such steps have the purpose of ensuring the proper operational definition of patients' characteristics, treatments actually applied, evaluation of outcomes, and record-keeping methods.

THE INFINITE-DATA CASE

In the planning phase of a study, few questions are more useful to consider than this: What could we learn from an unlimited amount of data obtained in the same way that we are planning to obtain ours in this study? Careful consideration of this question can lead to dropping a study, to improving it, or simply to clarifying issues of procedure and analysis, as in the examples discussed below.

Appropriate Subjects, Controls, and Data

In earlier days, medical students were sometimes used as volunteers to assess the risks of side effects from prospective new drugs. If a drug is intended to treat a disease affecting mainly elderly patients, and if younger subjects are expected to be used in a clinical trial, this question should arise before the study begins: What could unlimited data about the responses of healthy 25-year-olds tell us about the incidence of, say, nausea and vomiting in 70-year-old sick patients who will take this drug? The question is a good one to pose before data collection begins. Even though the answer to the question may be obscure, its obvious importance may lead to changing the investigational approach. Thus, giving thought to the infinite-data case can clarify what groups of subjects are appropriate for what aspects of the study at hand.

Such thinking can also help to define appropriate controls. One study involved a promising method for directly dissolving a clot in patients during the first two hours after a heart attack. The initial proposal was to apply the new method in all eligible patients and to use as controls those patients who arrived more than two hours, but less than eight hours, after a heart attack; this control group would be treated with current standard therapy. An infinite supply of data gathered in this way could at best resolve whether it was better to receive the new therapy within two hours or the standard therapy after two hours. Not even an infinitely large study could determine whether the new method was better than the standard one, either in the first two hours or in the next six.

Even an infinitely large study will not provide information about questions for which data are not collected. Thinking about analyzing the data as if they were already in hand and infinitely abundant can point both to unnecessary information that should not be collected and to key items of information that must be gathered.

Statistical Relationships and Regression

Laws of physics such as Ohm's Law, Newton's Laws of Motion, and Einstein's famous $E = mc^2$ allow one to calculate exactly the value of one variable that must accompany the stated value of another. But in medicine and everyday life such relationships are rare; instead we see "statistical relationships" that may hold true on average, but not case by case. Thus, tall people tend to be heavier than short people; older children tend to be taller than younger ones. Higher doses of a drug usually produce larger effects. A useful way to make this idea of a statistical relationship more amenable to quantitative treatment is the concept of regression. Think of two variables x (dose) and y (response). We define the regression of y upon x to be the curve that depicts at each value of x (dose) the *average* value of y (response) for those elements of the population having that value of x (receiving that dose). Now, though individual variability still attends the pair of variables x and y, a well-defined single curve relates the average of one variable to stated values of the other.

This idea of regression is far reaching, and has broad applicability. Generalizations to more than two variables lead to the concept of *multiple regression.*

The Limits of Associations

An observational study with infinite data can definitely demonstrate the presence of an association between two variables, such as lung cancer and smoking, without resolving questions of cause and effect. For example, an extensive study of adult men might show strong and roughly equal positive associations between height and weight and between girth and weight. We must draw on other information to support the proposition that by increasing the weight of a man we will increase his girth but not his height. To establish cause and effect typically demands recourse to knowledge outside the particular study.

When an experiment is carried out, treatments are imposed and subsequent events are followed; these procedures make causal inference much more direct, but dependence on outside knowledge is unlikely to be wholly absent. The point would be quickly illustrated by an experiment in which subjects were given large drinks of whiskey and water, rum and water, or brandy and water, and all showed signs of intoxication. It is "outside knowledge" that supports the conclusion that the effect was not due to the "common factor," water.

Confounding Variables

In a study discussed earlier in this section, the time elapsed after a heart attack and the method of therapy were confounded. Two variables are said to be *confounded* in a study if they appear in such a pattern that their separate effects cannot be distinguished. A common, often subtle, and sometimes ruinous form of confounding occurs when the personal choice of a patient (or physician or other key participant) can affect either side of a treatment comparison. The polio-vaccine trials (involving 2 million children) provide a surprising illustration. In that study, the incidence of polio was clearly lower among unvaccinated children whose parents refused permission for injection than among children who received the placebo after their parents gave permission.[2] As it turned out, families who gave permission differed from those who did not in ways that were related to susceptibility to poliomyelitis.

Personal choice also acts as an enemy of easy inference in questions of drug compliance. Studies with clofibrate[3] showed that subjects who took 80% or more of the prescribed dose had substantially lower mortality than subjects with poorer drug compliance; this evidence seemed to indicate that the drug was beneficial. But the same difference in mortality was observed between high- and low-compliance subjects whose medication was the placebo. Drug compliance, a matter of personal choice, was for some reason related to mortality in the patients in this study. Had there not been a placebo group, the confounding between the quantity of the drug actually taken and unknown factors related to survival might have gone unnoticed, and the reasoning "more drug, lower mortality; therefore, the drug is beneficial" might have gone unchallenged. As these examples suggest, consideration of the infinite-data case before the study begins should include efforts to identify points where personal choice may be confounded with variables under study.

"Exhausting Experience"

To think about the infinite-data case is to consider what could be learned from an infinitely large study of the kind contemplated. A closely related question is what could be learned by exhausting experience of the kind that the study will sample. Occasionally, this exhaustion of the data would involve only a finite set of observations. Thus, a sample of the current opinions of pediatricians in the United States on confidentially furnished contraceptive information for teenagers corresponds not to an infinite-data case but, rather, to the finite collection of the opinions of all pediatricians in the country on this topic. We could avoid concern about such special cases by speaking of the *all-possible-data case*. Some statistical writings use the term *population* to capture the ideas discussed here under the rubric of the infinite-data case.

A sometimes troublesome point is illustrated by the following example, which deals with motorcycle accident fatalities and helmet laws.[4] In Colorado, in the period 1964–1968, when the state had no law requiring helmets, there were 74 fatal motorcycle accidents (an annual rate of 6.3 per 10,000 registered motorcycles); in the period 1970–1976, after the enactment of a helmet law, there were 248 such accidents (an annual rate of 4.6 per 10,000 registered motorcycles); in the period 1978–1979, after the helmet law had been repealed, there were 137 deaths (an annual rate of 6.1 per 10,000). Since these figures include all the fatal motorcycle accidents in Colorado during those years, should we regard this information as itself exhausting experience?

Most statisticians would say no. They might say, for instance, that the deaths observed in these periods could be thought of as random outcomes of complex probabilistic processes; we happen to have relatively brief peeks at these processes; each death rate we have observed indicates the average level of risk per registered motorcycle in its period, but we must doubt that any of them exactly reflects that average risk. There is clearly a role for the concept of an infinite-data case in thinking about this problem. By observing indefinitely long periods (under unchanging conditions) *with* a helmet law and also *without* a helmet law, we might in principle learn the exact relationship between a helmet law and the risk of motorcycle accident death. Our actual finite data tell us, uncertainly, about that infinite-data case and about the actual level of risk in the three periods observed.

Overall, then, thinking about the data to be acquired in a study as if they were already in hand and as abundant as desired can identify problems, opportunities, and fruitful questions early enough to help most studies and (profitably) to abort some.

PROBABILISTIC THINKING

When unpredictable variation is large enough that it may affect conclusions, probabilistic thinking is likely to be helpful. In principle, the laws of physics plus a lot of elaborate instrumentation could permit us to treat the result of rolling a die as a deterministic matter, but at our usual practical level of analysis, that outcome is a chance matter to be regarded as probabilistic. Two similar patients with the same disease may have different outcomes. Perhaps that, too, is in principle deterministic (though much more complex), but at our usual level of analysis it is better regarded as probabilistic.

With an infinite number of observations we would learn, in the problem with the die, the probabilities that it would come to rest showing 1, 2, 3, 4, 5, or 6. (If it is a fair die, these probabilities will all be one sixth.) In more complicated situations, the infinite data would show the probabilities of more complex kinds of outcomes. Thus, if two diagnostic tests, A and B, are used and the outcomes measured are survival to one year or death in the same period, then the infinite-data case would answer all questions of this form: What is the probability of survival to one year for patients with an A score between a_1 and a_2 and a B score between b_1 and b_2? With more variables under study, the description of the possibilities grows rapidly more complex. The actual finite data can at best provide approximate answers to questions that could be answered precisely from the infinite-data set. A principal objective of probabilistic thinking is to appraise the closeness of that approximation by drawing on the finite data themselves for the appraisal.

Attention typically focuses not on the entire probability distribution, but on particular aspects of it. This idea becomes more concrete if we consider, briefly, some especially important elements of probabilistic thinking.

Sample Means and Standard Deviations

A statistic is a number computed from the observations in a sample. The sample mean (the familiar average, learned in grade school) is a statistic that tells about the "general size" of the sample's observations. Different samples drawn from the same infinite-data case will have somewhat different sample means, so any one sample mean must be thought of as only a probabilistic approximation of the mean that would be found if the full infinite-data case could be examined. How closely the sample mean approximates the infinite-data mean is a major concern of probabilistic thinking.

The standard deviation is a statistic that describes the degree of variation among the individual observations in the sample. If all had the same value, the standard deviation would be zero; the farther apart from one another (and from their mean) the individual observations are, the larger the standard deviation is. If the standard deviation of some sample is very small, then the sample average closely represents every individual value, whereas a large standard deviation tells us that this is not so. As a general rule, when random samples have small standard deviations, the sample means are more likely to be close to the all-data mean than when standard deviations are large. This principle points to the key role of the standard deviation in probabilistic thinking. It is an intuitively appealing principle; it says that if individual random observations are in close agreement, their average is likely to serve as a good estimate of the all-data mean.

Random Variation and the Size of Samples

It is a mathematical fact that in all cases of practical interest the differences among random samples of size n from a single population tend to be smaller when n is greater. Moreover, many important sample statistics from random samples are also increasingly similar with larger sample sizes. Therefore, the random variation of statistics can be reduced by using larger samples, so long as the processes of acquiring the data are not degraded in the effort to enlarge the sample. (Important practical issues are involved here. Doubling the sample size by allowing a particle counter to operate for twice as long is one thing. But doubling the sample size of a clinical study by extending its intake period from two years to four years may be quite another: quality control may be harder to maintain, changes in personnel and shifts in the patient population may be more likely, the treatment itself may change, and so on.)

Bias

If all our observations use one instrument that is out of adjustment, so that all readings are too high by four units, then our data have a bias of +4 units. A large sample size will neither increase nor decrease this bias; with sufficiently large samples, this bias will stand out (falsely) as a numerical fact having almost no sampling error. We can think of bias as a numerical discrepancy between the mean of some statistic from our intended infinite-data case and the mean for our actual infinite-data case. Of course, no one intends to use an instrument that gives readings four units too large, but if that happens, then the actual infinite-data case will incorporate this bias, and the sample data will approximate the biased figure.

Bias may be the most difficult problem in quantitative research. It can enter a study in many and subtle ways. Articles have been written on biases that affect clinical research.[5] The use of treatment and control groups can help sometimes; if all readings are four units too large (though not known to be), then in the difference between the mean for the treatment group and the mean for the controls, the bias cancels out. On the other hand, if the treatment group's measurements were made on instrument I and the control group's measurements on instrument II, any instrument bias would be confounded with treatment; large sample size would not reduce this bias.

Bias can enter not only through equipment but also in follow-up, identification of disease stages, treatment, history taking, record keeping, and patient responses. Patients referred from different sources often differ materially, and if different referral streams enter different treatment groups, then comparisons of treatments will be biased. Alertness on the part of the investigators and symmetry between treatment groups in all operational respects are the primary weapons for combating bias (hence the value of randomization and blinding). Bias must be fought in planning the study, in its execution, and in the analysis of the data.

INDUCTION

The very notion of learning from experience carries with it the idea that the experience comes from one set of instances and the learning is to be applied to other (often future) instances. This is the philosopher's problem of induction. Probabilistic thinking helps us to approach this problem. Sometimes it is possible to draw a sample of n individuals from a population so that every possible sample of size n has the same probability of being chosen; this is called a simple random sample. The laws of probability are directly applicable and enable us to make definite statements about the whole population on the basis of the statistics computed from the one random sample we have drawn. (More complicated schemes of sampling often have powerful advantages, but we don't treat them in this chapter.)

Inference from a Probability Sample

Two things need to be said about these inferences. First, they necessarily take a probabilistic form, such as "It is a 99-to-1 bet that the population mean lies between 20.6 and 21.3" or "It is a 19-to-1 bet that the population mean is negative." Other forms for stating statistical inferences exist; they also include a numerical statement about the population or infinite-data case and quantification of the degree of confidence with which that statement can be made. Second, these inferences depend for their integrity on the actual imposition of the probabilistic mechanism (e.g., a table of random numbers) whose mathematical properties then provide the inference. If two treatment groups have not been constructed as random subsets of a single group of eligible patients but instead have simply been found to be similar in some ways, then one may still go through the motions of statistical methods, but the conclusions are no longer logical consequences of the laws of probability. They are less direct, dependent on ad hoc assumptions, and altogether less reliable.

The Health Interview Survey of the National Center for Health Statistics exemplifies probabilistic reasoning from a finite sample (of about 40,000 households annually) to the whole population of the United States. That survey uses *probability sampling*, a modest extension of random sampling; all possible samples of size n have known (but not equal) probabilities of being drawn, and the statistical analysis uses that information.

A random or probability sample from a population is often subdivided, for instance, into males and females or smokers and nonsmokers; these subsamples are also random or probability samples of the males in the population, of the females, and so on.

Comparison of Differently Treated Groups as Found

Often statistical inference is attempted under circumstances that are much more adverse than comparing two subsamples of a random sample from a population. Results from a therapy used in recent years are frequently compared with results from the therapy used earlier (*historical controls*). Or results from operation I applied in hospital A are compared with results from operation II applied in hospital B. Inference is difficult and hazardous in such cases because many influential interfering variables may differ systematically in the populations furnishing the data. In principle, the difficulties could be reduced—or perhaps even eliminated—by successfully carrying out three steps: identifying the interfering variables; finding the values of these variables in the two samples; and adjusting appropriately for the values of these interfering variables.

Unfortunately, an investigator rarely has an effective command of any one of these three steps. Indeed, identifying all of the important interfering variables alone is likely to be a more complex issue than whether operation I is better than operation II. Attempting to make the measurements required to find the values for the variables may greatly complicate and burden the study, increase costs, and multiply opportunities for error. Adjusting for interfering variables depends heavily on external information that may, in fact, not be available. Successfully carrying through these three steps is unlikely to be feasible; hence, valid comparison of differently treated groups is typically difficult, though sometimes possible.

Clarification of the relation between lung cancer and cigarette smoking, for instance, was achieved through a host of studies stretching over years. For each study that found an adverse effect of smoking, it was possible to suggest biases that had not been controlled, thus casting doubt on the conclusions. By 1964 so many kinds of studies had been done—some free of one kind of bias, some of another—that consensus was reached that heavy cigarette smoking increased the risk of lung cancer. (Ultimately, the increase in risk was recognized to be about 10-fold.) This example demonstrates that induction in the absence of an applicable probability model is possible, but that in those circumstances it can be difficult, slow, and hard to defend against even inappropriate criticism.

Comparing Treatments in Randomly Constituted Groups

Symmetry was mentioned earlier as a device for controlling bias. The randomized study enforces symmetry by taking a suitable group of subjects and dividing them at random (e.g., with a table of random numbers) into two subgroups, one to receive treatment I and the other to receive treatment II. What does the randomization achieve? It ensures that (except for treatment) both subgroups have the same infinite-data case. Both are in this sense alike with regard to all relevant "other" variables—even though some of the important ones might be unrecognized and even though none may have been measured. The randomization does not ensure that the two subgroups will themselves be identical (any more than any two finite random samples from the same population will agree with each other or with their infinite-data case); rather, it ensures that no bias favoring one treatment or the other can operate. Equally important, randomization leads to a precisely quantified measure of the uncertainty arising from the differences that do occur between subgroups. Because of this, the randomization rigorously justifies statistical inference about the comparative efficacy of the treatments in the group of subjects studied. The method forgoes attempting to untie the Gordian knot of interfering variables but, instead, cuts through it in one stroke.

Readers of the Surgeon General's 1964 report, *Smoking and Health*,[6] will find among the 392 references cited in the chapter on cancer seven key observational (nonrandomized) studies published in 1954 (the report's references 38, 84, 138, 158, 175, 268, and 365). In that same year, 1954, the polio-vaccine trial—a randomized double-blind placebo-controlled experiment—definitively demonstrated protection by the vaccine, which cut the polio rate by a factor of about 2.5. That effect, much smaller than a factor of 10, was established once and for all by the study. When the randomized experiment is feasible, it can be very powerful indeed.

Not all studies can be done by assigning treatments to randomly constituted subgroups. First, conditions to be investigated may not be assignable at all. For example, people choose whether or not to smoke, and they are born with attributes such as their blood type. Second, there may be ethical obstacles; if patients can definitely be expected to benefit more from treatment I than from treatment II, that should bar their being assigned to treatment II. (Thus, the initial "suitable group" should consist of patients for whom both treatments are equally appropriate, insofar as is known.) Third, resources may be inadequate. Because irregular practices or systematic mistakes can make an experiment meaningless, great care is given to quality-control measures in clinical trials, and care often entails expense.

Internal and External Validity

The sample survey using probability sampling provides specific inferences about the whole population at the time of the survey; these conclusions are logical consequences of the laws of probability, and we say that they have high internal validity. If we apply these conclusions next year or to a somewhat different, though similar, population, we move away from a statistical inference to a different kind of inference, one that draws on our knowledge of the phenomena under investigation—smoking habits, income, health status, or other factors. In this situation, we must be concerned with the external validity of the conclusions.

These two kinds of inference (first, from the data to the corresponding infinite-data case and, second, from that infinite-data case to wider situations) arise not only with sample surveys but in clinical studies. The 1954 polio trial involved randomized comparison of placebo and vaccine in children in grades one, two, and three. Generalization of its conclusions to older and younger children belongs to virology and immunology, not to statistics.

How a study is carried out can affect its external validity. One study might compare two treatments in a large body of patients in a narrow age range in a particular large city. A different study, using the same number of patients, might compare those two treatments in several locations and might use wider age limits. The second study would pose fewer problems of external validity, though this gain would be won at a cost in complexity of statistical analysis; the second study, moreover, would require additional quality-control measures to ensure compliance with the protocol and adherence to standards. Investigators often must balance the demands of internal validity, including narrowly selected groups of subjects for study, against the demands of external validity, where broad representation of potential future subjects may be important.

In summary, induction is the process of reaching conclusions from one set of instances that can then be applied to other instances. The relationship can be especially direct if a probability sample is drawn from a population with the aim of describing the whole population. But even in such a straightforward situation, interpretation may be difficult, simply because the infinite-data case itself could rarely, if ever, settle questions about cause and effect. Comparison of treatments in differently established groups raises thorny questions, both theoretical and practical; inference in such cases is likely to be error-prone, difficult, and slow. Comparing treatments in randomly chosen subsets of a suitable group of subjects ensures that, except for treatment, both groups have the same infinite-data case; thus, bias—even from unrecognized interfering variables—is ruled out. If the suitable group of subjects is defined too narrowly, problems of external validity may prove troubling.

STUDY DESIGN

Statistical considerations merit attention at the time of planning a study fully as much as they inevitably claim attention at the time of analysis. Four statistical issues deserve particular care during study design: preventing bias, ensuring efficiency (a high information yield per observation), ensuring the integrity of the process (quality control), and determining the size of the sample.

Bias

Prevention of bias requires identifying possible interfering variables and then ensuring that their uncontrolled effects will not favor one treatment or another. Such variables must first be listed. Then any variable on the list can be coped with in one of two ways: its effects can be controlled—for example, the design might call for an equal age distribution in each treatment group; or its effects can be made symmetrical through randomization (which may or may not be followed by statistical adjustments, perhaps by regression methods). The key is to prevent any influential variable from becoming confounded with the effects of treatment.

Efficiency

A subfield of statistics called statistical design of experiments is largely devoted to devising ways to collect data that reduce statistical variation. One device exploits knowledge about interfering variables by applying regression methods (analysis of covariance). Another chooses closely similar subsets of the eligible population within which to compare the treatments; comparison of treatments in identical twins epitomizes this approach. The crossover design goes further, using both treatments in every subject, but results may be invalid if certain conditions do not apply to the physiologic processes under study.[7] (See also Chapter 5 of this book.) Statistical design of experiments has other devices in its kit as well, and may produce substantial economies in time, money, or other resources; it can also produce substantial improvements in both internal and external validity.

Integrity of the Process

Ensuring that the operational definitions really do apply in the data-collection process is necessary for a successful study. The process of operational definition, discussed earlier in this chapter, must be planned, and its execution needs to be provided for in the study protocol.

Sample Size

How many observations should we make? People often bring this question to a statistician (usually before the study begins, fortunately). For this question to be answered, more detail is needed; it resembles the question, How much money should I take when I go on vacation? One needs to ask, How long a vacation? Where? With whom?

Three questions must be answered before the sample size can be determined: How variable are the data? How precise an answer is required? How much confidence do you want to have in the answer? These questions are worth asking even if the sample size will be determined by the budget or the time available to do the study. Sometimes a planned study is dropped because sample size analysis shows that the study has little chance of providing a useful answer under the existing constraints of time or budget. Thus, if eligible subjects must have a disease D, with low prevalence, it may not be realistic to undertake the study if, say, 20 years would be needed to accumulate the required number of cases of this rare disease.

Another place that prevalence enters into consideration at the stage of study design is in screening. If one wishes to identify cases of disease D by applying a test to unselected members of the population, the practicality of the enterprise depends on the relation between the test's false-positive rate, r, and p, the prevalence of the disease in the population. A little reflection shows that if the prevalence p is 1 in 1000 and the false-positive rate r is 1 in 100, then the test will turn up about 10 false positives for each true positive turned up. Those testing positive then are 10 to 1 bets *not* to have the disease. The time to consider this possible difficulty is at the outset—the design stage. If p were 0.15 and r were 0.01, that same test might be quite serviceable, because true positives would outnumber false positives (among those who had positive tests) by about 15 to 1.

STATISTICAL REPORTING

Good statistical reporting aims for full, clear disclosure of what was done, what resulted, how the authors interpret the results, and why.

Describing the Data Acquisition

The operational definitions of all terms should be clear. The reader should not be left with doubts about how the subjects were selected, how they were assigned to treatments, what treatments were applied, how outcomes were measured, or in what order these steps were taken. DerSimonian et al.[8] reviewed reports of clinical trials published in four leading medical journals. Their criteria for full reporting required that the papers answer these six questions: What were the eligibility criteria for admission to the study? Did admission to the study occur before treatment was allocated? Was treatment allocated at random? What method of randomization was used? Were patients blind to the treatment they received? Were outcomes assessed by persons who were blind to treatment? All these are crucial in presenting the results of clinical trials.

Reporting the Data

The data should be summarized clearly in tables, in words, and in charts (frequently it is desirable to use all three). Missing data and extreme observations, both those retained and those excluded (and why), should be explicitly reported.

At minimum, the raw data should be carefully labeled and stored in a form that will allow others to understand and use them in the future. Data sets should be clearly defined and not melded into the next analysis or merged with new cases as they arrive; if a data set is in flux, as may happen in recently completing clinical trials, the date at which the database was locked for the reported analysis should be reported. Often it may be desirable to publish raw data or data files used in analysis of complex arrays. Public internet-based repositories exist for many types of data including DNA sequence data (GenBank, http://www.ncbi.nlm.nih.gov/Genbank/index.html), gene-expression data (GEO, http://www.ncbi.nlm.nih.gov/geo/), and phenotype-genotype correlation data (*db*GaP, http://www.ncbi.nlm.nih.gov/sites/entrez?Db=gap). Many journals allow internet posting of large supplemental data sets with the published article. If possible, the data should be archived on the journal's website to provide assurance to the community that no post-hoc alterations have been made to data sets. Most publicly funded research now has data access clauses embedded in the notice of grant award, so authors, editors, and database administrators should collaborate to allow access to data as appropriate. Good reporting will also include an explanation of the quality-control measures applied, the methods used for follow-up, and the auditing measures employed.

Describing the Analyses

The reader should be told not only what was done and how, but also what happened. Summary statistics should have the aim of revealing information to the reader. The methods of statistical analysis should be explained. The best way to do this is topic by topic—the same way that the analysis is usually carried out. This kind of reporting promotes understanding, specificity, and, incidentally, ease of writing. Sometimes a published paper lists statistical procedures in the Methods section—for instance, "We used chi-squared, the *t*-test, the *F* test, and Jonckheere's test." This style of reporting, if applied to the recipes used at a banquet, would list all the ingredients in all the dishes together and report the use of stove, mixer, oven, meat grinder, eggbeater, and double boiler.

Questions of Two Kinds

In addition to showing the data or generously detailed summaries of them, the statistical analysis should state each of the principal questions that motivated the study and discuss what light the data shed on those questions. (This is not the same thing at all as reporting just the results that are statistically significant.) To lend clarity to both significant and nonsignificant results, it is wise to use confidence intervals when feasible and to report the power of statistical tests.[9] Interesting statistical results that arise out of studying the data (rather than out of studying the principal questions that motivated the study) are necessarily on a different, and somewhat ambiguous, logical footing. A study may enable the investigator to look at scores or even hundreds of interesting questions involving various subgroups and kinds of response. Investigating all these questions, either systematically or implicitly, by careful scanning, will inevitably turn up some "interesting outcomes." But this inevitability serves as a warning that the particular interesting findings may not hold up under repetition. It is usually wise to regard such outcomes with considerable reserve, more as hypotheses than as established facts. It is especially important to be candid about the nature and amount of "data dredging" that has accompanied the analysis. The *New England Journal of Medicine* has published guidelines for the reporting of subgroup analyses.[10]

Any doubts about this message may be quelled by considering a thought experiment. In the first phase we might assess a person's literacy in English by asking that he or she spell any five-letter English word. In the second phase we might program a computer to use a random number generator, and produce a succession of letters of the alphabet chosen with probabilities for the various letters that correspond to their frequencies in written English. Such a text will surely contain some correctly spelled five-letter English words. (The sample at hand as this is being written shows "sites" as the 148th through 152nd letters.) It would be foolish to attribute any meaning to such a result. In a parallel vein, if only chance is at work, one must expect among 1000 significance tests to find 50 (5% of 1000) judged as significant at $p < 0.05$. Thus, post-hoc "significant findings" demand candor when they are reported and great reserve when they are interpreted.

Good statistical reporting can help users address the issue of external validity. The Hypertension Detection and Follow-up Program Cooperative Group reported comparative five-year mortality rates under two treatment regimens for patients with high blood pressure.[11] In a second paper,[12] the group explored how their basic finding held up in subgroups defined by age, by race and sex, and by years of follow-up. Such information can help readers to gauge the probable applicability of the study's basic result, that stepped care resulted in better survival experience than referred care.

Finally, good statistical reporting includes a discussion of the limitations and possible weaknesses of the study; this step can help to forestall unsound critical attacks on a study and to focus attention on any real problems that deserve further consideration.

REFERENCES

1. Sollman TH. A manual of pharmacology and its applications to therapeutics and toxicology. Philadelphia: WB Saunders, 1957:129.

2. Meier P. The biggest public health experiment ever: the 1954 field trial of the Salk poliomyelitis vaccine. In: Tanur JM, Mosteller F, Kruskal WH, et al., eds. Statistics: a guide to the unknown. 3rd ed. Pacific Grove: Wadsworth & Brooks/Cole, Advanced Books & Software, 1989:3–14.

3. Coronary Drug Project Research Group. Influence of adherence to treatment and response of cholesterol on mortality in the Coronary Drug Project. N Engl J Med 1980; 303:1038–41.

4. Krane S. Motorcycle crashes, helmet use and injury severity: before and after helmet law repeal in Colorado: Symposium on Traffic Safety Effectiveness (Impact) Evaluation Projects, May 29–31, 1981, Chicago, 1981:330 (Table 1). (Conducted by National Safety Council under contract no. DTNH22-80-C-01564).

5. Sackett DL. Bias in analytic research. J Chronic Dis 1979; 32:51–63.

6. Smoking and health: report of the advisory committee to the Surgeon General of the Public Health Service. Washington, D.C.: Government Printing Office, 1964:235–57. (Public Health Service publication no. 1103).

7. Brown BW Jr. Statistical controversies in the design of clinical trials—some personal views. Contr Clin Trials 1980; 1:13–27.

8. DerSimonian R, Charette LJ, McPeek B, Mosteller F. Reporting on methods in clinical trials. N Engl J Med 1982; 306:1332–7.

9. Freiman JA, Chalmers TC, Smith H Jr, Kuebler RR. The importance of beta, the type II error, and sample size in the design and interpretation of the randomized controlled trial: survey of 71 "negative" trials. N Engl J Med 1978; 299:690–4.

10. Wang R, Lagakos SW, Ware JH, Hunter DJ, Drazen JM. Reporting of subgroup analyses in clinical trials. N Engl J Med 2007; 357:2189–94. [Chapter 15 of this book.]

11. Hypertension Detection and Follow-up Program Cooperative Group. Five-year findings of the Hypertension Detection and Follow-up Program. I. Reduction in mortality of persons with high blood pressure, including mild hypertension. JAMA 1979; 242:2562–71.

12. *Idem.* Five-year findings of the Hypertension Detection and Follow-up Program. II. Mortality by race, sex and age. JAMA 1979; 242:2572–7.

CHAPTER 2

CZ

Some Uses of Statistical Thinking*

JOHN C. BAILAR III, M.D., PH.D.

ABSTRACT   Many researchers skillfully apply statistical concepts and methods appropriate for describing and summarizing the uncertainty of their results. In this context, p-values and confidence limits are especially important. However, these measures do not account for deviations from the presumed (and often implicit) model or for other nonrandom sources of error or uncertainty that affect the findings.

The need for a broader concept of statistical thinking is illustrated by four examples of unexpected uncertainty in research. These involve 1) studies of the Gulf War Syndrome (which illustrate the need for sound data in statistical analysis), 2) the relation between doses of a carcinogen and its effects (which illustrates the effect of an error in a critical assumption), 3) analyses of the carcinogenic potential of Tris (which illustrate uncertainty in generalizing results), and 4) the health effects of automotive emissions (which illustrate how a complex problem can be attacked as a sequence of somewhat simpler problems).

Actual uncertainty and error in empirical studies may well exceed the uncertainty estimated from the data in hand and the statistical model used for estimation and testing. A substantially broader view of statistics and statistical thinking could do much to improve quantitative analysis in science.

The original meaning of the term "statistics" promises much. The word is ultimately derived from the Latin word for "state," in the sense of a nation, and has been defined as the collection, analysis, interpretation, and presentation of masses of numerical data. Ultimately, statistics in this sense is the study of political facts and figures, where "political" is taken to mean matters that affect the body politic.

*Modified from a presentation in the Carolina Environmental Essay Series, Institute for Environmental Studies, University of North Carolina at Chapel Hill. Reprinted with the permission of the publisher.

Both scientific conclusions and technical decisions based on empirical data must include realistic appraisals of the likelihood that they are wrong. Unfortunately, we commonly underestimate the extent to which such decisions and conclusions are wrong. The scientific method gives special attention to uncertainty, which rather broadly covers all actual or possible sources of error, recognized or not, as well as the probabilities of errors of various types and sizes. This differs a little from common usage, in which the word "uncertain" reflects our recognition that we may be wrong in some way—for example, when we recognize that our information is inadequate or that we may have misinterpreted some observation. I have chosen to broaden the term to include unrecognized problems because the broader concept needs a name, and no other term seems more appropriate. Four examples illustrate what I mean by uncertainty resulting from unrecognized problems. These examples come from the fields of environmental hazards and medical research, but the concepts cover the whole range of academic disciplines, as well as everyday life.

Many scientists and users of science are already familiar with statistics in the formal development of a hypothesis and its negation (often designated *null* and *alternative hypotheses*), the calculation of p-values and confidence limits, and their interpretation. These matters are important and indeed often critical to scientific progress, but so are many other, less widely understood aspects of statistics. These include the initial development of research questions and strategies, devising and testing detailed protocols, the optimal use of such checks on bias as randomizing and blinding, measuring and maintaining the quality of data, selecting the most appropriate methods of analysis, and generalizing results to populations or outcomes not directly studied. Training, practice, and, sometimes, expert consultation about these additional facets of statistical thinking can often enhance research investigations and promote progress in science.

THE NEED FOR GOOD DATA

"Gulf War Syndrome" (GWS) has been said to affect many thousands among the 700,000 veterans of the Gulf War of 1991–1992. Among the many symptoms attributed to GWS are fatigue, malaise, headaches, bone and joint pain, difficulty sleeping, and skin rashes. There has been much concern that this syndrome is a result of some kind of exposure—perhaps chemical, including chemical warfare agents—that may have been common in the Persian Gulf area at the time these veterans were serving there. However, each of these symptoms may occur commonly in persons who did not serve in that war. The important question is therefore whether the frequency and/or severity of their symptoms is greater than that in military personnel and veterans who were not deployed to the Persian Gulf region in that conflict. The most important policy implications have to do with diagnosis and effective treatment, prevention in possible future conflicts, and compensation for what may be a service-connected disability. I am convinced that many veterans have suffered substantially from their service in the Gulf War; questions revolve about how many, with what severity, the cause and nature of the afflictions, and effective treatment (which depends critically on the cause and nature).

I have seen at least 20 research studies about GWS written by various broad-based scientific groups, all of which have concluded that no satisfactory evidence relates GWS to any unique physical exposure. A very few cite some weak evidence that the syndrome might be related to a specific exposure in the Persian Gulf theater, but also conclude that the evidence does not establish a physical cause for the problems. Given these expert opinions, why is there still so much uncertainty about the existence and nature of some specific GWS and about our society's response to it? Among the chief difficulties are the lack of a single definition of the syndrome (which seems to be whatever any research investigator—or even any veteran—wants to make it at the time), the lack of any suitable control group for comparison, and possible differences in reporting of symptoms between persons who do and those who do not believe they have the syndrome.

The problem of Gulf War Syndrome is inherently statistical, because we need to know outcomes and, from those, to determine risk factors and levels of risk for the occurrence of GWS. Our understanding of these matters will have substantial impact on the way we deal with veterans of that conflict, and perhaps with veterans of present and future conflicts. I am quite skeptical that any specific chemical exposure is a cause, in part because of evidence that U.S. veterans of every conflict at least as far back as the Civil War have complained of similar sets of symptoms, although we do not have good estimates of their frequency, and also because of some evidence that persons complaining of GWS had an elevated frequency of non-specific symptoms prior to deployment, and even prior to military service. It further appears that veterans of other wars from other countries have had similar problems. An active program of research is looking at many aspects of GWS, and it is possible that evidence for some identifiable physical cause will emerge, but it is my present impression that GWS is a version of a more general "war syndrome," or perhaps an even more general "stress syndrome."

Some of the biggest challenges to drawing sound conclusions from research on such syndromes, including GWS, lie in developing a generally accepted case definition, identifying suitable comparison groups (troops deployed to the Gulf had important differences from troops in the United States or deployed elsewhere), applying the case definition uniformly to patients and comparison groups, and avoiding recall biases. These are formidable challenges.

UNCERTAINTY FROM UNRECOGNIZED ERROR IN A CRITICAL ASSUMPTION

My second example of uncertainty in quantitative results has to do with the relation between the dose of a carcinogenic chemical and the probability that cancer will occur—that is, the shape of the dose-response curve. Most forms of cancer occur with some frequency or rate (called *background*) even when there is no specific chemical exposure ("dose"), and the critical scientific issue is the magnitude (sometimes zero) of any additional risk caused by small exposures. Because of the limited sensitivity of experiments of feasible size, direct observations at low doses are not generally useful, and one must make a reasoned inference from effects at higher levels of exposure.

For effects other than cancer, many dose-response curves appear to have a threshold. For example, small amounts of carbon dioxide in the air we breathe have minimal impact on health (indeed, they can be beneficial), but larger amounts are toxic and even lethal. Our metabolic systems can handle low salt intakes, but higher intakes appear to produce hypertension in susceptible persons. A little aspirin, or pesticide, or alcohol may have no serious acute effects on function, but moderately larger amounts can have large effects.

Figure 1 shows some possible dose-response curves. For each curve in the figure, the response (cancer, for example) is shown to be small (the background rate) at zero exposure; the four curves also show the same response at a "high" dose, but they differ at intermediate points. Curve A shows a true threshold; there is no response until the dose approaches the level designated "low" in the figure. Curve B has no threshold, but each intermediate point is below the straight line between the response rates at zero and high dose. Curve C is the straight line (that is, the response is proportional to the dose), and Curve D is entirely above the line. Clearly, risk at a "very low" dose, not much above zero, depends a lot on the true curve, but there is no direct way to tell which of these forms, if any, is close to the truth. Research studies suggest that carcinogens may sometimes have a threshold, but that more often they do not, implying that even the smallest exposure has some risk. And even a tiny individual risk, spread across millions of people, maybe of considerable concern. (The Food and Drug Administration commonly regulates to prevent food-borne risks estimated to be larger than one in a million over a lifetime; this translates into several deaths per year in the United States if the whole population is exposed.)

For a time, carcinogenesis experts—in industry, regulatory agencies, and universities—did assume, however, that whatever the true relation between exposure and carcinogenesis, the response at low doses would be no greater than proportional to that at higher doses. (The underlying biologic assumption was that responses lie below an exponential curve, but such curves are very

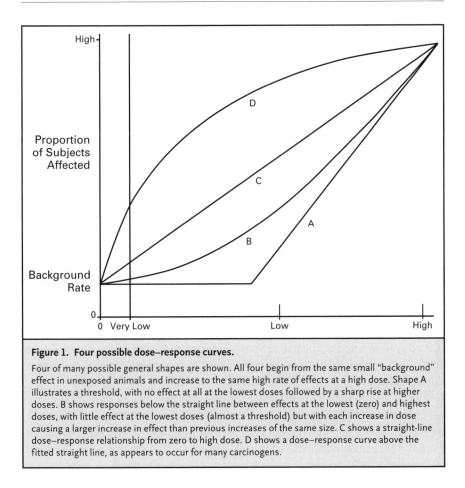

Figure 1. Four possible dose–response curves.

Four of many possible general shapes are shown. All four begin from the same small "background" effect in unexposed animals and increase to the same high rate of effects at a high dose. Shape A illustrates a threshold, with no effect at all at the lowest doses followed by a sharp rise at higher doses. B shows responses below the straight line between effects at the lowest (zero) and highest doses, with little effect at the lowest doses (almost a threshold) but with each increase in dose causing a larger increase in effect than previous increases of the same size. C shows a straight-line dose–response relationship from zero to high dose. D shows a dose–response curve above the fitted straight line, as appears to occur for many carcinogens.

nearly linear at low response rates, so this came to be called, incorrectly, the linear assumption, and risks are generally calculated as if the curve were linear.) In other words, they believed that one could determine the risk at some high exposure, and assume with confidence that if exposure to the chemical were reduced, say, 100-fold, the carcinogenic risk would also be reduced at least 100-fold, perhaps more, and possibly even to background (Curves A and B in Figure 1). Thus, a straight-line model (Curve C in the figure) was considered "conservative" of the public health, and risk assessment based on scaling-down effects at high doses was thought to set an upper bound on risk at much lower doses. A few dose-response curves seemed to flatten as dose increases, as in Curve D. This pattern was assumed to be uncommon, though it appears that this assumption was never checked against data.

Table 1. Some Plausible Reasons for Expecting a Straight-Line Model to Give Non-Conservative Estimates of Risk.*

1. Dose-related mortality from other causes

2. Direct interference of experimental methods with the causation of cancer

3. Saturation of enzyme systems

4. Population heterogeneity (genetic or environmental) in susceptibility to the carcinogen

5. Intervening mechanisms, such as cell killing at high doses

6. Carcinogens with high-dose cancer-suppressive effects

*From Bailar et al.[1] Reprinted with permission of the publisher.

That the straight-line model was ordinarily conservative was thus widely assumed, despite plausible biologic reasons for thinking that low doses might at times be more efficient than higher doses in terms of producing more cancers per unit of exposure. Table 1 lists some plausible biologic reasons for thinking that this may not always be true.[1] Extensive data available from the National Toxicology Program were used to test the straight-line (that is, effectively, exponential) model at moderate to high doses.[1] The straight-line model (Curve C) was fitted to data at zero dose (control) and the highest tested dose, and it underestimated risks at intermediate doses (generally at half the highest dose) almost as often as it overestimated risks.

Figure 2 shows experimental data for the induction of one kind of liver cancer by vinyl chloride. Data were collected for female rats fed at estimated doses of 0, 2400, 6000, and 10,000 parts per million (ppm), with only small variations from those figures in actual intakes. No cancers were found at zero dose, in line with decades of experience in the laboratory that have shown that this cancer is extremely rare in untreated animals (as it is in humans). This long-term history was used to assume that the response at zero dose was zero cancers. These doses are in the range that might be studied in routine investigations, and the top panel of the figure shows that a fitted exponential model for results at the target doses of 2400 and 6000 ppm (dashed) is well within the range of uncertainty in the data (expressed as vertical "error bars" in the figure). The results at 10,000 ppm might have been considered irrelevant or erroneous. The upper 95% confidence limit on the fitted exponential curve (solid) is also shown; it is rather close to the fitted line (dashed).

The bottom panel of Figure 2 shows additional data at much lower doses; it also shows the low-dose range of the upper 95% confidence limit (solid) from the upper panel of the figure. It is apparent that actual risks at doses up to, say, 50 ppm were many times higher than estimated from the fitted model. Low exposure levels such as these are generally most relevant to human risk, and

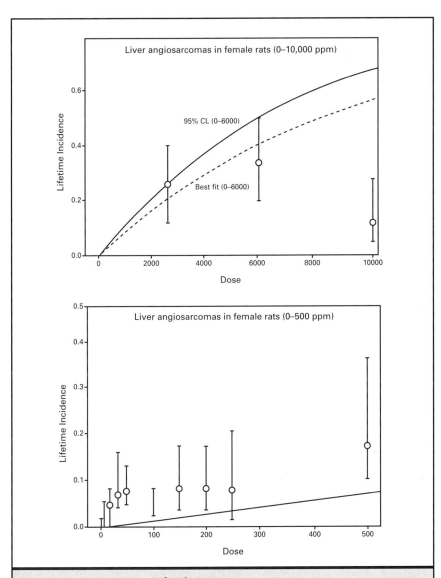

Figure 2. Liver angiosarcomas in female rats.

Observed rates of liver angiosarcoma in female rats at high doses (top) and low doses (bottom), with 95% confidence limits above and below the observed data. The top panel also shows the best fitting exponential model (effectively the straight-line model at low doses) and its upper 95% confidence bound. The bottom panel shows similar data at much lower doses, and the low-dose section of the 95% upper confidence bound (solid line) shown in the top panel. All of the low-dose best estimates, and most of the whole confidence ranges on the observed data, lie above the line fitted to the high-dose data. Originally from Maltoni et al.[2] Reproduced here from Bailar et al.[1] Reprinted with permission of the publisher.

Table 2. Examples of Cancer Rates Higher Than Forecast by Linearity in Dose-Response Studies of Animal Carcinogenesis. *

Chemical	Sex	Species and Strain*	Tumor Type	Route	Adjusted Lifetime Cumulative Incidence			p-value#
					Dose			
					None	Mid	High	
4,4'-methylene-dianiline·2HCL	M	b	Hepatocellular carcinoma	Water	0.22	0.66	0.70	0.025
1,2-dibromoethane	F	o	Oral, GI squamous carcinoma	Gavage	0.00	0.80	0.80	0.0002
1,4-dioxane	F	o	Fibroadenoma	Water	0.05	0.46	0.47	0.024
1,3-butadiene	F	b	Hemangiosarcoma	Inhalation	0.00	0.38	0.41	<0.00001
Carbon tetrachloride	M	b	Hepatocellular carcinoma	Gavage	0.07	0.98	0.98	0.008
Dimethylvinyl chloride	M	b	Oral, GI squamous carcinoma	Gavage	0.00	0.86	0.90	0.004
Cytembena	M	f	Mesothelioma, osteosarcoma	Peritoneal injection	0.05	0.74	0.68	0.00003
1,5-naphthalene-diamine	F	f	Endometrial stromal polyp	Food	0.07	0.28	0.27	0.04
Iodinated glycerol	M	f	Plasmacytic leukemia	Gavage	0.31	0.72	0.76	0.04
2-methyl-aziridine	F	c	Skin, breast adenoma	Gavage	0.00	0.81	0.83	0.02

* Species and strain: b-B6C3F1 mouse; f-Fischer 344 rat; o-Osborne Mendel rat; c-Charles river rat.

One-tailed exact p comparing the mid-dose result to the value obtained from an exponential model.

Data from Bailar et al.[1] Reprinted with permission of the publisher.

human risk might have been seriously underestimated if we had not had the additional low-dose data.

These extra data were available because the dose-response relations of vinyl chloride had been recognized as a problem needing special study. But is this failure to follow a straight-line (or exponential) model common? Table 2 lists some other chemicals for which the data show a risk at an intermediate dose that is close to that at the highest dose; risk assessments for each of these must be suspect because we cannot determine from the available information how rapidly the same dose-response curve rises at low exposures or where it has largely leveled out. For example, in the study of 1,2-dibromoethane, no unexposed animals developed squamous cell cancer of the oral cavity or

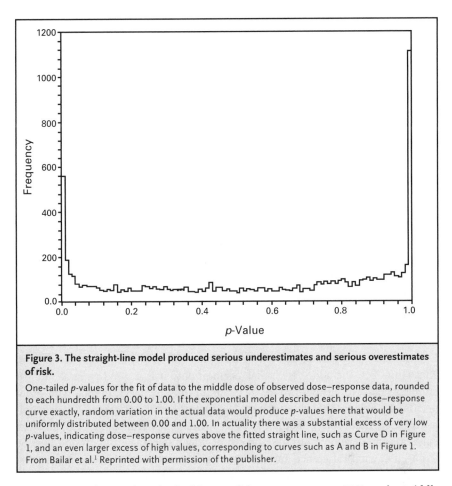

Figure 3. The straight-line model produced serious underestimates and serious overestimates of risk.

One-tailed *p*-values for the fit of data to the middle dose of observed dose–response data, rounded to each hundredth from 0.00 to 1.00. If the exponential model described each true dose–response curve exactly, random variation in the actual data would produce *p*-values here that would be uniformly distributed between 0.00 and 1.00. In actuality there was a substantial excess of very low *p*-values, indicating dose–response curves above the fitted straight line, such as Curve D in Figure 1, and an even larger excess of high values, corresponding to curves such as A and B in Figure 1. From Bailar et al.[1] Reprinted with permission of the publisher.

gastrointestinal tract, but the incidence of these cancers was 80% at the middle dose, and no higher at the highest dose. We have no way to estimate the risk at 1/10, or 1/100, or 1/1000 of the middle dose except to say that it probably does not exceed that found at the middle dose.

The data in Table 2 were selected post-hoc from many thousands of similar sets of observations from the U.S. National Toxicology Program. These estimates of lifetime incidence are based on rather small experimental groups (often 50 to 60 animals of each sex at each dose), so they are subject to considerable random variation, and by chance alone a few chemicals might give results like those in Table 2. Also, I chose these examples because they showed a particular kind of result (supra-linearity at low doses), so their individual *p*-values would tend to be small. The basic question, then, is not whether this large set of results includes some apparent violations of the assumed conservatism of the straight-line model, but whether the number of apparent violations in the entire data set is greater than can be attributed to chance.

My colleagues and I devised a statistical score to examine this question[1]: when the straight-line (i.e., exponential) model holds exactly, the score is about equally likely to take on any value between 0 and 1. (The score was the one-tailed p-value for the fit of the middle value to an exponential curve through the zero-dose and high-dose results.) If the straight-line model is truly conservative, many values of the test statistic will be close to 1.00, whereas if it underestimates low-dose risks, many values will be near 0.00. If the straight-line model is sometimes too conservative, sometimes too generous, and sometimes right on the mark, we will see a mixture of these outcomes: a peak near 0.00, another peak near 1.00, and an even spread of values between the extremes. Figure 3 shows that this is just what happened, and that the straight-line model seriously underestimated risks almost as often as it overstated them. Also, the underestimates of risk may be larger (as a proportion of the actual risk) than the overestimates, which cannot exceed 100%. Use of the straight-line model to estimate carcinogenic risk appears to be dangerous to the public health.

The more general lesson here is that we can all make assumptions that seem perfectly reasonable, but may be wrong. Widespread acceptance of some technical assumption does not guarantee even a good approximation to the truth. It is not easy to evaluate, or even to recognize, all of the assumptions used in analyzing data, including statistical assumptions. It is a good general rule for an investigator to write down all of the assumptions, check the list with other persons knowledgeable about the subject matter and the nature of the data collected (e.g., randomized laboratory experiments, clinical records, or population surveys), and develop a fair assessment of how much each assumption may be wrong and what difference such errors might make in conclusions. Such a list is likely to still be incomplete, but experience in thinking about various types of problems in assumptions and data, and how such problems affect conclusions, can improve interpretations and, not incidentally, protect them from some kinds of attack by critics.

UNCERTAINTY IN GENERALIZING RESULTS

My third example comes from the field of cancer risk assessment[3] and involves four estimates of the cancer hazard presented by a flame retardant commonly known as Tris.[4-7] The four risk assessments were all done within a period of about six weeks in 1977, and all four sets of investigators had access to essentially the same information.

Tris was introduced in about 1972 to reduce the risk of fire in fabrics, especially in fabrics used to make pajamas for infants. Later, however, the preliminary

Table 3. Cancer Incidence after Lifetime Feeding with Tris.*								
	Ratios of Number of Animals with Cancers to Number Treated, by Site of Cancer							
Tris: Parts per Million in the Diet	Kidney		Stomach		Liver		Lung	
	M	F	M	F	M	F	M	F
	Mice							
0	0/55	0/55	0/51	2/52	28/55	11/54	12/55	4/55
500	4/50	2/50	10/48	14/48	30/49	23/49	18/44	9/50
1000	14/50	2/50	13/50	22/49	23/50	33/50	24/50	17/50
	Rats							
0	0/54	0/54						
50	25/55	4/55						
100	29/55	10/55						

*Data from Brown et al.[4]

results of an animal study showed that Tris fed at high doses to mice and rats was a potent carcinogen. Thus, questions arose about the risk of sending children to bed in Tris-treated sleepwear. Table 3 shows the experimental results for the four cancer sites where the increase in cancer incidence was judged to be statistically significant in at least one species and one sex. (About 60 animals of each sex and species were tested at each dose, but a few died early and in some instances not all organs could be examined, so denominators vary.) Large and statistically significant increases were found in the frequency of cancer of the kidney in male mice and in both sexes of rats, the stomach and lung in both sexes of mice, and the liver in female mice. The increase in kidney cancer in rats is especially striking because the level of exposure was only one-tenth of that in mice, but the added risk of cancer was higher.

The four risk assessments all focused on kidney cancer, using the data in Table 3. Thus, differences in assessed risk must result from differences in how the data were extrapolated from this rodent bioassay to human beings. The size of the risk is critical here, because Tris was, beyond question, effective in reducing the flammability of woven fabrics, and almost as certainly reduced the number of injuries and deaths of children at risk of burns. Substitutes for Tris were available, but they did not have the same desirable chemical and physical properties.

Several kinds of problems arise almost immediately in trying to estimate the human risks of a carcinogen from a laboratory experiment such as that summarized in Table 3. Some of the largest, well recognized by risk assessors, are:

- Extending results from animals (mice and rats, in this case) to humans, who may respond to the same stimulus in different ways;

- Extending results from the high doses in the experiments to what were expected to be much lower doses in infants;

- Extending results from feeding (in the animals) to skin exposure (in humans), although it was recognized that some Tris might also be ingested by infants who chew on their pajamas;

- Extending results from a lifetime of exposure in rodents to exposure of humans over a period of perhaps 1 to 2% of their lifetimes.

Though each of these is a problem in toxicology or carcinogenesis, each is also a problem in statistics because it affects overall uncertainty about the meaning of the data for the specific problem at hand, and hence affects the scientific and statistical inferences that may be drawn from the data.

It should be no surprise that several scientists, all quite competent in this sort of work, made different assumptions, approximations, and guesses about these and other critical uncertainties. These differences are reflected in what the risk assessors presented as their best estimates of the lifetime risk of kidney cancer per million infants exposed: Brown, Schneiderman, and Chu[4] estimated 52 per million exposed children (upper 95% confidence level, and based on the mouse data); Harris[5] estimated 7 to 6300 per million; Hooper and Ames[6] estimated 17,000 per million; and the Consumer Product Safety Commission (CPSC) staff[7] estimated 160 per million (averaged over males and females).

The most critical points of difference among the risk analyses concerned the amount of Tris that would be absorbed from treated garments and the relation between risk to animals and risk to humans at similar exposure levels. These involved a host of subsidiary questions such as the decline in availability of Tris as garments are washed repeatedly, how many garments a child would wear, and the effects of age at exposure and duration of exposure. The nature of other differences among the risk assessors is illustrated by some of the decisions made by Hooper and Ames that:

- Twelve Tris-treated garments would be worn during the first year of life;

- Each garment had 5000 cm^2 of surface area, half of which would be in contact with the child at any one time;

- The amount of Tris available for absorption per cm^2 could be determined by the amount removed from polyester fabric (the fabric most commonly used) by solvents; for this they used a number halfway between the amounts of Tris removed from "high" surface Tris garments and those classified as "low," with adjustment for the amount removed by washing weekly for one year and calculated that 30 mcg/cm^2 of Tris was available for absorption; and

- Six percent of this available Tris is absorbed through the skin and 1% by mouthing the garment.

From such estimates and calculations, Hooper and Ames estimated that a child would absorb 70 mg/kg/year. They then assumed that cancer risk in children and in rats would be the same in terms of mg/kg/year. The other risk assessors went through similar processes but made other assumptions: for example, that the animal–human conversion should be in terms of surface area rather than weight; that the risk to humans should reflect the small fraction of the normal life span during which they were exposed (perhaps 2%, rather than the 100% in animals); or that mice would provide a closer estimate of human risk than rats.

Each group of risk assessors had a lively appreciation of the uncertainties in its estimate, and the problems were discussed at length, both in the risk assessment documents and in formal testimony before the CPSC. But errors were discussed in terms of a single order of magnitude—10-fold—rather than the substantially larger differences actually existing among the four estimates— a factor of roughly 300 (from 52 to 17,000) or even 2500 (from 7 to 17,000). Nor can the skeptical observer even be sure that these ranges bound the true value. If each "best estimate" is equally likely to fall above or below the true value, the chance that four independent estimates would all be too low is 1 in 16, or 6.25%. These estimates were not independent—the risk assessors communicated freely with each other, as we would want them to do, and they all had access to the same data—so the chance that all four are too low may be a good bit larger than 6.25%.

Despite these uncertainties, the control of the potential hazards of Tris was a success of risk assessment methods. By 1977, when Tris was recognized as a possible human carcinogen, an improved range of other flame retardants had been developed for use on clothing, and there was no evidence to show that they were hazardous. The CPSC commissioners found that even the lowest estimate of cancer risk for Tris—7 per million over a lifetime, or about 20 to 25 cancers per year if all infants in the United States wore Tris-treated sleepwear for their first year—was too high. As the CPSC commissioners moved to regulate the use of Tris, the industry itself voluntarily stopped using it on clothing and on fabric meant for clothing. These four quantitative assessments of health risk differed in many ways, including their conclusions about the size of the risk, but they contributed to the same decision.

THE HEALTH EFFECTS OF AUTOMOTIVE EMISSIONS

My last example has to do with controlling the health effects of automotive emissions. Solid evidence indicates that the very high levels of general air pollution sometimes seen in the past in many countries, particularly in air that was stagnant over large cities for long periods of time, increased both morbidity and mortality. The increases were sometimes quite large. Many cities and countries have had much success in cleaning up the air, and today's questions center on whether today's reduced pollution levels still have some small effects, and if so, whether they merit remedial action. Such questions require a quantitative estimate of the risk, specific for various population segments if possible. However, it would be highly infeasible and probably impossible to conduct a good research study linking the health of the population directly to tailpipe emissions. Fortunately, we can break this huge, shapeless question into smaller parts that are still difficult, but offer some hope of success. Specifically, what we want to know can be cast in a short series of linked questions:

- What is getting into the air from various sources, including automotive engines?

- How do emissions translate into personal exposures (including personal variations such as for persons living near a major roadway, or indoor versus outdoor locations)?

- What effects do those exposures have on human morbidity and mortality, with special attention to persons who may be at increased risk by reason of co-existing disease, genetic makeup, or concurrent exposures to potentially synergistic agents, or for other reasons?

Each of these questions is difficult to answer, and the linkages from one to the next are not easily established. The Environmental Protection Agency (EPA), which has responsibility for air quality in the United States, has constructed a series of rather elaborate statistical models to deal with various aspects of outdoor air pollution, including automotive emissions (for various classes of trucks as well as automobiles, and all types of fuels). Similar models have been developed in Germany and elsewhere. However, these models estimate emissions—and stop at that. We must take on faith that emissions translate into exposures, and that exposures translate into adverse health effects. One aspect of that faith is that most persons spend most of their time indoors, often with heating and air conditioning systems that may alter the composition of the outdoor air. But even emissions are difficult to measure, and there are numerous important matters for which one simply cannot obtain good data. For example, few persons seem to want to have their own cars selected for testing that takes several days, and many might not want to have monitoring instruments on-board in their cars—especially persons who know that they are driving high polluters. We do not know how owners' perceptions of their cars' possible problems may affect willingness to submit cars for testing, so test results may be correct for the cars tested but seriously inaccurate for the population of cars on the road.

Or, one might want to know the effect on engine emissions of some change in the design of a fuel injection system or a spark plug. Innovations can be put in test engines and their performance examined in detail in the laboratory, or even on the road. But there is no way to tell, today, what might be coming out of an engine built today but still on the road twenty years hence, possibly after it has been poorly maintained or seriously misused.

We might want to estimate or predict the impact of a revised program of inspection and maintenance of vehicles. Many persons are now familiar with the routine: We may wait for hours for our cars to be briefly tested and certified (we hope) as meeting regulatory standards for use on the road. In many states, testing includes sampling of the exhaust, and we blandly, or blindly, assume that those cars that fail to meet the test will be either repaired or taken out of service. There is good evidence that that is not true, at least in the United States. About two thirds of vehicles failing these state-mandated tests simply do not appear again in later testing records, nor is there evidence that they have been scrapped. Are they moved to a different state that has less demanding, or no, testing requirements? Are they converted to off-road uses? Are some in fact repaired but not retested? How many are still in regular use, not repaired and without the certification that the state requires? We do not know, but the EPA must model these and many other factors, and then use the model to set standards that are known to be very costly to consumers, on the assumption that the unmeasured health benefits are likely to exceed the highly visible costs.

Again, this matter is inherently and unavoidably statistical, because it deals with the analysis and interpretation of quantitative data, including data that are unavailable and must be guessed at in order to deal with a policy issue of considerable public importance. It shows, however, that dividing a complex problem into parts—a form of divide and conquer—can simplify analysis and interpretation. Here, the EPA has divided the problem into segments (in practice, many more than the three listed above), developed data, models, and analytic methods to solve each segment, and linked the segments together to develop overall assessments of health risks. Such an approach raises critical questions about both the reliability of conclusions about each part and the linkages among them, but I see no feasible alternative. To draw a direct line from automotive emissions to human health effects would require a vast, complex, and very expensive new data system that would be so unwieldy that quality in all its aspects could not be guaranteed. The EPA is well aware of the difficulties in its assessment of the "bottom line" and is appropriately cautious in proposing new regulations on the basis of somewhat uncertain estimates of risk.

USING STATISTICAL CONCEPTS

These four examples differ in obvious and important ways, but they have a few critical similarities. Each involves a serious and, in retrospect, obvious problem in statistical thinking; the investigators did not always recognize these problems. Each required the interpretation of a body of scientific and technical data that was large, complex, known to have some defects, and not precisely targeted at the question of present interest. Further, knowledgeable people subjected each of the four to extensive statistical analysis. And in the end, in each example the uncertainty generated by random variability was essentially trivial in relation to other uncertainties:

- With the Gulf War Syndrome the problem was the absence of good data, the likelihood of serious bias in what was available, and the general political atmosphere, which demanded answers when none were available.

- With carcinogen dose-response curves, general acceptance of a critical assumption introduced substantial uncertainty. The assumption was not validated against the data until 1988 (when it was found wanting), despite ready opportunities to do so.

- With Tris, the risk assessors had to make some judgment about the size of the added risk and to make it as useful as possible, despite huge uncertainties that were acknowledged by all parties.

- With automotive emissions, the problem was the very complex link between the engine and fuel that cause the problem and the ultimate, often long-delayed, health endpoints that might be affected.

The problems were apparent in these four examples because we had access to at least some data, from the same or other sources, showing contrary findings. That is not common in science, despite the general notion that the scientific method involves independent replication. Strict replication is actually rare in science; professional rewards such as advancement and tenure, as well as the sociology of science, produce substantial pressures to refute, but none to replicate. In my work as statistical consultant for the *New England Journal of Medicine,* I reviewed close to 400 papers each year. Nearly all of these had passed the rigorous standards of outside peer reviewers, and had also been judged by the *Journal* staff to be likely to meet other standards for publication, including scientific importance, interest to readers, ultimate relevance to medical practice, length, quality of writing, and balance of fields covered by the *Journal.* About half of the papers that came to me for statistical review were eventually published in the *Journal.* How many of these 400 papers, judged to be of high quality, would pass the test of independent confirmation? How many are really free of major, unrecognized problems in basic assumptions, or study design, or quality of data, or interpretation of findings, or generalization to other subjects? I do not know, but as time passes and as I see more and more scientific work that appears to be sound but is overturned by newer (and sometimes better) studies, some patterns seem to emerge. Many of the problems are what I regard as fundamentally statistical, and many of these statistical problems are subject to considerable amelioration. The solutions to these problems involve what I call statistical thinking, as did the four examples above—that is, they involve concepts, definitions, procedures, and ways of looking at scientific processes and data that focus on drawing inferences from information that is inevitably incomplete or subject to error. To the extent that information (not just the data from a particular experiment) is subject to error, the inferences are uncertain; and statistical thinking is the best way to anticipate, detect, measure, reduce, and otherwise manage such uncertainty.

Statisticians have some reason to be pleased with their long and successful history of educating themselves and others in some basic statistical matters. That success has not only been helpful in itself; it has been an essential base for moving forward. For example, statistical methods have led to substantial advances in many scientific fields, though the basic assumptions that underlie those methods are rarely satisfied exactly and the results are often misinterpreted or misused. We can now move on to the next level of sophistication, where uncertainty (and the statistical treatment of uncertainty) is even more important and generally different from the routine.

Statistical thinking, as embodied in the best practice of applied statistics, is the art and science of inference, as opposed to subject matter and technical content. Because the sources of uncertainty are so varied, statistics must concern itself with the full range of scientific activity—and indeed statistics can have much to offer at each step, from framing the initial questions for study, to designing an investigation and setting a protocol, to the collection and processing of data, to formal analysis, and ultimately to the drawing of generalizations to subjects and groups not studied.

Statistics, or inference, is the machinery of the scientific method. It is the cogs and wheels, the belts and pulleys, the presses and drills and furnaces that are left when we take away the specifics of problem and discipline and data. A few examples of these very general statistical tools and concepts are research design, data reduction, randomization, the special role of prior hypotheses, blind assessment of outcomes, and replication. These aspects of statistics were implicit in its original definition, but they have become a critical foundation for all of medical science and, indeed, for science in general. Statistics, like mathematics, can be studied in its own right, and again like mathematics, it can be applied to an enormous and varied range of problems.

LESSONS FROM THE EXAMPLES

These examples, and many others in health and in quite unrelated fields, have led me to recognize four features of statistical data available for use in almost any issue that has important policy implications.[8] First is that the data are likely to be vast. One could fill many shelves, even libraries, with material relevant to each of my four examples, and the scope of available material for some other problems would be even greater.

Second, the data tend to be highly complex, in the sense that the problem involves many scientific and technical disciplines as well as non-scientific fields, and no one person can be expert in all of them.

For example, full understanding of the Gulf War Syndrome would require deep knowledge of military operations, in general and in the Gulf Theater; the actual locations of the troops in the Gulf area and their possible exposures; the prevailing winds and weather near the sites of presumed exposure; the health-care systems for military personnel and veterans (including the civilian systems used by most veterans, and including medical healthcare record systems as well as medical care more generally); toxicology; biostatistics; epidemiology; survey statistics (especially response biases); and many other disciplines. Given that nobody can be expert in all of these disciplines simultaneously, how are we to deal with this complex situation? The answer is to use a multidisciplinary approach, in which people with a broad range of expertise and experience work together to solve the problem.

Third, most of the data and analyses that are available are of poor quality. My review of published and unpublished materials on each of the four problems discussed above, and many other topics, has shown uniformly that a small amount of good work has been done, but that poor work is far more common, and that a person who is not expert in the field and is not appropriately critical could be seriously misled. Even organizing and getting through a mountain of relevant literature, to determine what subset is worth detailed attention, can be a daunting task.

Fourth, most of what is available will not be appropriate anyway. My best example is estimation of the carcinogenic potential of a chemical that has been tested in animals but for which no human data are available. Laboratory experiments have an important role in this situation and will remain important because chemical compounds are often newly synthesized, or considered for new uses. Ideally, such compounds should not be manufactured and used in quantity if they present serious health hazards to unsophisticated users, but this means that our understanding of possible health risks must be derived from studies in other animals, tissue or organ cultures, the chemical structure of the compound, and other sources, before extensive human exposure occurs. The best substitutes for human data are data from long-term animal testing, but such studies have grave limitations. Because of limits on the feasible sizes of experiments, it is necessary to test small numbers of animals at high doses— but one must then extrapolate from high to low exposures as well as from animal species to humans. There may be additional extrapolations from lifetime exposure to intermittent or irregular exposure, or from one route of administration (such as food) to another (such as inhalation), as well as still other kinds of extrapolations. At the end, these uncertainties are compounded to a level where actual risks to humans, or even whether there is any risk at all, may be very uncertain. Repeated but independent risk assessments of the same chemical have commonly shown differences of 1000-fold or more. I do not recommend that we abandon such assessments, which are generally the best we can do, but risk assessors should (and commonly do) point to the inherent limitations on the precision of the estimates that can be produced. I firmly believe that, despite these problems, it is better to have a reliable summary of what is known, including uncertainties, than to just guess.

Consider these four features of data that I find are related to almost any policy issue—that they are vast, complex, of poor quality, and off-target anyway—and see whether you do not find echoes of them in your own fields of endeavor.

These considerations, based on my concern about the relation between statistics and policy, lead me to conclude that bias (in its broadest statistical sense) is almost invariably more important than randomness (or sampling variation), at least where the outcome matters very much. Statistics, in its original sense, is inherently an integrative discipline, but that sense has been largely abandoned. We may measure effects rather precisely in any one small, well-designed research study, but there will inevitably be important differences among separate studies of the same phenomenon. We should give substantial attention to what is already known about related areas of the subject, and there is often scope for considerable interpretation about the application of results to a specific situation.

ACKNOWLEDGMENTS

I am indebted to several colleagues for thoughtful and helpful comments, especially Drs. Marvin Schneiderman, Frederick Mosteller, Richard N. L. Andrews, and David Bates; and to the Editor of *Risk Analysis* for permission to reprint Tables 1 and 2 and Figures 2 and 3.

REFERENCES

1. Bailar JC, Crouch EAC, Shaikh R, Spiegelman D. One-hit models of carcinogenesis: conservative or not? Risk Analysis 1988; 8:485–97.

2. Maltoni C, Lefemine G, Gilberti A, et al. Vinyl chloride carcinogenicity bioassays (BT project). Epidemiologie Animale et Humaine. Proceedings of the 20th meeting of Le Club Cancerogenese Clinique, Paris, November 10, 1979.

3. Bailar JC III, McGinnis JM, Needleman J, Berney B. Methodological challenges in health risk assessment. Auburn House, 1993.

4. Brown C, Schneiderman M, Chu K. Estimation of human lifetime carcinogenic risk from exposure to Tris. Memorandum to the U.S. Consumer Product Safety Commission. March 21, 1977.

5. Harris RH. Estimating the cancer hazard to children from Tris-treated sleepwear. Memorandum to the U.S. Consumer Product Safety Commission. March 8, 1977.

6. Hooper NK, Ames BN. Letter to John Byington, Chair, U.S. Consumer Product Safety Commission. March 21,1977.

7. Bayard SP. Preliminary analysis of Tris-induced human lifetime risk to cancer based on data from the NCI lifetime animal study and BBS best estimate of lifetime human exposure. Letter to Robert M. Mehir. March 17, 1977.

8. Bailar JC. Inhalation hazards: The interpretation of epidemiologic evidence. In: Assessment of inhalation hazards, U. Mohr et al., eds., Springer-Verlag, pages 39–48, 1989.

CHAPTER 3
ℭ

Use of Statistical Analysis in the New England Journal of Medicine

SHILPI AGARWAL, M.B.B.S., GRAHAM A. COLDITZ, M.D.,
DR.P.H., AND JOHN D. EMERSON, PH.D.

ABSTRACT   Surveys of the statistical methods used by the authors of the 332 Original Articles in Volumes 298 through 301 (1978–1979), the 115 Original Articles in Volume 321 (1989), and the 97 Original Articles in Volume 350 (January–June 2004) of the *New England Journal of Medicine* reveal an increasing variety of uses of statistics. A reader whose statistical knowledge is limited to some simple descriptive statistics (percentages, means, and standard deviations) had full access to 27% of the articles in 1978–1979, but this access has declined to 12% in 2004. Physicians and others need a good basis in understanding statistical concepts and methods if they are to keep up with the literature. Among the surveys' 21 categories of methods, 66% of the Original Articles in 2004 used some form of survival analysis, followed in frequency by epidemiologic statistics (53%) and contingency tables (43%). Familiarity with sophisticated statistical methods, in addition to more-basic concepts such as power and t-tests (each reported by 36% of the 2004 articles), has become increasingly important for access to articles in the *Journal*.

The categories of statistical methods reported most frequently in the 2004 survey showed substantial increases from the earlier surveys. Survival methods increased from 11% in 1978–1979 to 32% in 1989 to 66% in 2004. Use of epidemiologic statistics increased from 9% to 22% to 53%. Use of contingency tables increased more gradually, from 27% to 36% to 43%. Reporting of power remained at 3% from 1978–1979 to 1989, but then rose to 36% in 2004. Overall, among Original Articles that reported using methods beyond descriptive statistics, the average number of such methods per article rose from 2.3 in 1978–1979 to 2.9 in 1989 and 3.8 in 2004.

From these data and reviews of statistical methods used in specialty journals, we conclude that Original Articles in general medical journals are making increasing use of statistical methods. The tabulations in this study should aid clinicians and medical investigators who are planning their continuing education in statistical methods, as well as faculty who design or teach courses in quantitative methods for medical and other health professionals.

In this chapter we report on the frequency of use of statistical techniques in the *New England Journal of Medicine* to answer such questions as the following: Will knowledge of a few elementary statistical techniques, such as chi-squared analyses and *t*-tests, assist readers in understanding the statistical content of a high percentage of research articles in the *Journal*? Which techniques are used most often and, therefore, could most profitably be part of the readers' statistical background? To aid clinicians and medical investigators who are continuing their own education, as well as persons designing courses in biostatistics for physicians and others, we report on components of the statistical content of Original Articles in Volume 350 (January–June 2004). To document the change in the use of various statistical methods over time, we also present parallel results from the Original Articles of Volume 321 (1989) and Volumes 298–301 (1978–1979).

METHODS

This chapter analyzes Volume 350 (January–June 2004), Volume 321 (1989), and Volumes 298–301 (January 1978–December 1979) of the *Journal*. For 2004 and 1989, all articles identified as Original Articles were reviewed, as the use of statistical methods is concentrated in those articles. Ninety-seven Original Articles in Volume 350 (2004) and 115 in Volume 321 (1989) were reviewed in detail.

The earlier review of Volumes 298–301 (1978–1979) included all articles identified in the table of contents as Original Articles, Medical Progress articles, Medical Intelligence articles, and Seminars in Medicine of Beth Israel Hospital, Boston.[1] Of those 760 articles, 332 were Original Articles.

Throughout these studies, two reviewers read the Methods sections and all tables and figures, and scanned other sections of the article for the pertinent information. For each article, the presence or absence of statistical methods in each of 21 categories, described below, was recorded and entered in coded form into a computer file. All reviewers were faculty members, postdoctoral fellows, or graduate students trained in both quantitative sciences and statistical applications to medical research.

Categories of Statistical Methods

Table 1 lists the 21 categories of statistical methods used and gives a brief description of their content. Although most categories in Table 1 need no further description, some categories required a judgment according to the following criteria.

Articles in the first category contain no statistical methods other than percentages, means, standard deviations, standard errors, and histograms. Thus, these articles lack the statistical content to belong to other categories. Only this category is defined so that it does not overlap with any of the others.

The *multiple comparisons* category includes any methods that adjust significance levels or *p*-values when several statistical comparisons are made. Chapter 8 of this book and Godfrey discuss these and related issues in some detail.[2, 3] *Cost-benefit analysis* requires a direct quantitative comparison of cost with benefits.

Considerations of *power* can arise in a number of ways; we looked for an indication that sample size was determined, in part, by considering the probability of detecting a specific effect or alternative hypothesis. A post-hoc analysis of power was considered an acceptable treatment, as were other, more-formal analyses. Significance tests or confidence limits, although useful, did not qualify as treatments of power. Freiman et al.[4] describe the importance and interpretations of power in medical research design.

When an article contained an examination or analysis of data in a scale other than that of the raw data (for example, as square roots or logarithms), we indicated that a *transformation* was used. We did not count the replacement of raw data with ranks or categories as transformation.

The last category ("other") includes specialized methods, each used in at least one article, that did not fit into the previously defined categories. For example, Lang et al.[5] examined the modeling of plasma glucose and insulin concentrations in human beings by fitting a sine curve to the "smoothed" time series. Another article[6] used the Kolmogorov-Smirnov test for goodness of fit. During 2004, we observed a great variety of other methods—for example, principal component analysis[7] and significance analysis of microarrays (SAM) and prediction analysis of microarrays (PAM),[8] used mostly in gene-expression studies or genetic epidemiologic research.

Occasionally, a particular method, although not used by the authors themselves, was mentioned when citing the work of others. We attributed such methods to the article concerned because we believe that an understanding of the method in question would enhance statistical understanding of the article.

Table 1. Categories of Statistical Procedures Used to Assess the Statistical Content of Articles.	
Category	**Brief Description**
No statistical methods or descriptive statistics only	No statistical content, or descriptive statistics only (e.g., percentages, means, standard deviations, standard errors, histograms)
Contingency tables	Chi-squared test, Fisher's exact test, McNemar's test
Multiway tables	Mantel-Haenszel procedure, log-linear models
Epidemiologic statistics	Relative risk, odds ratio, log odds, measures of association, sensitivity, specificity
Student's *t*-test	One-sample, matched-pair, and two-sample *t*-tests
Pearson correlation	Classic product-moment correlation
Nonparametric correlation	Spearman's rho, Kendall's tau, test for trend
Simple linear regression	Least-squares regression with one predictor and one response variable
Multiple regression	Least-squares regression with >1 predictor (includes polynomial regression and stepwise regression)
Analysis of variance	Analysis of variance, analysis of covariance, and *F* tests
Multiple comparisons	Procedures for handling multiple inferences on same data set (e.g., Bonferroni techniques, Scheffé's contrasts, Duncan multiple-range procedures, Newman-Keuls procedure)
Nonparametric tests	Sign test, Wilcoxon signed-rank test, Mann-Whitney test
Life table	Actuarial life table, Kaplan-Meier estimate of survival
Regression for survival	Cox proportional-hazards and logistic regression
Other survival analysis	Kruskal-Wallis test, log-rank test
Adjustment and standardization	Adjusted incidence rate and prevalence rate
Sensitivity analysis	Examines sensitivity of outcome to changes in parameters of model or in other assumptions
Power	Loosely defined; includes use of the size of a detectable (or useful) difference in determining sample size
Transformation	Use of data transformation (e.g., logarithms), often in regression
Cost-benefit analysis	Combining estimates of cost and health outcomes to compare policy alternatives
Other	Anything not fitting above headings, such as cluster analysis, discriminant analysis, Scatchard analysis, Jonckheere-Terpstra test, Gray's method, Poisson regression, Satterthwaite's correction, forest plot, Shapiro-Wilk test, principal components, nearest-shrunken-centroid method, significance analysis of microarrays (SAM), prediction analysis of microarrays (PAM)

Quality Control

Any discrepancies between reviewers were resolved by discussion. During 2004 this process resolved discrepancies for 3 items. During 1978–1979 reviewers examined 218 of the 760 articles in detail. For these articles, any discrepancies between the two independent reviewers were discussed and resolved. The remaining 542 articles were reviewed more briefly for the presence or absence of specific statistical procedures and techniques. The accuracy of the coding of these articles was determined by an independent examination of 96 of them. Discrepancies were found for 15 items in 11 articles. Another careful reading of those articles indicated that all but two errors involved overlooking a procedure.

Study Design

For the 97 Original Articles from Volume 350 (January–June 2004), the percentage distribution of types of study design was: randomized clinical trial, 46%; prospective cohort, 25%; case-control, 8%; case series, 14%; and case report, 7%.

The 115 Original Articles from Volume 321 (January–June 1989) were not classified by study design. For 1978–1979, we partitioned the 332 Original Articles into longitudinal (prospective or retrospective[9]) and cross-sectional designs. Longitudinal studies aim to elucidate a state of nature that changes or may change. Cross-sectional studies focus on phenomena that are thought to be static over the period of interest. The percentage distribution was: prospective, 55%; retrospective, 5%; and cross-sectional, 40%.

RESULTS

Table 2 summarizes the frequency of statistical methods used in Volume 350 (January–June 2004). Twelve percent of the articles used either no statistical methods or only descriptive statistics. Beyond those articles, most articles used more than one method, so that the 97 articles contained a total of 339 article-methods.

Survival methods, the most frequent category, were used by 66% of the articles. Epidemiologic statistics, at 53%, was the only other category above 50%. Four other categories were found in at least 25% of the articles: contingency tables, power, t-tests, and nonparametric tests. The remaining 11 specific categories were used in, at most, 12% of the articles. Fourteen percent of the articles used other statistical methods. Within the category of survival methods, we found that 37% of the 97 papers used life tables, 30% Cox proportional-hazard models, 26% log-rank tests, 21% logistic regression, and 6% the Kruskal-Wallis test.

Table 3 shows the percentage frequency of statistical methods used in Original Articles from Volumes 298–301 (1978–1979), Volume 321 (1989), and

Table 2. Statistical Content of 97 Original Articles in Volume 350 (January–June 2004) of the *New England Journal of Medicine*.

Procedure	N	Percent
No statistical method or descriptive statistics only	12	12
Survival methods*	64	66
Epidemiologic statistics	51	53
Contingency tables	42	43
Power	35	36
t-tests	35	36
Nonparametric tests	24	25
Transformation	12	12
Analysis of variance	11	11
Adjustment and standardization	9	9
Nonparametric correlation	6	6
Multiple regression	6	6
Simple linear regression	5	5
Multiway tables	4	4
Multiple comparisons	3	3
Pearson correlation	3	3
Cost-benefit analysis	1	1
Sensitivity analysis	2	2
Other methods	14	14
Total article-methods**	339	

*"Survival methods" includes the original categories of life table (36 articles), regression for survival (48), and other survival analysis methods (30).

**When the three categories of survival methods are distinguished, there are 392 article-method uses in 2004.

Volume 350 (2004) of the *Journal*. The percentage of articles reporting the use of no statistical methods decreased over time, and the use of survival methods rose from 11% in 1978–1979 to 66% in 2004. The use of epidemiologic statistics also increased greatly, from 9% to 53%, and reporting of power became much more common (36%). Other categories of statistical procedures showed smaller changes in reporting over time.

DISCUSSION

Nearly 88% of the 97 *Journal* articles surveyed in 2004 relied on some type of statistical analysis beyond simple descriptive statistics. These articles used survival methods most frequently (66% of all articles), followed by epidemiologic statistics (53%), contingency tables (43%), and power (36%). We are impressed with the varied combinations of methods employed, although this finding does depend on the initial definition of the categories.

Table 3. Statistical Content of Original Articles in Volumes 298–301 (1978 and 1979), Volume 321 (1989), and Volume 350 (2004) of the *New England Journal of Medicine*.

Procedure	1978–1979 N = 332 (percent of total)	1989 N = 115 (percent of total)	2004 N = 97 (percent of total)
No statistical method or descriptive statistics only	27	12	12
Survival methods[†]	11	32	66
Epidemiologic statistics	9	22	53
Contingency tables	27	36	43
Power	3	3	36
t-tests	44	39	36
Nonparametric tests	11	21	25
Transformation	7	7	12
Analysis of variance	8	20	11
Adjustment and standardization	3	9	9
Nonparametric correlation	4	1	6
Multiple regression	5	14	6
Simple linear regression	8	9	5
Multiway tables	4	10	4
Multiple comparisons	3	9	3
Pearson correlation	12	19	3
Cost-benefit analysis	1	0	1
Other methods	3	9	14
Total article-methods	637	311	339

Percentages do not add up to 100% because many articles used more than one form of statistical analysis.

† "Survival methods" includes the original categories of life table, regression for survival, and other survival analysis methods.

Comparing the results from 2004 and those from 1978–1979 and 1989 confirms our main findings of increasingly frequent and varied usage of statistical methods by *Journal* authors. If there was a trend in the 1980s, it was toward increased use of newer and more varied statistical techniques. Methods for analyzing survival data had the largest apparent gains; in particular, we noticed more use of regression techniques for analyzing survival outcomes. More generally, we found that *Journal* authors frequently use techniques of multiple logistic regression for analyzing binary responses. Increasing use of survival analysis through the 1990s is reflected in the reporting of this method in 66% of studies in 2004 in comparison to 11% in 1978–1979 and 32% in 1989. The increase in attention to power was also substantial: from 3% (1978–1979 and 1989) to 36% (2004). Use of epidemiologic statistics increased from 9% in 1978–1979 to 22% in 1989 and to 53% in year 2004.

We cannot conclude with certainty that the apparent shifts in the counts and percentages reflect changes in statistical practice. The observed changes may arise in part from differences in our own research methods. However, these findings further strengthen our main message that *Journal* authors use a wide array of statistical methods and that many Original Articles use varied combinations of these methods. A passing acquaintance with a few basic statistical techniques cannot give full access to research appearing in the *Journal*.

To assess differences in the use of statistical methods in general medicine journals and specialized journals, we identified reviews of statistical methods used in specialized journals. A 1995 study, comparing prevalence and use of statistical analysis, finds that rheumatology journals[10] tended to use fewer and simpler statistics than general medicine journals. A 1994 study of use of statistical analytic methods in the *AJR* and *Radiology*[11] shows that 44% of the major articles used no statistical methods or descriptive statistics only, reflecting the nature of imaging studies; further, 15% used only two methods, and 14% used three or more methods. On the other hand, a study of *Pediatrics* shows that statistical complexity has increased from 1982 to 2005, based on a review of all papers in Volume 115.[12] The number of statistical procedures per article increased (from 2.5 in 1982 to 3.9 in 2005), as did the range of inferential statistical procedures used.

A 1987 review of surgical journals shows that a reader who has knowledge of descriptive statistics has access to 44.5% of the articles,[13] whereas in 2002 only 18% of the articles in obstetrics and gynecology journals do not use any type of statistical method,[14] and by 2005 only 11% of general pediatrics articles do not use inferential statistics. We conclude that the Original Articles in general medical journals are using increasingly complex statistical techniques.

The use in medicine of a wide range of statistical methods gives clinicians and medical investigators good reason to continue their own education in statistics. The percentages presented in Table 2 may help them in identifying the statistical techniques they should master. This study reviews statistical techniques from the perspective of a general reader and makes no attempt to identify a hierarchy of statistical backgrounds, which may vary for physicians within each specialty. Furthermore, the *Journal* is oriented to clinical medicine in general, and professional specialization may influence the relative importance of the various statistical methods.

REFERENCES

1. Emerson JD, Colditz GA. Use of statistical analysis in the *New England Journal of Medicine*. N Engl J Med 1983; 309(12):709–13.

2. Ware JH, Mosteller F, Delgado F, Donnelly C, Ingelfinger JA. *p*-values. Chapter 8 of this book.

3. Godfrey K. Comparing the means of several groups. N Eng J Med 1985; 313:1450–6.

4. Freiman JA, Chalmers TC, Smith H Jr, Kuebler RR. The importance of beta, the type 2 error, and sample size in the design and interpretation of the randomized controlled trial: Survey of 71 "negative" trials. N Engl J Med 1978; 299:690–4.

5. Lang DA, Mathew DR, Peto J, Turner RC. Cyclic oscillations of basal plasma glucose and insulin concentrations in human beings. N Eng J Med 1979; 301:1023–7.

6. Ault KA. Detection of small numbers of monoclonal B lymphocytes in the blood of patients with lymphoma. N Engl J Med 1979; 300:1401–5.

7. Bullinger L, Döhner K, et al. Use of gene-expression profiling to identify prognostic sub-classes in adult acute myeloid leukemia. N Eng J Med 2004; 350:1605–16.

8. Valk PJM, Verhaak RGW. Prognostically useful gene-expression profiles in acute myeloid leukemia. N Eng J Med 2004; 350:1617–28.

9. White C, Bailar JC III. Retrospective and prospective methods of studying association in medicine. Am J Public Health 1956; 46:35–44.

10. Cardiel, MH. Type of statistical techniques in rheumatology and internal medicine journals. Rev Invest Clin 1995; 47(3):197–201.

11. Elster, AD. Use of statistical analysis in the AJR and Radiology: frequency, methods, and subspecialty differences. AJR 1994; 163(3):711–5.

12. Hellems MA, Gurka MJ, Hayden GF. Statistical literacy for readers of Pediatrics: a moving target. Pediatrics 2007; 119(6):1083–8.

13. Reznick RK. A rationale for teaching of statistics to surgical residents. Surgery 1987; 101(5):611–7.

14. Welch GE, Gabbe SG. Statistics usage in the *American Journal of Obstetrics and Gynecology*: has anything changed? Am J Obstet Gynecol 2002; 186(3):584–6.

Design

CHAPTER 4

♋

Randomized Trials and Other Parallel Comparisons of Treatment

NANCY E. MAYO, PH.D.

ABSTRACT   The strongest evidence for the benefits or risks of a treatment comes from assigning subjects by a random mechanism to one of two or more treatments and then following the groups in parallel over time. These features define the classic randomized clinical trial (RCT). RCTs are deceptively simple because they are theoretically straightforward, but, as with many things, the devil is in the details. By drawing on reports, primarily of intervention studies, from the *New England Journal of Medicine* (NEJM), this chapter surveys five critical issues of research design: (1) specifying the question; (2) choosing the method for assigning subjects to groups; (3) appraising the choice of outcomes; (4) weighing the statistical power of the study; and (5) recognizing a need to end a study early.

A vast amount of literature discusses the design and analysis of intervention studies, primarily randomized clinical trials. Other literature focuses on how readers can rate the quality of clinical trials.[1, 2] Few works, however, address the needs of both reader and investigator. To help fill this gap, this chapter and Chapter 9 discuss features of the design and analysis of randomized clinical trials that both investigators and readers need to know if they are to put the most into, and get the most out of, journal articles.

Trials, like other parallel designs, enroll groups of subjects during the same calendar period and follow them over the same time interval. Many parallel designs start with random assignment of subjects to two or more treatment groups. Outcomes in the groups are compared at the end of the study (between-group comparisons). Parallel designs do not focus on changes within treatment groups (within-group comparisons), nor do they include historical controls, studies in which the treatment is not under the direct control of the investigators, or those in which subjects are their own controls, as in a time-series or cross-over design (Chapter 5).

A parallel design aims to evaluate a deliberate intervention, often an innovation in treatment. The strongest evidence for the benefits or risks of a treatment comes from assigning subjects by a random mechanism to one of two or more treatments; these generally include either placebo treatment or the current standard treatment. The groups are then followed in parallel over time. These features define the classic randomized clinical trial (RCT).

This chapter surveys critical issues of research design by drawing on reports, primarily of intervention studies, from the *New England Journal of Medicine* (NEJM). This choice of topics followed a review of 76 reports (covering 73 RCTs) published in NEJM in 2003. Boxes for eight studies summarize important design features of these RCTs.

WHAT IS THE QUESTION?

In clinical medicine, research study of some treatment begins with patients who have an identifiable health condition and are in optimal settings (termed efficacy studies) before the treatment is tested in the wider world of more-typical patients and settings (termed effectiveness studies).[3] In efficacy studies the investigators try to ensure exact compliance with the study protocol as well as full adherence on the part of the participants, whether the intervention is pharmacological, behavioral, or surgical. In an RCT success depends on meticulous attention to detail at all levels, whereas in effectiveness studies, the participants are tested in their natural settings[3]; they may not get all components of the intervention optimally and may deviate from the regimen prescribed in the protocol. This distinction does not imply that efficacy studies are somehow "better" than effectiveness studies. Both are essential, and effectiveness studies must be done when interventions are likely to be disseminated and offered outside strictly controlled laboratory or clinical settings. Although presented as a dichotomy, the distinction between these two terms is not always clear. Table 1 summarizes some of the key differences between efficacy and effectiveness.

Table 1. Defining Features of Efficacy and Effectiveness Trials.	
Efficacy	**Effectiveness**
Ideal circumstances	Real-world circumstances
Perfect compliance	Compliance self-determined
No protocol violations	Protocol violations may occur
Endpoints on all subjects	Missing data and incomplete follow-up
Intention-to-treat analysis / per protocol analysis (subjects with missing data are often excluded)	Intention-to-treat analysis; missing data imputed

Typical efficacy studies offer the experimental interventions under circumstances that would maximize compliance. For example, two studies compared the efficacy of infusions of natalizumab vs. placebo for Crohn's disease[4] and for relapsing multiple sclerosis.[5] The protocols for both studies stipulated that patients would come to the hospital for intervention. Wainwright et al.[6] compared treatment with nebulized epinephrine or placebo on duration of illness of hospitalized infants with acute bronchiolitis. The intent of these three studies was to offer the experimental drugs under circumstances that would maximize adherence to the protocol as well as completeness of the data.

Interventions can be offered in ways that reduce barriers to adherence without going to the extreme of hospital admission. An example of a close-to-efficacy study targeted persons with opiate addiction.[7] Subjects had to come to physicians' offices on weekdays, and they received the study drugs in one of three formulations: buprenorphine alone, with naloxone, or with placebo. This design ensured good compliance, and urine samples showed that the medication was taken on 90% of scheduled days. Another close-to-efficacy study compared the effect of using ordinary vs. impermeable bed covers on symptoms of allergies.[8, 9] Research personnel installed covers for subjects' bedding without the subjects knowing which type of cover they had received. Though a few subjects dropped out, the procedures facilitated compliance with the use of the covers.

In 2003 the NEJM contained many articles on effectiveness studies including behavioral interventions such as diet for obesity,[10, 11] multifactorial team management for Type 2 diabetes,[12] and long-term drug therapies, including: aspirin for primary prevention of colorectal adenomas,[13, 14] finasteride for prostate cancer,[15] and hormone replacement therapy.[16, 17] In a study of anti-hypertensive therapy[18] for cardiovascular events, Wing et al. randomly assigned 6,083 hypertensive subjects 65 to 84 years of age to either diuretics or ACE inhibitors, with the primary care practitioners responsible for initiating therapy and ongoing management. Initiation of drug therapy was delayed in 15% of patients, and at the end of the study (median four years) only about 60% were still receiving the assigned therapy. As often happens in practice, persons switched medications, took new ones, or discontinued therapy completely. It is critical that clinical trials examine such problems, because they will surely affect treatment outside the research setting. Wing et al. found that persons assigned to ACE inhibitors had statistically significantly lower rates of cardiovascular endpoints than persons assigned to diuretics—illustrating that, under conditions of use in the community, these drugs are effective for preventing serious cardiovascular complications of hypertension.

Non-adherence to the intervention is one form of protocol violation; other violations arise when subjects are later found to be ineligible, take additional, non-protocol therapies, or fail to be evaluated for the endpoints of interest. In the study of anti-hypertensive therapy described above, the endpoints were disease occurrence or death, and though about 3% of subjects were lost to monitoring, endpoints were available for all.

One design strategy to make a trial close to an efficacy trial, even in a real-world setting, assigns all potential subjects to a short run-in phase and accepts into the study only those who comply with the protocol. For example, Sandler et al.[14] studied the use of aspirin for the prevention of colorectal adenomas. A 3-month run-in period assessed adherence to therapy and toxicity. Subjects who took at least 5 aspirin tablets per week were considered adherent. The results of the run-in phase eliminated 88 of 719 subjects (12%), 12 for non-adherence and the rest because of intolerance to aspirin. In a similar instance Meis et al.[19] injected an inert substance into women being considered for a trial of an agent to prevent pre-term delivery, and those who came back after this test injection were randomized. This type of study answers questions related to efficacy among persons who generally accept a recommended intervention.

A run-in period serves mainly to exclude non-compliant subjects, people who respond to the study situation itself even in the absence of an active ingredient ("placebo responders"), and those who do not tolerate the study intervention.[20] Studies that use a run-in period usually overestimate the effects of the intervention and minimize the risks. If the run-in period eliminates a large proportion of people (say, more than 10%), and it would be difficult to identify clinically those people who would be eliminated, the question of effectiveness may not be answered.

The CONSORT Guidelines[21] recommend the use of a diagram that outlines the numbers of persons: considered for the trial; eligible; randomized; treated; and followed to various time points. Figure 1 reproduces the CONSORT diagram for the study of Gaede et al.,[12] in which people with Type 2 diabetes received either multifactorial team management or usual care. A strength of this diagram is that it shows how many people refused the trial ($n = 37$) and how many were deemed ineligible, at least before metabolic testing ($97 + 7 + 5 + 9 = 118$). Of the 80 persons randomized to each group, only 63 and 67 persons completed the study, and reasons for non-completion are detailed. The primary endpoint was an event rate, and a survival analysis (intention-to-treat) permitted all 160 subjects to be included, up to the time when their individual follow-up observations ended. During the 8-year course of the study 27 people died (of various causes), and 3 withdrew (low for this type of study). Data on the metabolic endpoints were restricted to the 130 who completed the trial, as shown in the diagram.

It is often helpful to think of an RCT as comparing policies with respect to treatment rather than just the core treatments; the policy should recognize that the treatment is provided in a context and that it will not always be delivered

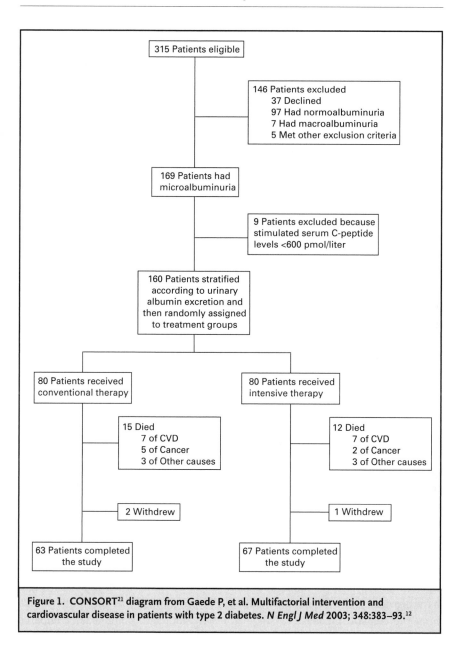

Figure 1. CONSORT[21] diagram from Gaede P, et al. Multifactorial intervention and cardiovascular disease in patients with type 2 diabetes. *N Engl J Med* 2003; 348:383–93.[12]

as recommended—or at all. Provisions for departures from protocol and other problems are a critical part of the policy, and this is the reason for intention-to-treat analysis. In efficacy studies the research environment ensures that protocol violations are rare, all or nearly all endpoints are reported, and the analysis examines effects in all subjects randomized. In effectiveness studies the number of subjects randomized, the number completing all phases of the study including the intervention, and the number with known endpoints can all be different, more nearly reflecting real life. This situation creates challenges for the analysis because the evaluation of the *treatment policy* should be based on "intention to treat": all subjects are to be included in the analysis according to their assigned study group, including any who received little or none of the intervention. The evaluation of the *treatment* itself involves only those subjects who received the intervention as specified (termed per-protocol analysis); the results of this analysis may not generalize if subjects remained on treatment because they were doing well, and switched treatment or dropped out because they were not. Though an effectiveness study with intention-to-treat analysis aims to reflect all the lumps and bumps of research, the need for complete and accurate follow-up is not diminished.

The ultimate aim of RCT designs is to contribute evidence for clinical decisions in real-world clinical practice. Thus, it is important to describe fully the practice environment of the study, including the potential for protocol violations and non-compliance. One criticism of RCTs is that, although optimally designed, they do not necessarily address questions that are important in clinical practice.[22] Many trials reported in the scientific literature address research questions required for drug approval and do not address questions important in clinical care.

Clinical practice rarely requires a comparison of some intervention against no intervention or against placebo. Knowing that some treatment is better than nothing may not be useful if there is already a standard treatment that is thought to be at least partially successful. Thus, most clinical questions relate to competing interventions, or an intervention compared to usual care. Gaede et al.[12] (see Box 1) provide a good example of a pragmatic clinical trial in which people with Type 2 diabetes were randomly assigned to receive either multifactorial team management or usual care. Two studies[23, 24] of the effect of combinations of parathyroid hormone and alendronate on bone mineral density might have provided more pragmatic evidence if a program of diet and exercise had been the control. Likewise, a study of opiate addiction could have compared drug therapy against a behavioral intervention rather than placebo alone.[7] A study of the μ-opioid agonist levorphanol for chronic pain[25] provided pragmatic evidence that high-dose opioid therapy resulted in a greater reduction in pain than low-dose, but with more side effects and no benefit to function, mood, or cognitive status—information of practical value for physicians and patients.

Hypothesis	Background implies one-sided: intensive, targeted intervention would result in lower rates of cardiovascular death, disease, and deterioration
Type of study	Effectiveness; 2-group parallel
Population	Type 2 diabetes and microalbuminuria
Intervention	Intensified, targeted, multifactorial management
Comparison	Conventional care
Outcomes	**Primary: Composite of mortality from cardiovascular causes, nonfatal myocardial infarction, coronary-artery bypass grafting, percutaneous coronary intervention, nonfatal stroke, amputation as a result of ischemia, or vascular surgery for peripheral atherosclerotic artery disease** Secondary: incidence of diabetic nephropathy, development or progression of diabetic retinopathy or neuropathy
Effect size	**35% reduction in expected rate of events** of 6% per year (reduction to 3.9%)
Sample size / Power	160 persons / 70% power; Type I error 0.05 (assumed to be two-sided)
Randomization	Simple
Blinding	Subjects not blinded; adjudicators of secondary endpoints blinded
Timeline for follow-up	Baseline, 4 years, and 8 years in conventional group; biochemical and clinical data every 3 months in intensive group
Missing data	2 withdrew in conventional group, 1 in intensive group
Analysis	Intention-to-treat; missing data excluded **Between-group: log-rank test; Cox proportional hazards** (time-to-event) to calculate hazard ratio, adjusted for age, duration of diabetes, sex, smoking status, and endpoint status at baseline Secondary: grouped survival model (binary regression with complementary log-log link), adjusting for age, duration of diabetes, sex, and endpoint status at baseline Other: analysis of covariance for measured variables, Mann-Whitney test, chi-squared test
Results / Conclusions	Intervention resulted in more people reaching established process and outcome targets: better pharmacotherapy, better control of bioclinical parameters leading, by end of study, **to a 50% reduction in risk of cardiovascular death and disease progression in intervention group**

Bold lettering refers to information for the primary outcome.

Box 1. A pragmatic trial of the impact of intensified, multifactorial team management for persons with type 2 diabetes.

Gaede et al. 2003[12]

One step helpful in "getting the question right" for RCTs is to use a format known as PICO[26]:

> PICO Question: Among people with specific characteristics defining the target Population, does a particular Intervention, in Comparison to a specified alternative intervention, usual care, or placebo, result in altered Outcomes?

The PICO format aims to develop evidence about interventions and comparison treatments that is strong enough to support firm conclusions about their relative merits. The boxes summarizing the studies used as examples in this chapter incorporate the PICO framework. Its structure helps to determine whether an article reports the elements required to decide whether the evidence provided is the evidence needed. (For assessing the evidence in research other than RCTs, see Chapter 6.)

ASSIGNING SUBJECTS TO GROUPS

The strength of the RCT design lies in the actions taken to ensure that estimates of treatment effect are free from many forms of bias. The process begins with the assignment of subjects to treatments, independent of their potential outcome. Randomization aims to ensure that subjects or investigators do not select the intervention that they think is likely to work best for this subject; this is in direct contrast to clinical medicine, where this aim is primary. *Simple randomization* gives each participant the same fixed, known probability of receiving any of the treatments and assigns participants independently of the treatment. In a typical two-arm trial (a comparison of one treatment with another or with placebo), simple randomization gives each individual a 50% chance of being assigned to the intervention arm; if there are three groups, each individual has a 33% chance of being assigned to a particular intervention arm. A disadvantage of simple randomization is that in small studies, say 20 subjects or fewer, it can produce serious imbalance between the groups.[27]

Blocking helps to equalize the numbers assigned to the treatment arms; with two treatments (arms) the randomization may use blocks of, say, 2, 4, 6, or 8 subjects, such that each treatment is assigned equally often within each block. For example, blocks of 6 in a three-arm trial would each assign two subjects to each treatment; only the last block, if it is incomplete, might deviate from this pattern, so that imbalance in treatment assignment cannot exceed two patients.

The sequence of treatments within each block is usually concealed from the investigators and subjects so that they cannot bias results by timing study entries to promote or avoid assignment to a specific treatment. Blocked randomization also helps to reduce the effects of any secular patterns that may affect study entry, procedures, or outcomes. Trials may start slowly in one or a few centers, and recruitment strategies and effects may change as skills with a new treatment improve, as early results are found to be promising, or as enthusiasm wanes. Blocking ensures that participants enrolling at different times and places are almost equally distributed among treatment groups.

Another advantage of randomization is that, in large samples at least, the groups will be balanced on important variables, unknown as well as known. However, when variables are known to affect outcome or study processes, it is prudent to ensure that these variables are not unequally distributed among groups, by *stratification*, with blocked randomization within strata. Even with only one or two stratification variables, the number of strata can be large. Consequently the number of subjects per stratum can be small, making the desired balance difficult to achieve. Stratification should therefore be reserved for critical variables. In a multi-institution RCT, stratification with randomization blocked by institution is strongly recommended. However, a study of a rare condition may require a large number of sites, with few subjects per site, so that stratification and blocked randomization by site may be impractical. More-complex randomization schemes are available to deal with special problems.[15, 16, 19, 27, 28] Their use is not without controversy, and they make the statistical analysis more complex.[27]

It is not necessary to randomize equally to treatment arms, as long as the probabilities are fixed; two of the studies[19, 29] from the 73 published in the NEJM in 2003 randomized persons with a ratio of 2:1 to the intervention group. In the Meis et al. study,[19] women at high risk of pre-term delivery were randomized with a 2:1 ratio to weekly injections of a progestational compound (17P) or placebo, to minimize the number of women in the placebo group who would receive painful injections weekly without any possibility of benefit.

Random is not a synonym for haphazard; randomization always requires a fully specified plan (e.g., stratification, blocking) and a device (e.g., a table of random numbers or a computer program). Today, randomization has been made easier and more secure through the availability of simple computer programs, many of which are available on public-domain websites. When the subject is ready, the randomization can be done in real time at a central location. A study staff member responsible for randomization signs on to a website, enters the group names and the size of the block (if any), and starts the program. One such website is www.randomization.com.

When subjects are assigned at random, their personal and prognostic characteristics are assigned at random with them. This approach ensures, barring bad luck, that the groups will be similar on all variables, known and unknown, measured or not. Bad luck or chance is always a possibility, particularly when sample sizes are not large, so the groups may be unbalanced on one or more variables. The investigator may look for imbalances by using the customary statistical tests of means or proportions, such as a t-test or a chi-squared test.

Since the groups are samples from the same population, the null hypothesis that the samples came from the same population is known to be true, and such "tests" do not have the usual interpretation of comparing populations. The resulting p-values, however, can identify variables that are far out of balance. If any variables with small p-values have a substantial role in explaining variation in the outcome, a prudent investigator would consider these variables in the analysis. Thus, an investigator may be concerned about a variable with a p-value of 0.20 because of its known relation with the outcome, yet choose to ignore a variable with a p-value less than 0.05 because this variable has little relation to the outcome, despite being measured (presumably for other reasons).

Properly designed and conducted RCTs are immune to selection bias, at least at the outset of the trial. If, however, as time goes on, subjects drop out for reasons related to the group assignment, selection bias creeps in. A defense against this is to analyze all subjects as if they did not drop out (or commit other types of protocol violations). Thus, intention-to-treat analyses shift the question from "Which is the best treatment?" to "Which treatment should be recommended, given the likely problems?" Geddes et al.[30] (see Box 2) randomized 48 persons with severe emphysema to receive lung-volume–reduction surgery or medical care; but, by the end of the study, deaths and loss to follow-up left only 32 persons (13 in the surgical group and 19 in the medical group). If people with the worst outcomes after surgery drop out, then the estimates of the effect of surgery on functional outcomes will be biased. As long as mortality is ascertained completely, this outcome will not be affected by dropouts, even if the dropout rate differs between the groups. However, outcomes other than death may be affected by differential missing data. If those with the poorest pulmonary function tended to drop out of the surgical group or died, then the average pulmonary function in the survivors would be higher than in the medical-care group, which had fewer deaths and fewer dropouts.

Subjects with poor outcomes are not always more likely to drop out; sometimes, those doing well are hard to follow. In an early study, Bailar et al.[31] showed that this happened with breast cancer, but there seem to be no similar studies for other diseases. Thus, drop-out bias can run either way.

Although properly conducted and analyzed RCTs eliminate some important sources of bias, so that the true effect of the intervention can emerge, RCTs are notorious for having restricted generalizability. This happens because subjects are selected who are most likely to benefit and least likely to be harmed. RCT investigators rarely randomize more than 20% of subjects with the disease or condition under study.[9, 32, 33] The information on the proportions of subjects screened for eligibility, accepted as eligible, and randomized is part of the uniform reporting criteria for RCTs developed by the CONSORT group. This information provides a perspective on the potential population impact (see Figure 1).

Hypothesis	Background implies two sided: lung-volume–reduction surgery could be beneficial or harmful in comparison to medical treatment
Type of study	Efficacy; 2-group parallel
Population	Individuals with severe COPD ($n = 48$)
Intervention	Lung-volume–reduction surgery
Comparison	Medical care
Outcomes	**Primary: Mortality, changes in FEV_1, shuttle-walking distance, and quality of life (SF-36*) at 6 months**
Effect size	0.75; based on a **30% improvement in FEV_1** with an expected mean value at baseline of 0.9 l ($\Delta = 0.3$ l.) with SD 0.4 l.
Sample size / Power	50 persons / 90% power; Type I error 0.05
Randomization	Simple, stratified by FEV_1 values and α-antitrypsin deficiency status
Blinding	Subjects not blinded; blinding of assessors not stated
Timeline	3, 6, and 12 months
Missing data	Missing pulmonary function and walking tests and interviews: 5 in surgical group, 1 in medical group; analysis was of survivors with complete data only
Analysis	(1) on-protocol only (1 person declined surgery after randomization); missing data excluded **Between-group at each point in time: Wilcoxon rank-sum test;** data not summarized over time; within-group: Wilcoxon matched-pairs signed-rank test for changes at each point in time from baseline; mortality rates compared using log-rank test and Cox proportional-hazards model.
Results / Conclusions	**FEV_1 greater for surgical group only at 3-month assessment.** Additional analyses not given in statistical methods section showed differences in FEV_1, lung volume, walking, and HRQL at all time points. Deaths: 5 in surgical group (3 early: ≤15 days; 2 late: >72 days), 3 in medical group (all ≥72 days). Survivors of surgical group had better outcomes than survivors of medical treatment. In selected persons with severe emphysema, **lung-volume–reduction surgery improved FEV_1, walking, and HRQL; effect on mortality uncertain.**

Bold lettering refers to information for the primary outcome.

Box 2. A trial comparing lung-volume–reduction surgery with medical care on the outcome of persons with severe emphysema.
Geddes et al. 2000[30]
*Medical Outcomes Study Short-Form-36—a standard HRQL questionnaire.

WHAT IS THE OUTCOME?

Best practice requires evidence to support patient management. The health effects of clinical practice go beyond survival or the control of specific conditions, and include patients' well-being and use of healthcare services. It is important, therefore, to identify all relevant outcomes, even though only one may be considered the primary endpoint for judging efficacy or effectiveness. Mortality may not be the most relevant endpoint if the patient's quality of life is severely compromised by the intervention, nor is a measure of survival alone helpful if mortality patterns are similar but morbidity and quality of life differ substantially.

In addition, it is useful and cost-effective to collect data that may explain outcomes or permit exploration of other relationships to develop new hypotheses. So what relevant outcomes could or should be measured?

A wide range of outcomes are recognized as relevant for the healthcare system to consider. In the past these were known as the five Ds: death, disease, discomfort, disability, and dissatisfaction[34]; destitution (which could be of the patient or of the healthcare system and translates into healthcare costs) was subsequently added.

Death is a common primary endpoint for clinical trials of pharmaceutical or surgical interventions for potentially lethal conditions; it is widely recognized as fundamentally important; it is accurately measured, and it is dichotomous, which facilitates statistical analysis and reporting of results. Other endpoints (including duration of survival) are often chosen because death may be uncommon, or long delayed. For the purpose of the study, death must be precisely defined: only deaths from the condition of interest, all deaths, or death within a fixed time interval after entry into the study. Also, a more-graded response provides more information. Ghosh et al.[4] (see Box 3) illustrated the use of a measure of disease activity (Crohn's Disease Activity Index) in a study of treatment with natalizumab. This index incorporates eight variables that span measurable gastrointestinal signs, need for drugs, hematocrit, and weight, as well as patient-reported outcomes such as pain and impact on activity and well-being. Response to treatment was defined as a reduction of 70 points or more (out of a maximum of 600 points).

The other four Ds—discomfort, disability, dissatisfaction, and costs of care—are highly relevant from the perspective of the patient and the healthcare system or payer. Two specific measurement paradigms go beyond death or disease endpoints: function and quality of life. The International Classification of Functioning, Disability, and Health (ICF)[35] provides a classification for impairments of body structure and function (e.g., muscle weakness, pain, fatigue, and mood), limitations in activities (e.g., walking, climbing, and self care), and restrictions on participation in usual roles (e.g., work, recreation and

Hypothesis	Worded as one-sided: 2 infusions of natalizumab at 6 mg per kg would result in a higher proportion of patients in clinical remission (Crohn's Disease Activity Index, CDAI < 150) than would 2 infusions of placebo.
Type of study	Efficacy; protocol violations: 4 patients received no infusions (deemed ineligible); 4-group parallel
Population	Persons with Crohn's disease who had CDAI between 220 and 450 (out of 600); 248 subjects at 35 study centers in Europe
Intervention	2 intravenous infusions 4 weeks apart: both at 6 mg of natalizumab per kg; both at 3 mg per kg; 1 at 3 mg per kg and 1 of placebo (3 groups)
Comparison	2 infusions of placebo
Outcomes	**Primary efficacy measure: CDAI; clinical remission;** clinical response: decrease in score of ≥ 70 points; *Serum level of C-reactive protein,* disease-specific HRQL, Inflammatory Bowel Disease Questionnaire *(IBDQ)*
Effect size	Clinical response: 40% in all 3 active drug groups vs. 15% in placebo group; response rate ratio (RR) = 2.67
Sample size / Power	60 persons per group ($\times$ 4); 80% power, Type I error 0.05 (two-sided)
Randomization	Site stratified, blocked (block size unspecified), computer-generated
Blinding	Subjects, investigators, clinical team, assessors
Timeline	Infusions 4 weeks apart; assessments at week 2, 4, 6, 8, and 12; primary outcome was remission at 6 weeks
Missing data	Primary endpoint at 12 weeks missing for 27 of 244 subjects (11%; 4 subjects did not receive either dose); last value carried forward used to impute missing data; declared not differential among study groups (statistical testing not reported)
Analysis	Intention-to-treat of 248 subjects; missing data imputed as last value carried forward.
	Remission and response **rates: Mantel-Haenszel chi-squared test (comparing each group vs. placebo)**; area under the curve for scores on CDAI; linear mixed modeling of repeated measurements for treatment effects on other endpoints (C-reactive protein, IBDQ) (parameters not shown)

Box 3. A trial testing the efficacy of natalizumab in reducing the severity and life impact of Crohn's disease. (continued next page)

Ghosh et al. 2003[4]

Results	**Remission: no difference at 6 weeks between 6 + 6 mg per kg and placebo groups,** but significant differences at week 4 and week 8; all three active drug groups had significantly higher remission rate than placebo group at week 4, and 3 + 3 mg per kg group also had significantly higher rate at weeks 6, 8, and 12.
	Response: all three active drug groups significantly higher response rate than placebo group at weeks 4, 6, and 8. Of a total of 30 contrasts 19 were significant at 0.05; 5 out of 30 were significant at 0.0017 (= 0.05/30)
	HRQL: at 12 weeks, scores on IBDQ were significantly higher only if 2 infusions active drug were given
	C-reactive protein (indicates degree of inflammation): significant decrease at 6 weeks in groups with 2 infusions of active drug and at 8 weeks in 3 + 3 mg per kg group (15 contrasts, 3 significant at 0.05)
	Adverse events: serious events were rare, and none were considered causally related to treatment; non-serious events were common, and incidence was similar in the four groups.
Conclusions	From abstract: *"[N]atalizumab increased the rates of clinical remission and response, improved quality of life and C-reactive protein levels and was well tolerated in patients with active Crohn's disease."* From text: *"the efficacy of natalizumab for reducing signs and symptoms of Crohn's disease appears to be at least similar to that of the tumor necrosis factor α-inhibitor infliximab"* (data not shown). Evidence of efficacy and tolerability in short term; value relative to other therapies remains to be tested.

Bold lettering refers to information for the primary outcome.

Box 3. A trial testing the efficacy of natalizumab in reducing the severity and life impact of Crohn's disease. (continued)
Ghosh et al. 2003[4]

leisure, schooling, and community and household roles and responsibilities). This model recognizes that interventions that are most often targeted at the impairment level should help patients achieve and maintain activity and participation, which in turn improves quality of life and often reduces the costs of future care.

Quality of life (QoL) is difficult to define, and any definition will miss dimensions that are important in some contexts (e.g., patient satisfaction with care versus level of function). One useful compromise is health-related quality of life (HRQL), defined by Patrick and Erickson[36] as "value assigned to duration of life as modified by impairments, functional states, perceptions and opportunities, as influenced by disease, injury, treatment and policy." A separate definition of global (not just health-related) QoL is offered by the World Health

Organization: "individuals' perception of their position in life in the context of the culture in which they live and in relation to their goals, expectations, standards and concerns."[37] The global construct of QoL is relevant in situations where the intervention has effects that affect or diverge from the patient's goals, expectations, standards, and concerns. Many treatments for advanced cancer have such far-reaching impacts, as do interventions providing components of palliative care, rehabilitation, or cognitive-behavioral therapy.

HRQL measures are increasingly used in trials, primarily to show that treatment-related increases in longevity or reductions in disease burden do not come at the expense of quality of life, either health-related or globally. However, neither QoL nor HRQL measures are relevant for acute conditions that are soon terminated by death or full recovery.

The timing of HRQL assessment is also important. For example, Geddes et al.[30] (see Box 2) did not measure HRQL until three months, after the short-term discomfort of lung-volume–reduction surgery should have dissipated. Ghosh et al.[4] (see Box 3) used a HRQL measure specific for Crohn's disease to monitor the effects of treatment on symptoms and the ability to participate in life's roles throughout the course of the study.

Costs of care are also highly relevant, particularly when the treatments have roughly equal disease outcomes. Here it is customary to consider both direct and indirect costs. Direct healthcare costs are costs to the healthcare system or person for such things as medical visits, drugs, tests, procedures, hospitalizations, alternative medicines, physiotherapy, etc. Direct non-healthcare costs are incurred for over-the-counter medications or health supplies, health activities, needed household help, and transportation, as well as for other out-of-pocket expenses. Indirect costs arise from such sources as days lost from work or household management because of illness, treatment, or caring for an ill family member.[38, 39] Measuring the costs of illness and care is difficult,[40] and generally requires substantial support from a health economist. Costs are not the same as charges, which are often much easier to measure than costs, but are less relevant for many purposes.

Two economic measures may be useful. *Cost-effectiveness* measures dollars per unit of clinical gain, such as cost per year of life gained; *cost-benefit* measures the benefit (years of life gained, or quality-adjusted life years) in monetary terms and, therefore, compares dollars to dollars.[41, 42] These concepts are closely related but distinct, and each is useful for appreciating the human and monetary costs of care.[43, 44]

Nathoe et al.[45] reported on the cost-effectiveness of on- and off-pump coronary bypass surgery (CABG) for patients considered at "low risk" for complications. Because randomization was expected to balance associated "non-cardiac" healthcare costs, direct medical costs were estimated only for activities associated with the procedure, in-hospital after-care, cardiac follow-up, and complications such as myocardial infarction or stroke. A cost per unit of resource used was available for each of the 16 services, and the sum yielded an estimate of total cost for each group. For example, operating time for staff was estimated at 3.82 hours for on-pump and 4.17 hours for off-pump. The unit cost per hour was $332; one day of stay in an ICU had a cost of $1057, and one day of stay on the ward was $247. The total cost associated with on-pump CABG was $14,908 compared with $13,069 for off-pump CABG. Is the difference, $1,839, significant? A first question is whether these figures are equally accurate. Are the inevitable errors likely to be about the same? If they are, statistical analysis may be appropriate. Costs do not follow a normal distribution and have very large standard deviations, as they cannot fall below zero and have no definite upper limit. Thus, a simple p-value for comparing two means is likely to be inappropriate because the data do not meet important assumptions; the usual result of ignoring critical assumptions is that two interventions are deemed "significantly" different when they are not. Various transformations can partially correct this problem.[46] Nathoe et al.[45] took a different approach to assess whether the difference of $1,839 was meaningful. They factored in quality of life by using a utility measure.[47] This measure provides an overall value for the strength of the preference an individual has for a given health state. When linked to life expectancy, it yields a measure called quality-adjusted life years (QALY). The difference in QALY for the two groups was very small, only 1%, in favor of the more expensive on-pump procedure. Thus, to produce a difference of one QALY would require expenditure of an estimated $183,900 for on-pump procedures. It has been estimated that "society" is willing to pay only $20,000 for 1 QALY, so $183,900 greatly exceeds society's willingness to pay.[48–50] Cost data are complex to collect[40] and analyze, and relating costs to quality of life is highly specialized and generally beyond the capacity of investigators who do not have special training and experience in that field.

In designing a trial the investigators must identify all relevant outcomes so that they can make an informed decision on what to include and why. Some endpoints may help to explain why other endpoints occurred and may help in identifying additional treatment targets. For example, Woodcock et al.[9] (Box 4) found that impermeable bed covers did not reduce the severity and life impact of asthma despite reducing dust mites. On the other hand, Sandham et al.[51] (Box 5) found that use of pulmonary artery catheters did not result in closer matching of intervention to therapeutic targets, providing an explanation for why catheters had no effect on surgical mortality or morbidity. Gaede et al.[12] (Box 1) found that therapeutic goals in the treatment of diabetes were more often met by intensive multifactorial team management, and this intervention was also associated with a lower mortality. Table 2 lists impacts of the active ingredients of the two interventions on various outcomes and illustrates how

Table 2. Illustration of a Model for Linking Treatment Effect to Intermediate or Surrogate Markers and Subsequently to Outcomes.

Trial Ingredients	Data Shown in Report
Groups	
Intervention group: Intensive team management	80 subjects; strict treatment goals
Conventional group: Primary care management	80 subjects; standard treatment goals
Treatment Effect	
Intervention changed behavior of:	
subjects and	intensive group had a diet of more carbohydrates and less fat
clinical team	significant differences between groups in use of ACE inhibitors, angiotensin II receptor antagonists, statins, aspirin, vitamin/mineral supplements
Intermediate or Surrogate Markers	
Intervention lowered risk factors for end-organ disease	Lower blood pressure, lower blood glucose, lower cholesterol, lower urinary albumin excretion; increased % of subjects in intervention group at pre-determined target for these clinical variables
Outcomes	
Intervention group had lower rate of death from or development of cardio- or peripheral vascular disease (CVD or PVD) and	Graph of time to meeting CVD or PVD endpoint
lower rate of development or progression of damage to kidney, eye, or nerves	Graph of relative risk (RR) of development or progression with 95% confidence intervals; RR of nephropathy, retinopathy, and autonomic neuropathy all ≤ 0.42 (and statistically significant); RR of peripheral neuropathy equal to 1.09.

Data from Gaede, et al.[12] on the effect of multifactorial team management on diabetes outcomes

measuring a range of outcomes can provide useful material for explaining the impact of the intervention on the primary outcome. For example, multifactorial management was hypothesized to change behavior of both patients and the clinical team in ways that would improve bioclinical markers of disease severity, which would lead to better outcomes in terms of rates of nephropathy, retinopathy, and neuropathy. The investigators presented data supporting this chain of events: patients changed diet; clinicians prescribed recommended drugs; bioclinical markers improved; and rates of end-organ disease were lower.

Hypothesis	Worded as one-sided: use of allergen-impermeable bed covers would improve asthma control
Type of study	Effectiveness as 31 in intervention group and 12 in control group removed bed covers ($p = 0.003$); 2-group, parallel in 2 phases, I for disease impact, II for drug use reduction
Population	Adults with asthma, shown after a run-in period to be able to comply with daily outcome recording; $n = 1122$ (732 mite-sensitive)
Intervention	Allergen-impermeable mattress, pillow, and quilt covers
Comparison	Look-alike placebo covers
Outcomes	**Primary (*Phase I*): morning peak expiratory flow rate** disease severity: use of beta-agonists, rate of exacerbation impairment: evening peak flow, symptoms participation: number of days of work missed disease-specific HRQL: St. George's Respiratory Questionnaire **Primary (*Phase II*): proportion who discontinued inhaled corticosteroids** reduction in dose of inhaled corticosteroids *intermediate outcome – reduction in dust mite concentration*
Effect size	**Primary (*Phase I*) - 20/112 l/min = 0.18** **Primary (*Phase II*) - 50% increase** (25% to 37.5%) in proportion of patients in whom **corticosteroid therapy could be discontinued**
Sample size / Power	750 mite-sensitive people; 90% power; Type I error 0.05
Randomization	Adaptive to achieve balance within practice and according to pet ownership, smoking status, and mite-specific IgE levels
Blinding	Subjects and assessors
Timeline	12 months with assessments at pre-randomization, 6 months (*Phase I*), and 12 months (*Phase II*)
Missing data	Primary endpoint missing for 14% in each group
Analysis	Intention-to-treat with missing data excluded; described according to measurement scale of outcomes; overall and restricted to mite-sensitive patients; **primary outcome (*Phase I*): analysis of covariance** with average morning peak flow in 4 weeks preceding 6-month evaluation as outcome, adjusted for baseline average peak flow; expressed as **adjusted between-group differences and 95% confidence intervals; primary outcome (*Phase II*): chi-squared test**; Mann-Whitney U test on proportionate reduction in dose of inhaled corticosteroids
Results / Conclusions	Dust mite concentration reduced at 6 months; **no impact on any health outcome. No evidence that covers are effective** as a single intervention to reduce severity and impact of asthma

Bold lettering refers to information for the primary outcome.

Box 4. A trial testing the effect of impermeable bed covers on reducing the severity and life impact of asthma.
Woodcock et al. 2003[9]

Hypothesis	Background implies two-sided: pulmonary catheters could be beneficial or harmful
Type of study	Close-to-efficacy as protocol violations in <6% in each group; 2-group parallel
Population	1994 elderly (≥60 years), high-risk surgical patients
Intervention	Pulmonary catheters to meet treatment goals
Comparison	No pulmonary catheters
Outcomes	**Primary: mortality—in-hospital from any cause;**
	Secondary: 6-month mortality, 12-month mortality, and in-hospital morbidity (myocardial infarction, left ventricular failure, arrhythmia, pneumonia, pulmonary embolism, renal insufficiency, liver insufficiency, sepsis)
	Intermediate outcomes - achievement of therapeutic goals
Effect size	Absolute difference in **mortality** of 5 percentage points (10% vs. 15%)
Sample size / Power	1000 persons per group; 90% power, Type I error 0.05
Randomization	Simple, stratified by type of surgery and ASA class, blocked by center
Blinding	Subjects and clinicians not blinded; assessors reading radiographs blinded by taping over area where catheter was or would be
Timeline	Until hospital discharge with follow-up to 12 months
Missing data	Primary endpoint on all; mortality at 12 months missing in <9% in each group; persons with missing data included up until last known date of follow-up
Analysis	Intention-to-treat (analyzed in the group to which they were assigned regardless of cross-over violations; persons not having surgery excluded); baseline prognostic variables compared. Differences in proportions were compared using Fisher's exact test or chi-squared test; **primary outcome: logistic regression,** to investigate effects of center and baseline prognostic variables; survival analysis using Kaplan-Meier survival curves. Subgroup analyses expressed as risk differences and 95% CI.
Results / Conclusions	Treatment goals difficult to achieve even with catheters; **no positive or negative impact of pulmonary catheters on any mortality** or morbidity endpoint except more occurrences of pulmonary embolism in catheter group ($n = 8$ vs. $n = 0$).

Bold lettering refers to information for the primary outcome.

Box 5. A trial to test the benefit of physiological monitoring using pulmonary artery catheters in reducing surgical mortality and morbidity.
Sandham et al. 2003[51]

If an outcome is directly observable, it is generally best not to rely on self-report. However, there is increasing recognition of the need to include patient-reported outcomes (PROs)[52] that cannot be observed clinically. These include measures of symptoms, satisfaction, and function, as well as patient ratings of health status or HRQL. These measures have been criticized as "subjective" rather than "objective," implying that they may be biased, but a better distinction would be "self-report" vs. "directly observable." Self-report measures provide an accurate representation of outcomes that are determined solely by the patient's own perceptions: What the patient perceives is, by definition, the datum required. In this sense the response is not biased.[53] Thus, symptoms such as pain or nausea would best be assessed using self-report, as there is no other way to observe their presence or measure their severity. A notable exception is that pain ratings for infants have been developed by making direct observations of facial and crying patterns.[54]

Outcomes in recent reports of RCTs in the NEJM have included mortality, disease occurrence and severity, complications, functional impact, emotional distress, health-related quality of life, and healthcare costs. The variety of both outcomes and measurement scales in these reports requires a variety of analyses, which can make the reports challenging for the reader. Among the 73 RCTs published in the NEJM in 2003, more than half ($n = 39$) included one or more outcomes measured on a continuous scale, including 22 in which the primary outcome was continuous. The intent of this section has been to help the reader identify the range of constructs that are affected by medical interventions, but the choice of outcomes also affects the statistical analysis and the needed sample size, topics that are explored in Chapter 9.

The choice of outcomes dictates another essential component of outcome measurement in RCTs, *blinding*, also known as masking. A fundamental protection against bias is to have the assessors of outcome unaware of the treatment assigned to each patient ("blind"), so that possible prejudices about the impact of intervention cannot affect their measurements. Clinicians caring for a patient may also be kept in the dark about treatment assignments ("double blind") to avoid inadvertent disclosures to patients and to protect the objectivity of clinical observations. Of course, some outcomes are immune to observer influence; for example, mortality should not be affected by knowledge of group assignment. Blinding of study subjects is crucial when using patient-reported outcomes but is less important when a physiological measurement or survival is the outcome. Assessment of other disease outcomes, however, may include some degree of medical judgment, and hence it is standard practice to have external experts decide on the presence or absence of clinical conditions when these define the outcome. Even such endpoints as disease progression or occurrence of an event may be subject to some degree of bias, and a few measurements (e.g., weight loss) may be affected if knowledge about the assigned treatment alters the patient's state of mind.

The most effective way to keep study subjects blind is to offer a look-alike standard treatment or placebo; this is possible mainly for pharmaceutical interventions. In a 2002 study of arthroscopic surgery for osteoarthritis of the knee,[55] subjects were randomized to arthroscopic debridement, arthroscopic lavage, or a sham debridement without insertion of the arthroscope. Subjects in the sham arm were prepared for the procedure, three small skin incisions were made, the motions and sounds of the procedure were simulated, and the subjects spent the night in the hospital (as did subjects in the other arm). This subterfuge was essential because the only way to assess benefits was by self-report.

The terminology referring to blinding is sometimes confusing. Different experts may be blind to different kinds of outcomes, and several may be blinded in one study—the investigator in charge, the physician caring for the patient, the pathologist, and the person assessing the patient. Terms such as single, double, and triple blind are not used consistently; they indicate only how many people were blind, and do not identify what was concealed from whom.[56, 57] In reading reports of RCTs it is important to ascertain who was blinded and the impact of less than perfect blinding on the size and direction of the treatment effect, as not all outcomes are affected by unblinding.

But does blinding really matter? Consider a 1999 trial of bed rest versus usual activity for sciatica.[58] As the authors eloquently state, in the absence of total amnesia, the subjects knew to which group they had been assigned. Likewise, in a study comparing osteopathic spinal manipulation to standard care for back pain,[59] subjects knew their treatment. A systematic review of RCTs of treatment for hip or knee osteoarthritis[60] concluded that it was difficult or impossible to blind *subjects* in 34% of surgical trials and 78% of rehabilitation trials, in contrast to 0% of oral drug trials. It was also difficult or impossible to blind evaluators in 52% of surgical trials and 76% of rehabilitation trials.

In addition to having experts judge feasibility of blinding for this review,[60] two experts also judged the impact of unblinding using explicit criteria based on the intervention, control situation, and outcome. The impact on validity of the assessment was considered nil in 65% of the trials. In contrast, the impact of unblinding of *subjects* was considered nil for 86% for pharmacological trials. Unblinding of the *outcome assessor* posed a greater risk of biased measurement for non-pharmacological trials, with only 56% considered unbiased (compared with 90% of pharmacological trials).[60]

WEIGHING IN ON POWER

The greatest limitation on the design of RCTs is usually not money, investigators, or facilities, but number of subjects. If too few subjects are recruited into the trial, other design features cannot compensate, and the trial will fail. Recruiting an adequate number of subjects reduces the risk of missing evidence that an intervention is effective. This risk of "a Type II error" is the probability the investigator takes of accepting the null hypothesis (no difference between groups) when there is, in fact, an effect of a specified size. Statistical power is one minus this probability.

In designing a trial the investigator needs to identify what "signal" or minimum change is clinically meaningful, and whether the intervention is likely to be potent enough to produce an effect of this magnitude. The development of most of the standard measures in the health field has provided guidance on the size of clinically meaningful changes.[61] A pilot study or the literature can be used to estimate variability. Specification of power for an RCT must generally be a compromise involving such things as available resources (including potential subjects) and clinical significance of an effect of a specified size.

The sample size must also provide enough power to study other important endpoints, even if they are for explanatory or exploratory purposes, including comparisons of subgroups that have been identified *a priori* as requiring specific evidence. However, few studies have adequate power to detect effects in subgroups, as a four-fold increase in sample size is needed to test interactions[62] between treatment group and some factor of interest.

The power of a study is often set at 80%, which means that an investigator takes a 20% chance of failing to detect an effect of a specified size; but power of 80% may not be appropriate for all questions. If the unknown (but real) advantage of the innovation is larger than the specified size, the study has higher power, sometimes much higher. Certainly, if a study is mounted to evaluate a high-cost, high-risk intervention, then taking a 20% chance of failing to detect a conservatively specified effect might be a wise decision. However, if the evaluation concerns interventions that may be widely adopted, an investigator may wish to be very sure that study results do not show, falsely, that usual practice is less effective than the intervention, especially when the current treatment has minimal harm and is already widely applied. In such circumstances the investigator may choose power of 90% or 95% to reduce this risk, at the price of a substantial increase in sample size. As a large proportion of a study's budget goes to infrastructure, the incremental costs associated with increasing sample size, except for the extra delay for recruitment, may be small. Wing et al.[18] compared two pharmacological approaches to management of hypertension, ACE inhibitors and diuretics. As both approaches were in wide use, it was important to reduce the chance of concluding they were not different if one or other of these regimens was superior, and so 90% power was used rather than 80%. With 90% power; a sample size of 3000 per group was estimated to be required to detect a 25% difference (the "specified" difference) in the rate of cardiovascular events over a 5-year period.

Power is only one element in deciding on sample size. The investigator's risk of reaching a false-positive conclusion also plays a major role. This risk, conventionally termed Type I error, is the ordinary level of statistical significance. By convention, this value is often set at 0.05; that is, the investigator takes a 5% risk of rejecting the null hypothesis (no difference between groups) when the null is actually true.

Significance level and power are closely linked. The significance level determines the "critical region" (discussed in Chapter 8), which consists of results of the statistical test that are incompatible with the null hypothesis. For a specified size of effect, the power is the chance that the result is in the critical region. Thus, decreasing the significance level (say, from 0.05 to 0.01) shrinks the critical region and hence also reduces the power.

Another factor affecting power and the Type I error is the number of outcomes that are subjected to statistical testing. Because clinical trials are so costly to set up and run, often a considerable amount of data is collected on study subjects in order to be able to fully understand the effects seen, but also to take advantage of the trial infrastructure to ask other questions. Fairclough[63] describes a useful framework for considering the various hypotheses posed in a trial.

Hypotheses may be classified as confirmatory (equivalent to primary or secondary outcomes), explanatory (which may explain why certain outcomes did or did not occur),[9, 51] and exploratory (to gain deeper understanding of the effects of the intervention on other variables).[63, 64] The level of Type I error is most important for confirmatory outcomes. If the study has more than one primary outcome, and they are not highly correlated, the overall significance level of 0.05 might be partitioned among them; for explanatory and exploratory outcomes, the investigator need not adhere rigidly to a total of 0.05. Wainwright et al.[6] studied the use of nebulized epinephrine for infants with bronchiolitis (Box 6); they reported two primary outcomes and two secondary outcomes (all confirmatory), and the significance level for each was set at 0.01 (close to 0.05/4).

Studies often seek evidence for whether one treatment is better than another, rather than just whether the effects of the treatments differ. In this situation it is customary to set up the alternative hypothesis as two-sided (the treatments differ), but declare significance only when the difference is in the hoped-for direction (the new treatment is better). Thus, a two-sided significance level of 0.05 yields a one-sided significance level of 0.025, and a result is significant only if its one-sided p-value is less than 0.025. This approach focuses on the real uncertainty that exists at the outset of a trial[65] and avoids the abuse of statistical testing that might occur if decisions about one-tail testing were not in the original protocol.

Sample size is also driven by the ratio of "signal to noise": that is, the magnitude of difference in outcomes between groups ("signal") and the background variability ("noise") for this construct. The term "effect size" quantifies the ratio of signal to noise; for outcomes measured on a continuous scale, it

Hypothesis	Two-sided: nebulized epinephrine could be beneficial or harmful in comparison to placebo
Type of study	Efficacy; 2-group parallel; stopping rule if evidence of superiority of active drug after 50 subjects randomized at primary site
Population	Infants hospitalized for bronchiolitis ($n = 194$)
Intervention	Three 4-ml doses of 1% nebulized epinephrine 4 hours apart
Comparison	Look- and smell-alike placebo
Outcomes	**Primary: Length of hospital stay; time to ready-for-discharge** Length of time receiving supplemental oxygen among those on oxygen Respiratory effort calculated using an arbitrarily weighted summative index developed by authors for this study (Severity Score)
Effect size	**0.5 (medium effect size);** not supported by estimates of effect or variability
Sample size / Power	200 infants / 85% power; Type I error 0.01
Randomization	Stratified by site, blocked with block size = 50
Blinding	Subject, treatment team, and evaluators
Timeline	Admission to hospital discharge (days)
Missing data	Endpoints on all
Analysis	Intention-to-treat; **Between-group: analysis of variance with logarithmic transformation** for skewed distribution of time variables; ratios (treatment/placebo) calculated for all variables (95% CI that includes 1 indicates no difference between groups); general linear modeling to estimate impact of group on time variables adjusted for hospital, use of supplemental oxygen, and severity score
Results / Conclusions	Stopping rule not met: **No difference between groups on length-of-stay or time to discharge-readiness;** for those receiving supplemental oxygen and intravenous fluids, time to discharge-readiness was longer in epinephrine group ($p = 0.02$). **No evidence for the use of epinephrine for the treatment of bronchiolitis in hospitalized infants**

Bold lettering refers to information for the primary outcome.

Box 6. A trial of nebulized epinephrine for hospitalized infants with acute bronchiolitis.
Wainwright et al. 2003[6]

is the difference divided by a measure of variability of either the difference or the baseline.[66] This ratio can theoretically take on any value, but in studies of interventions in clinical populations the signal seldom exceeds the noise; that is, most effect sizes are less than 1.0. Cohen[67] has classified effect sizes as trivial (0.0 to 0.2), small (0.2 to 0.5), moderate (0.5 to 0.8), and strong (0.8 and above). Strong effect sizes (that is, large differences between groups with little variability) are easy to detect and require few subjects. Small effect sizes require large numbers of subjects and, often, sophisticated statistical analysis.

Interventions are evaluated to make changes that are clinically meaningful or relevant. Thus, an effect size should be anchored in some change that is clinically meaningful, declared in advance of the study. The common terms are minimal clinically important difference (MCID) and minimal detectable difference (MDD).[68, 69] In deciding on the effect size, the investigator must also consider the potency of the intervention to produce this impact. Some of the largest effects are induced by surgery; effects of pharmaceutical agents or behavioral interventions like diet are usually smaller. One endpoint in the Women's Health Initiative (WHI) was HRQL, and the authors[17] assessed effect sizes as part of the study (see Box 7). The effect sizes for hormone replacement therapy (HRT) were all very small, less than 0.11, which would be considered trivial by Cohen's criteria, although some of these effects were statistically significant. Thus, a very large study could conclude that there were differences because a p-value ducked under the 0.05 threshold, but the differences may not have any clinical relevance. It is important to declare in advance of statistical testing the effect size being sought, in order to distinguish significant effects from important effects. Studies need to detect important differences, not any differences. From the data presented in the report on HRQL from the WHI study,[17] it is unlikely that very many subjects (fewer than 1%) would have achieved a clinically important difference on the physical-limitations scale of the Rand-36, which is 25 points out of 100.

Woodcock et al.[9] chose their sample size to be fairly sure (power 80%) of finding a 20 l/min increase in peak flow among asthmatics using impermeable bed covers (Box 4). Data at hand indicated that the standard deviation of peak flow measurements in this population was 112, yielding an effect size of 0.18, considered trivial by Cohen.[67] The results of the study showed that peak flow increased by only about 10 l/min (SD: 93 l/min), so the effect of the impermeable bed covers was not statistically significant and perhaps not clinically important.

Although these are important parameters to declare and to rationalize, the most important feature determining sample size is the measurement scale of the primary outcome variable. Different sample size methods must be used for comparing means (continuous outcomes) and proportions (categorical outcomes). Many free-access internet sites provide sample size (or power)

Hypothesis	Background implied two-sided: HRQL could be better or worse in hormone-replacement group in comparison to placebo
Type of study	Effectiveness as women took drugs unsupervised; 74% of women in HRT group and 80% of women in placebo group took at least 80% of prescribed pills; 9.7% and 6.6%, in HRT and placebo respectively, discontinued use; 2-group parallel with a 4-week placebo lead-in to test compliance
Population	16,608 post-menopausal women aged 50 to 79 with an intact uterus
Intervention	HRT with estrogen plus progesterone
Comparison	Look-alike placebo
Outcomes	Impairments: Menopausal symptoms (arbitrarily weighted and summed into a score); depressive symptoms (CES-D); sleep disturbance (WHI Insomnia Rating Scale); cognition (MMSE)
	Primary: generic HRQL using the RAND-36 (SF-36 with different scoring algorithms)
	QOL component: satisfaction with sexual functioning
Effect size	Not stated *a priori; a posterori* effect sizes were all less than 0.2 (trivial effect), and this magnitude was compared with the smallest increment of change possible on each scale
Sample size / Power	Type I error 0.004 (0.05/13); Bonferroni* correction because 13 outcome variables were assessed for impact of HRT
Randomization	Stratified by site and age, blocked with random block size
Blinding	Subject and treatment team
Timeline	Randomization to 12 months
Missing data	HRQL data missing for approximately 9% per group at 12 months
Analysis	Intention-to-treat with missing data excluded;
	Simple linear regression: Change in each of the 8 RAND-36 subscales and other 5 outcomes modeled as a function of study group; multiple linear regression to explore moderating effects of baseline variables (age, body-mass index, moderate or severe vasomotor symptoms, menopausal symptoms, sleep disturbance, previous use of HRT, and history of cardiovascular disease) and their interactions with study group
Results / Conclusions	**Small but statistically significant effect of HRT on 3 of the 13 outcomes** (physical functioning and bodily pain subscales of RAND-36 and sleep disturbance); no moderating effects of any baseline variables. Subgroup analyses for younger women and those with moderate to severe night sweats and hot flashes showed improvement with HRT but no effect on HRQL. No meaningful effect of HRT on patient-reported outcomes.

Bold lettering refers to information for the primary outcome.

Box 7. Impact of hormone replacement therapy (HRT) on HRQL from the Women's Health Initiative trial.

Hays et al. 2003[17]

* Bonferroni correction is a conservative way of adjusting for the effect of multiple comparisons; Type I error is made stricter by dividing by the number of comparisons, e.g., $0.05/n$.

estimation programs. However, this ease of access should not be confused with simplicity, because the calculation of sample size is rarely as straightforward as these sites make it appear, for reasons that are discussed in Chapter 9. It is necessary to have enough subjects to answer the question, but not so many as to expose more people than necessary to inferior treatments once there is evidence that one treatment is inferior to the other. In practice, the projected sample size for a study is always a compromise among effect size, variability in outcomes, statistical power, and the selected significance level. Basic calculations of sample size are useful in planning a study, but a more precise estimate is usually required for funding and for ethical reasons.

The measurement scale is important for determining sample size because it influences the amount of variability in the measurement. Measurement scales are of two types, continuous and discrete (including dichotomous). A continuous measure can, in concept, take on any value within its range, limited only by the precision of the instrument used. For example, birth weight can be measured with considerable precision, and the measurement contains much more information than in a dichotomy (such as less than 3500 g vs. 3500 g or more). Discrete scales can have only specific values, of several types: dichotomous, categorical (with more than two categories, ordered or unordered), and numerical. Mortality is a common outcome collected in clinical trials—the value is dichotomous: dead or alive. Sample size calculations for such data are relatively easy. Categorical scales with more than two levels (polychotomous) can be ordinal (ranked) or nominal (no ranking). An example of an ordinal outcome is self-reported rating of health, commonly measured as Excellent, Very Good, Good, Fair, or Poor. An example of a non-ordinal outcome is discharge destination: home, another acute-care hospital, skilled nursing facility, long-term care, or inpatient rehabilitation center. Another type of discrete scale has numerical values—an ordinal and interval variable; for example, the number of episodes of rhinitis following installation of impermeable bed covers.

Categorical scales generally provide less information than related continuous scales. This property influences the magnitude of an effect that the study can demonstrate. On a categorical scale a "change" requires that the subject be in another category; on a continuous scale a "change" can be any measurable amount (though, of course, small changes may not be meaningful). This relation between change and variability is the key reason why studies of dichotomous outcomes often require sample sizes much larger than studies that use continuous outcomes.

A study of intensive intervention for persons with type 2 diabetes[12] illustrates this idea (Box 1). The targeted change in glycosylated hemoglobin was to lower it to a level below 6.5%. Table 3 shows that intensive treatment led to greater average change in glycosylated hemoglobin (–0.5%) than did usual

Table 3. Illustration of the Role of the Measurement Scale of the Outcome (Continuous or Categorical) in Assessing the Significance of the Group Difference.

	Continuous Outcome Change from baseline: Mean (SD*)		Categorical Outcome Proportion on target (<6.5%)	
Glycosylated hemoglobin (%)	Intervention	Usual Care	Intervention	Usual Care
	−0.5 (1.7)	0.2 (2.4)	15%	3%
p-value	<0.001$^{\Psi}$		0.06	
Between-group difference (Δ)	0.7		12%	
SD§ (adjusted)	2.0* (0.93)$^{\Psi}$		29%	
Effect size: Δ/SD (adjusted)	0.41$^{\#}$ (0.75)$^{\Psi}$		0.275	
Power (adjusted)	64% (81%)$^{\Psi}$		44%	

*SE reported in table, converted to SD by multiplying SE by $\sqrt{67}$ and $\sqrt{63}$, respectively (SE = SD/√n); proportions estimated from bar graph.

$^{\Psi}$$p$-value for the between-group comparison of mean changes is derived from an adjusted analysis with adjustments for age, duration of diabetes, sex, endpoint status at baseline, and baseline glycosylated hemoglobin; as the adjustment factors explain some of the variation in the outcome, the estimated variability (0.93) is less than the measured variability (2.0), resulting in a larger effect size (0.75 vs. 0.41). The power of the study is 81% with adjustment and 64% without. As adjustment does not have the same effect on reducing the variability of categorical outcomes; no such benefit is derived, but even without adjustment the power to detect differences between categorical variables is less than for differences in continuous variables.

§SD (unadjusted) of the control group is used as the reference: for proportions, SD is calculated as $\sqrt{p(1 − p) / n}$; as a chi-squared test was used in the analysis, only unadjusted effect size and power are presented.

$^{\#}$Effect size here is approximated by the standardized response mean, which is based on difference between groups on change and the standard deviation of the change (SD$_{change}$).

Data from Gaede et al.[12] on the effect of multifactorial team management on diabetes outcomes

care (+0.2%), and the difference between these (0.7%) was highly significant (p <0.001). If the outcome is expressed as a proportion rather than a mean, 15% in the intervention group met the target compared with 3% in the control group. With 67 and 63 subjects in the intervention and control groups, respectively, the power to detect a difference of this size (12 percentage points) was only 44%. When there is a choice, it is better to report and test the continuous outcome, though the categorical measure may be useful in showing how many people would need to be treated in order to get one person to reduce his or her glycosylated hemoglobin by the targeted amount—the number needed to treat (NNT, discussed in more detail in Chapter 9).

In addition to Type I and Type II errors and the measurement scale of the outcome, sample size is determined by the form of the planned analysis. A dichotomous outcome, such as dead or alive, can be analyzed by a simple test of the equality of two proportions, using a chi-squared test, logistic regression, or a survival model that includes time to death (a continuous variable). Each of these will have its own sample size requirements, as they estimate different parameters.

Other sample size considerations arise when subjects are not truly independent of each other because of some natural or forced clustering of subjects within other important variables. Clustering may arise, for example, in surgical trials where each surgeon may treat several subjects. One way to reduce this dependence is to randomly assign subjects to surgeons, as well as treatments. Surgeon-to-surgeon differences in outcome may be large, if training, experience, or technique is likely to vary and influence outcomes (including adverse events). Multi-center studies can impose a similar clustering effect if, for example, some centers tend to treat patients with more-advanced disease (including referrals) than others; it is possible for the best hospitals to have the worst unadjusted outcomes if their patients, on average, have prognoses below the average for the study. The dependence induced by these forms of clustering reduces the effective sample size. That is, the analysis has less precision than a simple random sample of the same size. An investigator embarking on a study that may involve clustering effects should gather as much information as possible on the nature of the clusters and consult a statistician for the sample size calculations and subsequent analysis. Puffer et al. and Donner et al.[70–73] give an in-depth examination of clustered randomized trials.

RECOGNIZING A NEED TO END A STUDY EARLY

Sample sizes specified in research protocols are estimates based on numerous assumptions. Sometimes those assumptions turn out to be wrong, and the trial is stopped early. (Extension past the projected estimate is almost never possible.)

Most large clinical trials include one or more interim analyses in order to identify (1) unexpected harmful events; (2) unexpectedly strong beneficial effects; (3) futility, in that no difference is likely ever to be established; and (4) data quality issues that must be corrected if the trial is to continue. A decision to stop a trial is not taken lightly and should be based on many factors, including: covariate imbalances among groups; the impact of unblinding; consistency across subgroups, sites, and primary and secondary outcomes; and missing data.

When an interim analysis yields data suggesting that a statistically significant difference will never arise (even if the hypothesized effect was observed in the rest of the sample), a trial may be stopped.[74]

Interim analyses are required if the trial is to detect these unexpected effects when only a fraction of the intended sample size has been enrolled, but this step raises a complication. The usual statistical tests are designed to determine whether findings are outside the usual boundaries at the end of the study, and different statistical procedures are needed to determine whether findings are outside such limits at any of multiple points during the study. Essentially, the differences between groups are tested with a smaller significance level than the usual 0.05 (that is, significance in an interim analysis requires a p-value substantially more extreme than 0.05), in such a way that the overall rate of Type I error for the study (if it continues) is 0.05. The literature of clinical trials discusses such issues under the topic of "stopping rules." A good starting point for further information on stopping rules and monitoring of clinical trials is Chapter 14 in the text by Friedman, Furberg, and DeMets.[27]

Part of the WHI study of hormone replacement therapy (HRT)[75] was stopped early because of an excess occurrence of breast cancer. Coronary heart disease outcomes and a global index also indicated an adverse effect in the HRT group, although neither crossed the boundary for stopping. At the time that the study was halted (May 2002), the proportions of women with coronary heart disease were 37% for HRT and 30% for placebo. (At follow-up to July 2002, these proportions were 39% and 33%, respectively.[76]) With the large sample sizes (>8,000 women per group), this difference was highly significant.

The Colorectal Adenoma Prevention Study conducted by Sandler et al.[14] was also terminated early, when a planned interim analysis revealed a substantial reduction in new adenomas among people assigned to aspirin (17%) compared to people assigned to placebo (27%). The interim data were considered so strong that additional recruitment would be superfluous.

Trials are also terminated early when it is unlikely that any difference between groups will be observed. For some questions, terminating because of "futility" may provide the satisfactory evidence upon which to base treatment—for example, if the intervention being tested is new and would not be adopted or approved without evidence of substantial benefit. However, for some other types of interventions, especially those already in practice, stopping without reaching a definitive conclusion about negative effects may result in their continued use under the evidence that they seem to be as good as the alternative, when in fact they may be less good or even harmful. This was the situation for the WHI comparison of HRT to placebo.[75, 76] The fifth interim analyses revealed more negative outcomes in the HRT group, but the boundary for stopping was not crossed. If HRT had been a new intervention, the trial might have been stopped earlier because of futility. However, as HRT was a widely used therapy for the distressing symptoms of menopause, arriving at a conclusion that HRT was no more effective than placebo in its impact on other serious health conditions (e.g., heart disease and breast cancer) would not have served the public well. It was essential that the trial continue, to determine whether HRT might be harmful. This boundary was crossed after the tenth interim analysis.

A more-complicated situation arises from concern about the need to stop enrollment for one particular subgroup that may be showing strong benefit or harm. The complication is that subgroup analyses often point to spurious associations. The risk of a Type I error (saying that interventions are not equal when they are), or even getting the direction of a difference wrong, increases with the number of subgroups being examined. Trials can usually be subdivided in many ways—by age, sex, extent of disease, etc.—and if these subgroups have not been identified in advance, and the analysis adjusted appropriately, the risk is very great that chance alone will cause one or more of them to show benefit or harm at some point in the trial.

This issue arose with the National Emphysema Treatment Trial (NETT)[77] (see Box 8), which tested the impact of surgical reduction of lung volume on mortality, exercise capacity, and quality of life in a sample of more than 1100 persons with emphysema. The protocol specified that the trial would stop if interim analyses revealed an estimate of mortality for which the lower bound of the 95% confidence interval exceeded 8%. In addition, certain baseline factors were considered to be prognostic, and mortality rates were regularly monitored within strata defined by these characteristics. One such analysis revealed that the risk of mortality among patients with the most severe disease was higher with surgical intervention than with medical care.[77, 78]

A very informative paper by Lee et al.[78] on the circumstances surrounding the stopping of the NETT summarized several important methodological issues related to terminating enrollment in a subgroup. Several criteria were identified at trial outset as indicating prognosis for benefit or risk; other criteria were added later. As a result, high-risk subgroups were not identified at baseline but through multiple comparisons of different variables and their interaction with group. Because this process took time, randomization of subjects with these high-risk characteristics was put on hold. This delay required excellent communication with the sites, as well as a change to the software to prevent a randomization number being issued. Thus, Lee et al. highlighted the importance of pre-specifying subgroups to avoid criticisms arising from "multiple comparisons, insufficient statistical power, inappropriate statistical analyses, or lack of biological plausibility" (p. 331).[78] An additional concern was that the title of the article submitted to the NEJM to explain the stopping of the trial for the specific subgroup, "Patients at high risk of death after lung-volume–reduction surgery,"[79] led to confusion in the press and public. The media message was that this type of surgery was harmful to all or to those with severe emphysema; the subgroup message was missed. Lee et al.[78] outlined better procedures for

Hypothesis	Background implies two sided: lung-volume–reduction surgery could be beneficial or harmful in comparison to medical treatment
Type of study	Efficacy; 2-group parallel
Population	Individuals with severe COPD successfully completing pulmonary rehabilitation run-in phase; $n = 1218$
Intervention	Lung-volume–reduction surgery
Comparison	Medical care
Outcomes	**Primary: mortality** at mean 29 months post surgery
	Impairment: Maximal exercise capacity at 2 years; pulmonary function, dyspnea
	Activity: Distance walked in 6 minutes (6MWT)
	Disease-Specific HRQL: St. George's Respiratory Questionnaire
	Generic HRQL: Quality of Well-Being
Effect size	**Not stated for mortality; for maximal exercise capacity, increase of 10 watts in maximum workload considered clinically meaningful**
Sample size / Power	Projected 2500 people; based on expected **mortality of 8%** in medical group; this sample size would provide sufficient power to distinguish between 8% for medical group and 4.5% mortality in surgical group; Type I error 0.05
Randomization	Stratified by site
Blinding	Neither subjects nor assessor blinded
Timeline	90 days; 6, 12, and 24 months; and up to 5 years (mean 29 months)
Missing data	On functional and HRQL outcomes for deceased; deceased assigned the lowest category; missing assigned the next-to-lowest category.
Analysis	Intention-to-treat; missing data assigned as not improved
	(1) **Mortality: Risk ratio** (unadjusted), not survival analysis owing to non-proportional hazard assumption because of increased early mortality risk in surgical group
	(2) Impairment: % of persons making increase of 10 watts or more on test of exercise capacity, tested using Fisher's exact test; between group comparison of distribution of change using Wilcoxon rank-sum test
	(3) Functional and HRQL outcomes dichotomized as improved or not and analyzed using logistic regression; subgroups identified by logistic regression with interaction between group and pre-identified covariates
Results / Conclusions	**Overall, no mortality benefit from surgery**
	Exercise capacity improved: at 6, 12, and 24 months proportions with improvements > 10 watts were 28%, 22%, 15% for persons with surgery compared with 4%, 5%, 3% for persons in medical group; persons with upper-lobe emphysema and low exercise capacity benefited; persons with non–upper-lobe and high exercise capacity were at higher risk of mortality.

Bold lettering refers to information for the primary outcome.

Box 8. A randomized trial comparing lung-volume–reduction surgery with medical therapy for severe emphysema.

National Emphysema Treatment Trial (NETT) Research Group 2003[77] stopping a trial, including pre-specifying the subgroups and communicating an unambiguous scientific message.

When no interim analysis is planned, but events during the conduct of the trial put the wisdom of continuing in question (accrual is slow; results of other studies become known), the investigators would usually conduct an analysis to see whether there is much chance that continuing the study will demonstrate a significant and important difference. They must, of course, use the information available at the time to assess the probability that a statistical test at the end of the study would find a difference, assuming that the minimum effect that the study was designed to find held for the remainder of the study. Van der Tweel and van Noord[74] provide a good conceptual summary of this issue, as well as sufficient statistical details for applying the information.

Not all types of trial require that the protocol include a stopping rule, especially when the intervention is not likely to do harm or when the intervention is not expected to become widely used. Interventions that are new and require evidence of both safety and efficacy before being approved for general use would generally have a stopping rule.[80] Stopping rules are also desirable in studies of approved or existing interventions, procedures, or practices that are being evaluated for further evidence of risk/benefit ratio, and applications in situations not adequately covered in prior trials. Stopping rules are not usually required for trials of behavioral interventions (including psychosocial and rehabilitation interventions) unless there is concern about possible harm or the "intervention," if beneficial, could be applied readily through educational advice or a simple organizational change. Among the 73 trials published in the NEJM in 2003, 52 trials (71%) did not report a stopping rule. Of the 21 trials that reported a stopping rule (29%), eight were stopped because the intervention was better,[7, 14, 15, 19, 28, 81–83] four were stopped because the intervention was worse,[84–87] two were stopped because of no difference,[88, 89] and seven continued as planned,[6, 24, 90–93] except for one trial with changes to the protocol.[94] Thus, a stopping rule was actually used in two-thirds of this small and select sample.

The design features discussed in this chapter—specifying the question, assigning subjects to groups, choosing outcomes, powering the study, and recognizing a need to end a study early—are only part of the challenges that an investigator faces in bringing a trial to conclusion. Chapter 9 presents issues encountered with the analysis of clinical trials. Together, the two chapters on design and analysis provide enough detail for a reader to fill out the checklist presented in Table 4. Anyone reviewing a clinical trial for educational purposes should find this checklist a useful tool for identifying elements that are critical to evaluation of interventions.

Table 4. Checklist of Important Components of an RCT.

Component	What to look for
Hypothesis	Test of differences or equivalence
Type of study	Efficacy or effectiveness; required for approval or to guide current practice (pragmatic trial); indication for stopping
Population	Who, how many, and special characteristics
Intervention	What are the active components?
Comparison	Should differ only on active component(s) or new treatment compared to standard treatment
Primary outcome	Distinguish this from other outcomes; measurement scale of the outcome; measurement scale used in analysis
Spectrum of outcomes	Mortality, morbidity (new diseases, severity, complications), impairments, activity limitations, participation restrictions, health-related quality of life, cost
Effect size	Difference in means or proportions with an estimate of variability
Sample size / Power	How many subjects were required to detect minimal difference with what level of power?
Randomization	What method was used?
Blinding	Was blinding of treatment possible? Who did not know the group assignment? Could knowledge of group assignment have affected measurement of outcome?
Timeline for assessments and/or follow-up	Number and timing of assessments
Missing data	Missing completely at random (administrative error); missing at random (can be predicted by other variables); missing not at random (a specific subgroup missing that cannot be identified by existing data)
Analysis	Intention-to-treat or on protocol What is done with missing data: excluded or imputed? Was there an adjustment for covariates? Specific statistical methods used for each outcome How were the effects summarized over time?
Results	Do the data presented match the analysis?
Conclusions	Do they flow from the results reported?

REFERENCES

1. Verhagen AP, de Vet HC, de Bie RA, et al. The Delphi list: a criteria list for quality assessment of randomized clinical trials for conducting systematic reviews developed by Delphi consensus. J Clin Epidemiol 1998; 51(12):1235–41.

2. Balk EM, Bonis PA, Moskowitz H, et al. Correlation of quality measures with estimates of treatment effect in meta-analyses of randomized controlled trials. JAMA 2002; 287(22): 2973–82.

3. Last JM. A dictionary of epidemiology. 4th ed. New York: Oxford University Press; 2001.

4. Ghosh S, Goldin E, Gordon FH, et al. Natalizumab for active Crohn's disease. N Engl J Med 2003; 348(1):24–32.

5. Miller DH, Khan OA, Sheremata WA, et al. A controlled trial of natalizumab for relapsing multiple sclerosis. N Engl J Med 2003; 348(1):15–23.

6. Wainwright C, Altamirano L, Cheney M, et al. A multicenter, randomized, double-blind, controlled trial of nebulized epinephrine in infants with acute bronchiolitis. N Engl J Med 2003; 349(1):27–35.

7. Fudala PJ, Bridge TP, Herbert S, et al. Office-based treatment of opiate addiction with a sublingual-tablet formulation of buprenorphine and naloxone. N Engl J Med 2003; 349(10):949–58.

8. Terreehorst I, Hak E, Oosting AJ, et al. Evaluation of impermeable covers for bedding in patients with allergic rhinitis. N Engl J Med 2003; 349(3):237–46.

9. Woodcock A, Forster L, Matthews E, et al. Control of exposure to mite allergen and allergen-impermeable bed covers for adults with asthma. N Engl J Med 2003; 349(3):225–36.

10. Foster GD, Wyatt HR, Hill JO, et al. A randomized trial of a low-carbohydrate diet for obesity. N Engl J Med 2003; 348(21):2082–90.

11. Samaha FF, Iqbal N, Seshadri P, et al. A low-carbohydrate as compared with a low-fat diet in severe obesity. N Engl J Med 2003; 348(21):2074–81.

12. Gaede P, Vedel P, Larsen N, et al. Multifactorial intervention and cardiovascular disease in patients with type 2 diabetes. N Engl J Med 2003; 348(5):383–93.

13. Baron JA, Cole BF, Sandler RS, et al. A randomized trial of aspirin to prevent colorectal adenomas. N Engl J Med 2003; 348(10):891–9.

14. Sandler RS, Halabi S, Baron JA, et al. A randomized trial of aspirin to prevent colorectal adenomas in patients with previous colorectal cancer. N Engl J Med 2003; 348(10):883–90.

15. Thompson IM, Goodman PJ, Tangen CM, et al. The influence of finasteride on the development of prostate cancer. N Engl J Med 2003; 349(3):215–24.

16. Hodis HN, Mack WJ, Azen SP, et al. Hormone therapy and the progression of coronary-artery atherosclerosis in postmenopausal women. N Engl J Med 2003; 349(6):535–45.

17. Hays J, Ockene JK, Brunner RL, et al. Effects of estrogen plus progestin on health-related quality of life. N Engl J Med 2003; 348(19):1839–54.

18. Wing LM, Reid CM, Ryan P, et al. A comparison of outcomes with angiotensin-converting–enzyme inhibitors and diuretics for hypertension in the elderly. N Engl J Med 2003; 348(7): 583–92.

19. Meis PJ, Klebanoff M, Thom E, et al. Prevention of recurrent preterm delivery by 17 alpha-hydroxyprogesterone caproate. N Engl J Med 2003; 348(24):2379–85.

20. Pablos-Mendez A, Barr RG, Shea S. Run-in periods in randomized trials: implications for the application of results in clinical practice. JAMA 1998; 279(3):222–5.

21. Moher D, Schulz KF, Altman D. The CONSORT statement: revised recommendations for improving the quality of reports of parallel-group randomized trials. JAMA 2001; 285(15):1987–91.

22. Tunis SR, Stryer DB, Clancy CM. Practical clinical trials: increasing the value of clinical research for decision making in clinical and health policy. JAMA 2003; 290(12):1624–32.

23. Black DM, Greenspan SL, Ensrud KE, et al. The effects of parathyroid hormone and alendronate alone or in combination in postmenopausal osteoporosis. N Engl J Med 2003; 349(13):1207–15.

24. Finkelstein JS, Hayes A, Hunzelman JL, et al. The effects of parathyroid hormone, alendronate, or both in men with osteoporosis. N Engl J Med 2003; 349(13):1216–26.

25. Rowbotham MC, Twilling L, Davies PS, et al. Oral opioid therapy for chronic peripheral and central neuropathic pain. N Engl J Med 2003; 348(13):1223–32.

26. Birch DW, Eady A, Robertson D, et al. Users' guide to the surgical literature: how to perform a literature search. Can J Surg 2003; 46(2):136–41.

27. Friedman LM, Furberg CD, DeMets DL. Fundamentals of clinical trials. 2nd ed. Littleton: PSG Publishing Company, Inc.; 1985.

28. McConnell JD, Roehrborn CG, Bautista OM, et al. The long-term effect of doxazosin, finasteride, and combination therapy on the clinical progression of benign prostatic hyperplasia. N Engl J Med 2003; 349(25):2387–98.

29. Hadziyannis SJ, Tassopoulos NC, Heathcote EJ, et al. Adefovir dipivoxil for the treatment of hepatitis B e antigen-negative chronic hepatitis B. N Engl J Med 2003; 348(9):800–7.

30. Geddes D, Davies M, Koyama H, et al. Effect of lung-volume–reduction surgery in patients with severe emphysema. N Engl J Med 2000; 343(4):239–45.

31. Bailar JC III, Lowry R, Goldenberg IS. A note on follow-up of lost patients. Natl Cancer Inst Monogr 1961; 6:123–7.

32. Lovato LC, Hill K, Hertert S, et al. Recruitment for controlled clinical trials: literature summary and annotated bibliography. Control Clin Trials 1997; 18(4):328–52.

33. Sociodemographic and clinical predictors of participation in two randomized trials: findings from the Collaborative Ocular Melanoma Study COMS report no. 7. Control Clin Trials 2001; 22(5):526–37.

34. White KL. Teaching and research in medical care: commentary. Am J Public Health Nations Health 1969; 59(Suppl 1):66–8.

35. World Health Organization. International classification of functioning, disability and health. 2nd revised ed. Geneva, Switzerland; 2001.

36. Patrick DL, Erickson P. Health status and health policy. New York: Oxford University Press; 1993.

37. The World Health Organization Quality of Life assessment (WHOQOL): position paper from the World Health Organization. Soc Sci Med 1995; 41(10):1403–9.

38. Warner KE, Hutton RC. Cost-benefit and cost-effectiveness analysis in health care. Growth and composition of the literature. Med Care 1980; 18(11):1069–84.

39. Drummond MF, Stoddart GL, Torrance GW. Methods for the economic evaluation of health care programmes. Oxford: Oxford University Press; 1987.

40. Goossens ME, Rutten-van Molken MP, Vlaeyen JW, van der Linden SM. The cost diary: a method to measure direct and indirect costs in cost-effectiveness research. J Clin Epidemiol 2000; 53(7):688–95.

41. Torrance GW, Stoddart GL, Drummond MF, Gafni A. Cost-benefit analysis versus cost-effectiveness analysis for the evaluation of long-term care programs. Health Serv Res 1981; 16:474–6.

42. Chiba N, Gralnek IM, Moayyedi P, et al. A glossary of economic terms. Eur J Gastroenterol Hepatol 2004; 16(6):563–5.

43. Moayyedi P, Mason J. Cost-utility and cost-benefit analyses: how did we get here and where are we going? Eur J Gastroenterol Hepatol 2004; 16(6):527–34.

44. Drummond MF, Stoddart GL, Torrance GW. Cost-utility analysis. In: Methods for economic evaluation of heath care programmes. New York, Toronto: Oxford University Press; 1986 p. 112–67.

45. Nathoe HM, van Dijk D, Jansen EW, et al. A comparison of on-pump and off-pump coronary bypass surgery in low-risk patients. N Engl J Med 2003; 348(5):394–402.

46. Zhou XH, Melfi CA, Hui SL. Methods for comparison of cost data. Ann Intern Med 1997; 127(8 Pt 2):752–6.

47. Kind P. The EuroQol instrument: An index of health-related quality of life. In: Spilker B, ed. Quality of life and pharmacoeconomics in clinical trials. Philadelphia: Lippincott-Raven Publishers; 1996 p. 191–201.

48. O'Brien BJ, Gertsen K, Willan AR, Faulkner LA. Is there a kink in consumers' threshold value for cost-effectiveness in health care? Health Econ 2002; 11(2):175–80.

49. Birch S, Gafni A. Cost-effectiveness ratios: in a league of their own. Health Policy 1994; 28(2):133–41.

50. Russell LB, Gold MR, Siegel JE, et al. The role of cost-effectiveness analysis in health and medicine. Panel on Cost-Effectiveness in Health and Medicine. JAMA 1996; 276(14):1172–7.

51. Sandham JD, Hull RD, Brant RF, et al. A randomized, controlled trial of the use of pulmonary-artery catheters in high-risk surgical patients. N Engl J Med 2003; 348(1):5–14.

52. Acquadro C, Berzon R, Dubois D, et al. Incorporating the patient's perspective into drug development and communication: an ad-hoc task force report of the Patient-Reported Outcomes (PRO) Harmonization Group meeting at the Food and Drug Administration, February 16, 2001. Value Health 2003; 6(5):522–31.

53. Hadorn DC, Sorensen J, Holte J. Large-scale health outcomes evaluation: how should quality of life be measured? Part II—Questionnaire validation in a cohort of patients with advanced cancer. J Clin Epidemiol 1995; 48(5):619–29.

54. Johnston CC, Sherrard A, Stevens B, et al. Do cry features reflect pain intensity in preterm neonates? A preliminary study. Biol Neonate 1999; 76(2):120–4.

55. Moseley JB, O'Malley K, Petersen NJ, et al. A controlled trial of arthroscopic surgery for osteoarthritis of the knee. N Engl J Med 2002; 347(2):81–8.

56. Montori VM, Bhandari M, Devereaux PJ, et al. In the dark: the reporting of blinding status in randomized controlled trials. J Clin Epidemiol 2002; 55(8):787–90.

57. Devereaux PJ, Manns BJ, Ghali WA, et al. Physician interpretations and textbook definitions of blinding terminology in randomized controlled trials. JAMA 2001; 285(15):2000–3.

58. Vroomen PC, de Krom MC, Wilmink JT, et al. Lack of effectiveness of bed rest for sciatica. N Engl J Med 1999; 340(6):418–23.

59. Andersson GBJ, Lucente T, Davis AM, et al. A comparison of osteopathic spinal manipulation with standard care for patients with low back pain. N Engl J Med 1999; 341(19): 1426–31.

60. Boutron I, Tubach F, Giraudeau B, Ravaud P. Blinding was judged more difficult to achieve and maintain in nonpharmacologic than pharmacologic trials. J Clin Epidemiol 2004; 57(6):543–50.

61. Finch E, Brooks D, Stratford PW, Mayo NE. Physical rehabilitation outcome measures. 2nd ed. Hamilton: BC Decker Inc.; 2002.

62. Brookes ST, Whitely E, Egger M, et al. Subgroup analyses in randomized trials: risks of subgroup-specific analyses; power and sample size for the interaction test. J Clin Epidemiol 2004; 57(3):229–36.

63. Fairclough DL. Summary measures and statistics for comparison of quality of life in a clinical trial of cancer therapy. Stat Med 1997; 16(11):1197–209.

64. Fairclough DL. Design and analysis of quality of life studies in clinical trials. Boca Raton, FL: Chapman & Hall/CRC; 2002.

65. Moye LA, Tita AT. Defending the rationale for the two-tailed test in clinical research. Circulation 2002; 105(25):3062–5.

66. Liang MH. Evaluating measurement responsiveness. J Rheumatol 1995; 22(6):1191–2.

67. Cohen J. Statistical power analysis for the behavioral sciences. 2nd ed. Hillsdale, NJ: Lawrence Erlbaum Associates; 1988.

68. Norman GR, Sloan JA, Wyrwich KW. Interpretation of changes in health-related quality of life: the remarkable universality of half a standard deviation. Med Care 2003; 41(5):582–92.

69. Wyrwich KW, Bullinger M, Aaronson N, et al. Estimating clinically significant differences in quality of life outcomes. Qual Life Res 2005; 14(2):285–95.

70. Puffer S, Torgerson D, Watson J. Evidence for risk of bias in cluster randomised trials: review of recent trials published in three general medical journals. BMJ 2003; 327(7418):785–9.

71. Zou GY, Donner A, Klar N. Group sequential methods for cluster randomization trials with binary outcomes. Clin Trials 2005; 2(6):479–87.

72. Donner A, Klar N. Statistical considerations in the design and analysis of community intervention trials. J Clin Epidemiol 1996; 49(4):435–9.

73. Donner A, Klar N. Methods for comparing event rates in intervention studies when the unit of allocation is a cluster. Am J Epidemiol 1994; 140(3):279–89.

74. van der Tweel I, van Noord PA. Early stopping in clinical trials and epidemiologic studies for "futility": conditional power versus sequential analysis. J Clin Epidemiol 2003; 56(7):610–7.

75. Rossouw JE, Anderson GL, Prentice RL, et al. Risks and benefits of estrogen plus progestin in healthy postmenopausal women: principal results from the Women's Health Initiative randomized controlled trial. JAMA 2002; 288(3):321–33.

76. Manson JE, Hsia J, Johnson KC, et al. Estrogen plus progestin and the risk of coronary heart disease. N Engl J Med 2003; 349(6):523–34.

77. National Emphysema Treatment Trial Research Group. A randomized trial comparing lung-volume–reduction surgery with medical therapy for severe emphysema. N Engl J Med 2003; 348(21):2059–73.

78. Lee SM, Wise R, Sternberg AL, et al. Methodologic issues in terminating enrollment of a subgroup of patients in a multicenter randomized trial. Clin Trials 2004; 1:326–38.

79. National Emphysema Treatment Trial Research Group. Patients at high risk of death after lung-volume–reduction surgery. N Engl J Med 2001; 345(15):1075–83.

80. DeMets DL, Pocock SJ, Julian DG. The agonising negative trend in monitoring of clinical trials. Lancet 1999; 354(9194):1983–8.

81. Ridker PM, Goldhaber SZ, Danielson E, et al. Long-term, low-intensity warfarin therapy for the prevention of recurrent venous thromboembolism. N Engl J Med 2003; 348(15):1425–34.

82. Andersen HR, Nielsen TT, Rasmussen K, et al. A comparison of coronary angioplasty with fibrinolytic therapy in acute myocardial infarction. N Engl J Med 2003; 349(8):733–42.

83. Goss PE, Ingle JN, Martino S, et al. A randomized trial of letrozole in postmenopausal women after five years of tamoxifen therapy for early-stage breast cancer. N Engl J Med 2003; 349(19):1793–802.

84. Belfort MA, Anthony J, Saade GR, Allen JC Jr. A comparison of magnesium sulfate and nimodipine for the prevention of eclampsia. N Engl J Med 2003; 348(4):304–11.

85. Heeschen C, Dimmeler S, Hamm CW, et al. Soluble CD40 ligand in acute coronary syndromes. N Engl J Med 2003; 348(12):1104–11.

86. Lawrence J, Mayers DL, Hullsiek KH, et al. Structured treatment interruption in patients with multidrug–resistant human immunodeficiency virus. N Engl J Med 2003; 349(9):837–46.

87. Ramsey SD, Berry K, Etzioni R, et al. Cost effectiveness of lung-volume–reduction surgery for patients with severe emphysema. N Engl J Med 2003; 348(21):2092–102.

88. Harrison MR, Keller RL, Hawgood SB, et al. A randomized trial of fetal endoscopic tracheal occlusion for severe fetal congenital diaphragmatic hernia. N Engl J Med 2003; 349(20):1916–24.

89. Tallman MS, Gray R, Robert NJ, et al. Conventional adjuvant chemotherapy with or without high–dose chemotherapy and autologous stem-cell transplantation in high-risk breast cancer. N Engl J Med 2003; 349(1):17–26.

90. Pitt B, Remme W, Zannad F, et al. Eplerenone, a selective aldosterone blocker, in patients with left ventricular dysfunction after myocardial infarction. N Engl J Med 2003; 348(14):1309–21.

91. Askie LM, Henderson-Smart DJ, Irwig L, Simpson JM. Oxygen-saturation targets and outcomes in extremely preterm infants. N Engl J Med 2003; 349(10):959–67.

92. Grier HE, Krailo MD, Tarbell NJ, et al. Addition of ifosfamide and etoposide to standard chemotherapy for Ewing's sarcoma and primitive neuroectodermal tumor of bone. N Engl J Med 2003; 348(8):694–701.

93. Pfeffer MA, McMurray JJ, Velazquez EJ, et al. Valsartan, captopril, or both in myocardial infarction complicated by heart failure, left ventricular dysfunction, or both. N Engl J Med 2003; 349(20):1893–906.

94. Crowther MA, Ginsberg JS, Julian J, et al. A comparison of two intensities of warfarin for the prevention of recurrent thrombosis in patients with the antiphospholipid antibody syndrome. N Engl J Med 2003; 349(12):1133–8.

CHAPTER 5

Crossover and Self-Controlled Designs in Clinical Research

JOHN C. BAILAR III, M.D., PH.D.,

THOMAS A. LOUIS, PH.D., PHILIP W. LAVORI, PH.D., AND

MARCIA POLANSKY, D.SC.

ABSTRACT In crossover studies each patient receives two or more treatments in sequence. This research design can produce results that are statistically and clinically valid with far fewer patients than would otherwise be required. It is not appropriate for some kinds of comparisons, and it is fragile, in the sense that many things can go wrong.

Before choosing a crossover design, an investigator should be prepared to demonstrate that carryover effects will not interfere with analysis, that drop-out rates will be low, and that the underlying disease is stable. A parallel study with covariate adjustment may be a strong competitor, and we recommend careful consideration of the trade-offs between statistical power and fragility.

We investigated several important features of the design and analysis of eight crossover studies that appeared in Volumes 344 to 354 of the *New England Journal of Medicine*. Overall, the studies seem substantially stronger in both design and analysis than 13 crossover studies we examined earlier, but important improvements in practice are still possible.

In any clinical trial the investigator studies the responses to treatment of a sample of patients for the purpose of inferring which treatment to prefer in a wider group or population. This chapter revises and updates a published paper[1] that was reprinted in the first two editions of this book. Chapter 4 discusses issues bearing on the strength of scientific inferences from parallel comparisons of clinical treatment. Such studies assign each patient to only one of two or more treatments and compare responses in the various groups. This chapter extends the discussion to crossover studies, in which each patient receives two or more treatments in sequence, and outcomes in the same patient are contrasted. One of the treatments may be a placebo or no treatment. To illustrate this chapter, we examined eight crossover studies from Volumes 344 to 354 (2001–2006) of the *New England Journal of Medicine.*[2–9]

We also comment briefly on self-controlled studies, in which patient status during or just after some treatment (including placebo or no treatment) is compared with status before or longer after treatment. For both types of study we highlight the clinically relevant issues for researchers and readers and refer them to the statistical literature (e.g., Senn[10]) for mathematical details.

PARALLEL VERSUS CROSSOVER DESIGN

In a two-treatment crossover study each patient's response under treatment A is compared with the same patient's response under treatment B, so that the influence of patient characteristics that determine the general level of response can be "subtracted out" of the treatment comparison. Crossover designs are most appropriate in the study of treatment for a stable disease (i.e., where there may be variations over time but no trend, and present status is not unusual for the enrollees) and a transient treatment effect. (Stable situations are studied in all eight of the *Journal* articles we examined.) Also, the crossover design reduces variance, but it does not alter average effect sizes. Though a condition of interest may be rare (e.g., McArdle's disease), the outcome under study must be frequent enough among patients with the condition, and sufficiently different between treatments, to be seen in a small sample.

If variation in patient characteristics accounts for much variation in response, a crossover design based on a small sample of patients can provide the same statistical accuracy as a larger parallel study. Nevertheless, the decision to use a crossover design cannot rely solely on this potential saving in sample size, because powerful designs are also potential disasters. Their success balances on a narrow base of scientific and statistical assumptions. An investigator choosing between parallel and crossover designs should consider five factors that determine the effectiveness of the crossover design (see box). We define these terms and discuss these five issues in detail after giving an example that illustrates the attractiveness of the crossover design.

Some Critical Features in Crossover Studies

1. carryover and period effects on treatment outcomes
2. treatment sequence and patient assignment
3. crossover rules and timing of measurements
4. dropouts, faulty data, and other data problems
5. statistical analysis and sample size

Table 1 lists information relating to some of these factors for the eight cross-over studies* we examine here. We consider a study to be a crossover study only if both treatments are realistic candidates for clinical use and if either could be administered after the other. Therefore, although treatment and control readings were taken in a study of a single treatment, we would not classify it as a crossover study unless the use of no treatment at all was a realistic clinical alternative. Also, many medical/surgical studies do, in a sense, have crossovers from medical to surgical therapy, but these often compare immediate surgery with the strategy that calls for medical treatment followed, if necessary, by surgical treatment. We classify such studies as parallel comparisons (Chapter 4). One variety of crossover design that we did not encounter in this series involves treatment of paired or multiple organs, such as teeth or limbs. By assigning one member of each matched set of organs to each treatment, the investigator may be able to compare responses within an individual. The strengths and weaknesses of the paired-organs design are similar to those of an ordinary crossover design, though the analog of carryover effects—in which treatment on one side may affect responses on the other—may be a greater concern than in ordinary crossover studies.

Example

The following example illustrates the power of the crossover design and potential problems associated with it.

With just four diabetic patients, Raskin and Unger[11] demonstrated a difference between the effects of two insulin-infusion regimens. As part of the experiment, they monitored urea nitrogen excretion for 48 hours—first while patients were receiving intravenous insulin and somatostatin, and again after switching the same patients to intravenous insulin, somatostatin, and glucagon. The data shown in Table 2 are the rates of urinary excretion of urea nitrogen in each of four patients while they were receiving insulin and somatostatin, and again after the investigators added glucagon to the insulin and somatostatin.

If these eight measurements had been obtained in eight patients in a study with a parallel design, the difference in mean nitrogen excretion rate (3 g per 24 hours) would not have been statistically significant. The standard error of the difference in means would be 2.76 (see Table 2). Using instead the within-patient differences as the basis of the data, we obtain exactly the same mean difference (3 g per 24 hours) but with a standard error of 0.4. These differences produce a paired t-statistic of 7.5 with 3 degrees of freedom, providing strong

* The *New England Journal of Medicine* staff kindly identified these eight studies for us from Volumes 344 through 354; we do not claim that they are all such studies that appeared in those volumes of the *Journal*.

Table 1. Characteristics of Eight Crossover Studies in the New England Journal of Medicine.

Reference	Subjects completed/ randomized; number of centers	Method of treatment assignment	Crossover rule	Blinding	Washout, or test for order effects?	Approach to analysis*	Disease or subjects	Treatments	Primary outcome variable(s) and p-value	Number of secondary variables
Cazeau 344:873–80	48/58, 15 centers	Randomized blocks, size not specified	Fixed time	Patients only	Carryover test	Intention-to-treat	Heart failure with 1-V conduction delay	Biventricular pacemaker; 3 mos inactive (40 bpm), 3 mos active	Distance walked in 6 minutes, $p < 0.001$	5
(Study group) 345:956–63	126/143, 18 centers	Randomized blocks, size not specified	Alternation	Double	Carryover test	Patients who completed study†	Parkinson's disease	Bilateral deep-brain stimulation of subthalamic nucleus or pars interna	Motor score, $p < 0.001$ for each implantation site	16
Batterham 349:941–8	12/12, 1 center	Random, not further specified	Treatments at separate sessions	Double	1 week washout	Intention-to-treat	Obesity	Peptide YY$_{3-36}$	Caloric intake in standardized setting, $p < 0.001$	7
Wilschanski 349:1433–41	24/32, number of centers not clear	Random, not further specified	Fixed time	Double	Washout#	Patients who completed study†	Cystic fibrosis with CFTR stop mutations	Gentamicin to nasal mucosa	Nasal potential difference, $p = 0.005$; amiloride response, $p = 0.1$, isoproterenol response, $p < 0.001$	1
Vissing 349:2503–9	12/12, 2 centers	Random, not further specified	Treatments at separate sessions	Patients only blind to sequence	Short-lived treatment	No losses	McArdle's disease	Oral sucrose	Perceived exertion, $p < 0.001$, heart rate $p < 0.001$	6

Table 1. Characteristics of Eight Crossover Studies in the *New England Journal of Medicine* (continued)

Study	Randomization	Timing	Blinding	Washout	Analysis	Condition	Treatments	Results	Ref.
Gilron 352:1324–34	Random, balanced Latin square	Fixed time	Double	Carryover test. 3-day washout	Per protocol	Neuropathic pain	Morphine, gabapentin, gabapentin-morphine combination, placebo	Mean daily pain intensity, $p < 0.001$	7
Simantirakis 353:2568–77	Random, not further specified	Fixed time	None	Carryover test	No losses	Obstructive sleep apnea-hypopnea	Atrial overdrive pacing vs. continuous positive airway pressure	Apnea-hypopnea index, $p < 0.001$ for CPAP and $p = 0.87$ for AOP	8
Berry 354:697–708	Random, not further specified	Fixed time	Double	4-week washout	Intention to treat‡	Refractory asthma	Etanercept vs. placebo	Effect of methacholine on FEV_1, $p = 0.05$; quality of life score, $p = 0.02$	10

Simplified descriptions of study protocols; some were much more complex than shown.

*Intention-to-treat analysis assumed when number of subjects completing the study equaled the number randomized.

†Intention-to-treat analysis not feasible or appropriate.

‡Part of a larger study; not clear which statistical methods applied to the crossover phase.

#No untreated washout, but assessment of responses after 14 days of treatment may have served that purpose.

TABLE 2. Urinary Excretion of Urea Nitrogen in Four Diabetic Patients.*			
	Treatment		
	IS	ISG	Difference[†]
Patient No.	Grams of urea nitrogen/24 hours		
1	14	17	+3
2	6	8	+2
3	7	11	+4
4	6	9	+3
Mean	8.25	11.25	+3.0
S.E.M.	1.90	2.00	0.40

*Data adapted from Table 1 of Raskin and Unger.[11] IS denotes intravenous insulin and somatostatin, and ISG denotes intravenous insulin, somatostatin, and glucagon.

[†]The S.E. of the difference between the means of ISG and IS would be $2.76 = \{(1.90)^2 + (2.00)^2\}^{1/2}$ if the study had used two separate study groups, each with four patients.

evidence for the hypothesis that the change from insulin and somatostatin in the first period of the experiment to insulin, somatostatin, and glucagon in the second period raised the level of nitrogen excretion.

These results could be interpreted either as supporting a difference between the effects of insulin and somatostatin on the one hand, and insulin, somatostatin, and glucagon on the other, or as supporting a difference produced by the order of administration (the combination of insulin and somatostatin was always used first). The study provides no information on, or control for, the effects on response of treatment sequence or of changes in disease state. Although diabetes is a fairly stable disease and the study design included a washout period between treatment regimens, a stronger study would have resulted if they had treated a random half of the patients first with insulin and somatostatin and the other half first with insulin, somatostatin, and glucagon. Patients could have been selected on the basis of low urea nitrogen values, and regression to the mean (by which random variation is likely to be a major factor in unusually high or low values, so that later values are less extreme) could have accounted for the observed difference. Also, no matter how powerful the design, studies based on data from only four patients may have relatively little clinical impact until they are confirmed with larger samples.

If the order of treatments made no difference, and the variation in response remained as in Table 2, a parallel comparison would require about 14 times as many patients to achieve the same level of statistical significance (about 56 patients divided equally between treatment groups). Even if no reduction of variance were obtained, the crossover design would require only half the number of patients to produce the same precision as a parallel comparison because each patient in a crossover study would contribute information on both treatments, but each patient would be under study longer than in a parallel design.

This reduction in sample size (patients) can be crucial in the study of treatment for an uncommon condition with a long and complex course. For example, Vissing and Haller[6] evaluated the use of oral sucrose in the treatment of twelve patients with McArdle's disease. The authors show the time course of the mean levels of perceived exertion and heart rate, each with small standard errors at each point, so that the effect of sucrose is evident even with just twelve patients.

KEY FACTORS

The five factors listed earlier as determining the effectiveness of the crossover design need to be considered carefully before any crossover study is initiated. We give some general guidelines on their consideration, and in this section we continue our discussion of them as they apply to the eight studies listed in Table 1.

Carryover and Period Effects

Both period and carryover influences are called *order effects*.

Carryover Effects. Therapeutic or toxic effects of the first treatment may persist (i.e., carry over) during the administration of the second. Investigators can often minimize this influence by appropriately delaying the second treatment (until after a washout period). For example, Batterham et al.[4] enrolled 12 obese and 12 lean subjects in a comparison of caloric intake after infusion of peptide YY_{3-36} (PYY) vs. saline, with one week between treatments. Each participant, obese or lean, showed a short-term, substantial decrease in caloric intake, with little variation in the percentage decrease among subjects or weight groups. The investigators found no effect of treatment on intake 12–24 hours after infusion, so a one-week interval seems adequate to wash out any effects of one treatment before administration of the other.

Period Effects. The disease may progress, regress, or fluctuate in severity during the period of investigation. Such variation may call for more-complex crossover designs. For example, Soter et al.[12] dealt with the complex course of systemic mastocytosis by switching treatment several times for each patient, with varying intervals between the crossover points. The effects of any systematic trends or cycles should have balanced out in the design.

These effects complicate interpretation and analysis, and weaken the scientific and statistical basis for choosing a crossover design. Carryover effects are the most troublesome, for they suggest that the activity of a subsequent treatment depends on the previous treatment. With proper design, both types of order effects can be assessed and removed from the treatment comparison.

The assessment of order effects must be based on a statistical model. If the relative advantage of one treatment over another depends on which treatment the patient received first, then the difference in mean responses of treatment groups during each period will vary from period to period. The technical term for this variation of treatment effect is *treatment-by-period interaction*. If such an order effect is similar to or greater than the average treatment effect, the various treatment sequences should be considered distinct test regimens (that is, the comparison of interest is AB vs. BA, not A vs. B). In this situation the design is no more powerful than that of a standard parallel comparison and can be less powerful or invalid. Brown[13] has shown that estimating and adjusting for order effects requires a sample size greater than that needed for a parallel comparison. Therefore, unless order effects are known to be negligible, the crossover design loses some of its advantages.

As shown in Table 1, the authors of the eight crossover studies in our sample tried, to various extents and in various ways, to control order effects by balanced sequencing and carefully timed measurements, but their reporting of this aspect of study design often lacked detail. Lack of carryover effects seems probable in most of the studies, but period effects could have been present. Readers of these reports could evaluate them more easily if the authors had included additional detail, such as an estimate and confidence interval for the treatment-by-period interaction.[14, 15] This interaction summarizes all order effects that may be present. A descriptive summary of the interaction can be provided by a simple two-by-two table cross-classifying average treatment response and period.

Treatment Sequence and Patient Assignment

The investigator must assign each patient to an initial treatment, and if there are more than two treatments or more than one administration of the treatments, he or she must specify the sequence. If all patients receive treatment according to the same fixed sequence, A followed by B, comparisons must be based on the assumption that the effects of the second treatment (B) after the first (A) do not differ from the effects that treatment B would have if it were given first. Such an experiment would provide no data for assessing this assumption. If disease or treatment characteristics cause B after A to be a fundamentally different treatment from B alone (e.g., chemotherapy after radiation vs. chemotherapy alone), no comparison of the treatments alone can be made. If some patients receive the sequence AB and others BA, then information is available on this issue.

If patients become available for study over time, there are four basic ways of assigning them to treatment sequences: (1) by random assignment among the sequences; (2) by use of the same fixed sequence for all patients; (3) by deterministically balanced assignment—for example, giving the first patient AB and the second BA, then repeating as often as needed; and (4) by uncontrolled, haphazard assignment—using sequences neither fixed in advance nor governed by a randomization procedure. Of these, only random assignment protects against conscious and unconscious bias. All eight papers in our sample used some form of randomization. This is a distinct improvement over practice as reported in our 1984 paper,[1] in which 7 of 13 papers reported randomization, but 4 used the same fixed sequence for all patients, 1 used a deterministically balanced assignment, and 1 assigned treatments haphazardly.

Crossover Rules and Timing of Measurements

An a priori-specified crossover rule strengthens the scientific and clinical validity of a study. Investigators commonly employ one of two types: switch treatments after a specified length of time (*time-dependent*), and switch when indicated by the clinical characteristics of the patient (*disease-state-dependent*). These rules have different impacts on the magnitude and interpretation of order effects and on the general scientific strength of the study.

As with other aspects of designed experiments, the timing of measurements should be described in detail in the research protocol. The most scientifically acceptable switch points depend only on elapsed time. Initiating a treatment after diagnosis of a disease, and withdrawing it or changing treatments when symptoms disappear, make it difficult or impossible to interpret observed treatment effects. Indeed, it almost surely violates the requirement that patients be able to "re-qualify" for the study before administration of the second (and subsequent) treatments. In the current set of eight papers at least seven used time-dependent crossover rules, including two with a washout period long enough to erase most biologically plausible carryover effects. This may be a small improvement over the 13 papers we reported in 1984, where 10 had time-dependent crossover rules and 1 a disease-state-dependent rule; in 2 the rules governing crossover were not clearly reported.

Whenever possible, crossover points should be concealed from both patients (blinded) and observers (doubly blinded). Knowledge of a switch can influence reported treatment response, its assessment, or both, so that blinding the crossover point can reduce the influence of any subjective order effects.

Dropouts, Faulty Data, and Outliers

Although dropouts and implausible data points are problems for any study, their effects may be large in a study with a crossover design, because each patient contributes a large proportion of the total information and because the design is sensitive to departures from the ideal plan. For example, consider again the study of diabetic patients[11] summarized in Table 2. If Patient 1 drops out during the first treatment period, only three patients remain to provide useful data. The mean difference between the two treatment regimens is still 3.00 g, but its standard error is now 0.577, and the t-statistic (with 2 degrees of freedom) equals 5.2, with a p-value of 0.03. Although the result is still statistically significant, the p-value has risen dramatically from the original 0.006. If the initial result had been less definitive, this loss of just one patient would have altered the conclusions of the study. A single dropout in the comparable parallel study (with 28 patients in each group) should have relatively little influence on the conclusions.

Dropout rates can be high in crossover studies, because the study design requires that patients receive at least two treatments and thus each participant remains in the trial for longer periods of time than in a parallel design. However, partial information on a patient completing one treatment and then dropping out can be used in estimating the treatment effects in Period 1, provided that dropping out is not related to treatment response. A high dropout rate greatly weakens any study, and the initial sample size should be sufficiently large to compensate for this effect. The studies in our sample were generally short, and most used treatments not likely to have important side effects—conditions that favor the success of a crossover design. However, dropout rates can be serious. Cazeau et al.[2] reported results for only 46 of 58 patients randomized; they are meticulous in reporting the reasons for dropout, so that readers can judge whether results may have been compromised. The report on Parkinson's disease[3] says that 143 patients were enrolled, 134 had the bilateral implants under study, and 127 provided follow-up data 6 months after implantation, but it is not clear when or why some of the patients dropped out. Wilschanski et al.[5] give reasons why 7 of their 32 subjects dropped out; Gilron et al.[7] used a sophisticated assignment algorithm (a balanced Latin square design) for their four-arm study, and report that 16 of their 57 subjects withdrew during the treatment periods. Such losses, in four of the eight studies examined here, can be quite serious, especially when sample sizes are so small, because they introduce bias into the results, upset the balance of many assignment algorithms, and increase the variance in results. Study reports should include the number of dropouts and reasons for each dropout.

Another problem in some studies is *outliers*—deviant data points that seem questionable but cannot be excluded as definitely wrong. Such points should be reported, whether or not they are used in the analysis, and conclusions should not be sensitive to them. Protection against such sensitivity can be obtained either by setting aside deviant data or by using techniques developed to be "resistant" to bias from omitting data points.[16, 17] Investigators do not always report outliers (though they should), so the fact that none were reported in these eight studies may not mean as much as it could.

Statistical Analysis and Sample Size

Observations made repeatedly in the same patient tend to be more similar than those made in different patients. Statistical analyses that take this relation into account are more complicated, but potentially more powerful, than those that are appropriate for a parallel comparison. Most important, the patient and not an individual measurement is the basic unit of statistical analysis.

One can think of the analysis as comparing the results of the treatments of a single patient and then combining these comparisons across patients. When only two measurements are compared (as in the study of Raskin and Unger[11]), the paired t-test provides a widely applicable procedure. In many studies, however, each patient contributes three or more observations, including a sequence of observations over each treatment period, and a different statistical analysis is necessary. In the present series, four of the reports[3, 5, 6, 8] used a repeated-measures analysis of variance, one[7] used a linear mixed model, and one[9] used a one-way analysis of variance. Though none of the reports gave sufficient detail to tell whether these methods were used to best advantage, they can be powerful multivariate tools for extracting the maximum information from a sample. The remaining two papers might have benefited from some form of multivariate analysis.

Multivariate regression and analysis-of-variance techniques model the association (correlation) among the measurements for a single individual and use this association in computing standard errors of comparisons. Also, the techniques allow adjustment of p-values for multiple tests on the series of measurements. In effect, they operate by linking together the results of several paired t-tests. They yield statistical tests and estimates of treatment and order effects to enable the investigator to assess the success or failure of the crossover design and to compare responses to treatment.

A comparison of this set of 8 reports with the 13 in the first and second editions of this book suggests that the crossover design is used less commonly than before, but that it is used in a substantially better way. For example, all 8 of our studies used randomization (compared with 7 of 13 in our earlier series), all paid some attention to period and carryover effects (compared with just 1 of the original 13), and double-blinding was used to better effect. However, although all of the recent reports included acceptable statistical analyses, each failed to report some potentially important information. This may be a reflection of the general tendency in medical journals to shorten Methods sections, which now often omit (or relegate to a supplementary appendix) information critical to a full evaluation of the results reported.

A remarkable feature of Table 1 is the general tendency of p-values for tests of the primary hypotheses to be very low; most were less than 0.001. Candidate explanations include: The investigators did not trust the power of the crossover design, or they anticipated dropouts that did not occur and wanted to be sure that they would have convincing data and so used a larger sample size than necessary; they overestimated variances in their observations and hence overestimated sample size requirements; treatment effects were greater than expected; or additional considerations drove the recruitment of patients (e.g., an intention to study subgroups of patients, concern about secondary endpoints, or a desire to detect relatively uncommon complications of treatment). Whatever the reason or reasons, the considerable strength of the crossover design may not have been fully exploited.

In medical research, clinical studies generally have one or two primary hypotheses, but secondary hypotheses may be more numerous. As shown in Table 1, the authors of these eight crossover studies made substantial use of their data in examining secondary hypotheses, but small samples can rarely separate the effects of primary and secondary hypotheses because the outcomes are too few to permit detailed study of possible interactions. None of the eight reports examined relationships between primary and secondary outcomes, so the reports on secondary analyses are on even weaker ground than such analyses in larger, parallel comparisons.

FURTHER COMPARISONS WITH PARALLEL DESIGNS

If neither time nor treatment order affects the response to the treatments under study, pairing each patient with himself or herself (that is, a crossover design) and analyzing the data properly can markedly reduce the influence of characteristics of study subjects on the treatment comparison. This pairing represents the ultimate form of statistical adjustment for such characteristics (Chapter 4). However, even when the disease and treatments are satisfactory for a crossover trial, the choice between such a trial and a parallel comparison can be difficult. Although a crossover design has the potential advantage of economy and of providing a direct comparison of treatments in the same patient, the parallel design allows more straightforward analysis, its efficacy depends less on assumptions about the disease process, and it generally produces a lower dropout rate because each patient provides fewer measurements in a shorter time. In addition, the use of baseline measurements and statistical adjustments can substantially increase the precision of a parallel design, sometimes making the required number of patients only slightly larger than for a crossover study. Generally, similar adjustments to crossover studies have little impact. An assumption in the crossover approach is that the roles of confounders are the same for both treatments and at both treatment times.

In a choice between parallel and crossover designs, the burden of proof is on those favoring the crossover design to show that it can succeed in improving on the parallel design; such proof may often be forthcoming. Evidence supporting an expectation of success with a crossover design in a particular study would include previous studies validating the absence of carryover effects, low dropout rates, and a relatively stable disease process. Even in such situations a parallel design adjusted for previously specified covariates can be a strong competitor. We recommend that a design be chosen only after careful consideration of research goals, the disease process, and the trade-off between power and fragility. Such consideration requires a collaborative effort among clinical, laboratory, and statistical scientists.

PATIENTS AS THEIR OWN CONTROLS

In many research studies (called "self-controlled") patients serve as their own controls before, during, or after treatment.[1] Many crossover and parallel studies include an element of self-control, but some clinical investigations rely entirely on self-controls. Such research designs incorporate many of the features of crossover studies, but new problems arise, as we discuss after presenting three examples of self-controlled studies. In one, Peck et al.[18] evaluated the effect of 13-*cis*-retinoic acid on severe acne by examining changes in disease status; it appears that the acne was of such duration and intractability in each patient that substantial spontaneous improvement was unlikely to interfere with treatment evaluation.

In another example[19] patients with hypertension that had been found on screening were followed to determine whether informing them that they had elevated blood pressure was reflected in increased absenteeism for illness. Each patient's work record after diagnosis was compared with the patient's previous record. (Other parts of this study used crossover and parallel designs; we do not discuss those aspects here.)

Packer et al.[20] used a self-controlled design to investigate the clinical reaction of patients with congestive heart failure to the abrupt withdrawal of nitroprusside. Previous research had established that nitroprusside produced rapid hemodynamic and clinical improvement in patients with congestive heart failure, but some results had suggested that the sudden termination of treatment caused adverse clinical reactions. The self-controlled design seems ideal for the study of this problem, and it is hard for us to see how either a crossover or parallel design, usually considered more powerful, could have been employed.

Each of the five critical issues in crossover studies discussed above applies with undiminished force to self-controlled studies. Some additional issues in self-controlled studies (though not unique to them) need to be considered, especially lack of symmetry, the nature of the problems, the study of patients with refractory disease, and the absence of direct comparisons.

Lack of Symmetry

A critical difference between crossover and self-controlled studies is the latter's fundamental lack of symmetry between observations during treatment and those during control periods. These observations often differ in such matters as duration, nature, and intensity of clinical studies, and decision rules about when to modify or switch treatments. Such differences can lead to substantial bias (for example, in opportunities to observe untoward developments in the disease process) that may tilt results toward or away from the treatment under study. For example, in the study of Peck et al.[18] of the effect of 13-*cis*-retinoic acid on severe acne, the scope and duration of observation before and after therapy did not match the intensity of study during the treatment period. In well-designed crossover studies this problem does not arise, because such effects are balanced between treatments and become part of the random error.

Nature of the Problems Studied

Another general difference between self-controlled and crossover studies is in the nature of the problems studied. Self-controlled studies are more often used at early points in the clinical development of new treatments, with more attention to multiple laboratory measurements than to one or two measures of clinical outcome. Although this measuring of multiple outcomes is not necessarily a weakness in self-controlled designs, it does mean that methods of analysis must be carefully tailored to exploit the data. One difficulty is the *multiple-comparisons problem*, addressed in Chapter 8. Another is the optimal multivariate analysis of numerous dependent variables, as well as covariates. We have found that expert help in multivariate statistical methods is rarely evident in self-controlled studies, though it might often lead to substantially more productive use of the data.

Study of Patients with Refractory Disease

A third common difference from crossover studies is the focus of many self-controlled studies on patients whose disease had responded inadequately to standard therapies.[1] This may result, in part, from the use of this design at early stages of investigation in human subjects and the ethical considerations that lead to the enrollment of patients with refractory disease. Several problems arise in studies of such patients. One is that intense, prolonged (though perhaps incompletely effective) treatment may require a prolonged washout or recovery period, whereas the patient's clinical problems demand prompt relief. Another problem arises from regression toward the mean—the tendency of an extreme value when it is re-measured to be closer to the mean, because the original value was likely to have been extreme, at least in part, by chance. If patients are enrolled in a self-controlled study of some new regimen when standard treatments appear to be losing efficacy (that is, when the patients' conditions tend to be worse than their own averages), some general improvement may occur that has nothing to do with improved therapy. This problem can sometimes be addressed by using a first set of measurements after a washout period to establish patient eligibility for enrollment in a self-controlled study and a second set, after a further stabilizing period, to establish baseline levels.

Patients whose disease fails to respond to standard treatment may include those with variant or more aggressive forms of the disease or those whose general conditions have deteriorated so that even a new, effective treatment is of little avail. Thus, such patients may not provide a fair test of the capabilities of a new treatment, but the value of studying such patients in the early development of a new treatment is often compelling. The main advantage is the reduced risk of compromising the wellbeing of patients by withholding standard treatments, which in these patients are already known to have little effect. Although studies of non-responders can rarely provide definitive conclusions about the efficacy of a treatment in more-responsive disease, they can provide information of considerable value in planning further studies (e.g., randomized controlled trials) that are designed to give unambiguous answers to questions about broad treatment recommendations.

Absence of Direct Comparisons

Self-controlled trials estimate the changes expected when a patient receives a treatment, so long as the criteria for treatment are similar to those for study eligibility. Investigators may need this information in the early stages of testing a new treatment to help decide whether or how to continue studying the treatment.

Self-controlled studies do not provide more-direct information about how a new treatment compares with standard therapies. Rather, one must combine the results of self-controlled studies with those of other studies, though this is often difficult because of inevitable differences in study design and conduct. The demographic composition of the patient groups may differ, or the disease may be more severe in one group than another. Often, one cannot even determine the direction of such differences, because investigators have used subjective or partly subjective assessments of clinical status, or they have not used the same set of objective measurements to establish a diagnosis or to monitor disease progress. Different investigators may even use different outcome variables to assess the effects of treatment. The reader must consider all these matters to obtain a valid assessment of the relative merits of two treatments, though it is generally not clear how to do so, and there is rarely any way to tell whether the adjustments were appropriate and adequate. Thus, despite the clear value of self-controlled studies in the initial investigation of new treatments, one must usually use a randomized controlled trial or some other powerful research design to determine with assurance whether the new treatment should be recommended for general use.

REFERENCES

1. Louis TA, Lavori PW, Bailar JC, Polansky M. Crossover and self-controlled designs in clinical research. N Engl J Med 1984; 310:24–31.

2. Cazeau S, Leclercq C, Lavergne T, et al. Effects of multisite biventricular pacing in patients with heart failure and intraventricular conduction delay. N Engl J Med 2001; 344:873–80.

3. The Deep-Brain Stimulation for Parkinson's Disease Study Group. Deep-brain stimulation of the subthalamic nucleus or the pars interna of the globus pallidus in Parkinson's disease. N Engl J Med 2001; 345:956–63.

4. Batterham RL, Cohen MA, Ellis SM, et al. Inhibition of food intake in obese subjects by peptide YY_{3-36}. N Engl J Med 2003; 349:941–8.

5. Wilschanski M, Yahav Y, Yaacov Y, et al. Gentamycin-induced correction of CFTR function in patients with cystic fibrosis and CFTR stop mutations. N Engl J Med 2003; 349:1433–41.

6. Vissing J, Haller RG. The effect of oral sucrose on exercise tolerance in patients with McArdle's disease. N Engl J Med 2003; 349:2503–9.

7. Gilron I, Bailey JM, Tu D, et al. Morphine, gabapentin, or their combination for neuropathic pain. N Engl J Med 2005; 352:1324–34.

8. Simantirakis E, Schiza SE, Chrysostomakis SI, et al. Atrial overdrive pacing for the obstructive sleep apnea-hypopnea syndrome. N Engl J Med 2005; 353:2568–77.

9. Berry MA, Hargadon B, Shelley M, et al. Evidence of a role of tumor necrosis factor α in refractory asthma. N Engl J Med 2006; 354:697–708.

10. Senn S. Cross-over trials in clinical research. 2nd ed. Chichester, UK: John Wiley & Sons Ltd., 2002.

11. Raskin P, Unger RH. Hyperglucagonemia and its suppression: importance in the metabolic control of diabetes. N Engl J Med 1978; 299:433–6.

12. Soter NA, Austen KF, Wasserman SI. Oral disodium cromoglycate in the treatment of systemic mastocytosis. N Engl J Med 1979; 301:465–9.

13. Brown BW Jr. The crossover experiment for clinical trials. Biometrics 1980; 36:69–79.

14. Hills M, Armitage P. The two-period cross-over clinical trial. Br J Clin Pharmacol 1979; 8:7–20.

15. Wallenstein S, Fisher AC. The analysis of the two-period repeated measurements cross-over design with applications to clinical trials. Biometrics 1977; 33:261–9.

16. Hoaglin DC, Mosteller F, Tukey JW, eds. Understanding robust and exploratory data analysis. New York: John Wiley & Sons, Inc., 1983. [Wiley Classics Library edition, 2000.]

17. Mosteller F, Tukey JW. Data analysis and regression: a second course in statistics. Reading, MA: Addison-Wesley, 1977.

18. Peck GL, Olsen TG, Yoder FW, et al. Prolonged remissions of cystic and conglobate acne with 13-*cis*-retinoic acid. N Engl J Med 1979; 300:329–33.

19. Haynes RB, Sackett DL, Taylor DW, et al. Absenteeism from work after detection and labeling of hypertensive patients. N Engl J Med 1978; 299:741–4.

20. Packer M, Meller J, Medina N, et al. Rebound hemodynamic events after the abrupt withdrawal of nitroprusside in patients with severe chronic heart failure. N Engl J Med 1979; 301:1193–7.

CHAPTER 6

cs

The Series of Consecutive Cases as a Device
for Assessing Outcomes of Interventions

LINCOLN E. MOSES, PH.D.

ABSTRACT   An important part of the medical literature consists of reports of
series of cases. Typically, a series has been accumulated over time and consists of
all patients meeting certain criteria over a specified interval. Ordinarily, if assessing an intervention, the report entails comparison—either explicit, between sub-
classes in the series, or implicit, between the whole series and ordinary expectations and experience. Interpretation of the series report depends on the author's
clarity about the definitions actually applied, the integrity of counting (who was
excluded and why), and the consistency of diagnosis, outcome measurement, and
other factors. In addition, such variables as age, parity, and stage of disease may
influence outcomes; thus, information concerning these factors may be needed
for confident interpretation of the series. Acceptance of a reported series result at
face value is, therefore, unlikely to be justified, and interpretation typically calls
for analysis. If the necessary ancillary information is not reported, the implications of the results may remain obscure.

An air of serving the common good clings to the process of reporting
as general information the results of one's own extensive experience.
Medicine enjoys a long tradition of such literature, and valuable results
have sometimes ensued. Moreover, a large share of medical knowledge has
been accumulated in just this way, through the publication of reports on series
of cases. The purpose of this chapter is to examine the usefulness and limitations of series for assessing the safety and efficacy of medical interventions.
Two historical examples help clarify the issues involved: the first demonstrates
results with a new technique; the second compares outcomes between two differently treated subsets of a single series of patients.

In 1847 John Snow published an epochal work, *On the Inhalation of the Vapour
of Ether in Surgical Operations*.[1] Snow described the equipment he had devised, the
procedure he had used, and 75 operations (52 at St. George's Hospital and 23

at University College Hospital) performed before September 16, 1847, in which he had delivered ether anesthesia.

These two series (with four and two deaths, respectively) were doubtless, in the eyes of the author and his readers, harbingers of the future. For a modern reader they also serve as a window on the past; in each of the 75 operations, neither the thorax nor the abdomen was entered. The two series showed that Snow's apparatus was effective in vaporizing ether for patient inhalation and that, with the new apparatus and procedure, anesthesia was induced in all patients, all patients revived from the anesthesia, and the surgery was performed more easily than without it. These results helped to dispel the mistrust of ether that had been engendered by inept applications in England in 1846.

In 1836, drawing from his practice over the years, Pierre Louis published an account of 77 patients with pneumonia uncomplicated by other disease.[2] He classified them by whether or not they had survived the disease and by when in the course of their illness he had begun bleeding them. Early bleeding turned out to be associated with reduced survival. The series of observations was an important part of his attack on bleeding as a panacea.

These accounts, though much abbreviated, show some of the characteristics of the series as a source of information in medicine. First, a series typically contains information acquired over time. Second, the patients in a series are all similar in some essential way: all the patients in Snow's series received ether, though with various operations; all those in Louis's series had the same disease (and physician) but varied in the way they were treated. Third, all the patients in a defined class are discussed: Snow described all administrations of ether on or before September 16, 1847; Louis described all patients with pneumonia for whom he had records indicating no other disease and whom he had bled. Fourth, a comparison is involved; it may be direct, as in the study by Louis, or indirect, as in Snow's study. Thus, fairness of comparison becomes a crucial issue. (Louis assured his readers that the two groups, survivors and decedents, were as alike in the initial severity of their disease as he could make them by including and excluding cases from his files.) Finally, the reported series, whatever its value as evidence, may or may not be influential. Louis was a member of the faculty at Paris, which lent weight to his report. (The influence of his report contrasts notably with the small impact of James Lind's beautifully controlled experiment demonstrating the curative power of lemons in scurvy. Lind was a naval surgeon without high standing, and his study did not affect the policy of the Royal Navy until some 40 years later.)

Just as a series can advance correct understanding, so it can promote the pursuit of bad leads. Presumably, most once-popular but later-discarded therapies were initially supported by series of favorable cases. Even in recent times, there was support for the use of a portacaval shunt for the treatment of esophageal varices and gastric freezing for the treatment of ulcers.

In this chapter, the aim is to analyze the strengths and weaknesses of series as sources of information for appraising the efficacy and safety of diagnostic and therapeutic interventions. Perhaps there are straightforward ways to distinguish the trustworthy from the spurious, misleading information that is sometimes conveyed in a series.

WHAT IS A SERIES?

I shall apply the term "series" to a study of the results of an intervention that has certain characteristics. First, it is longitudinal, not cross-sectional; postintervention outcomes are reported for a group of subjects known to the investigator before the intervention. Second, all eligible patients in some stated setting over a stated period are described. These eligible patients are seen as alike: they may have a common disease, they may have received the same treatments, or they may share some other essential characteristic. Series may have other important design factors; comparison groups may be present or absent, for example, and the research may have been planned either before the data were acquired or afterward.

Not every published series reports outcomes of interventions; descriptive features of patients with a certain disease might be reported in a series, for example. But here I shall deal with those series that do report the outcomes of an intervention applied to all eligible subjects, who are chosen according to criteria that depend only on pretreatment status. The actual data collection may go forward in time according to a research plan, or it may be undertaken after all cases are complete. Intermediate or mixed cases can also occur. The data are regarded as if the subjects were first identified on the basis of eligibility, then treated, and then observed with respect to outcome.

Much of the older medical literature consists of articles that meet this description. Feinstein[3] reviewed all issues of the *Lancet* and the *New England Journal of Medicine* appearing between October 1, 1977, and March 31, 1978. Of the 324 "structured research papers" that he identified, 47 (15%) contained reports on series (with "transition cohorts" and "outcome cohorts") as I use the term. This proportion of articles was approximately equaled by the 53 papers (16%) that reported clinical trials. Bailar et al.[4] reviewed all Original Articles published in the *Journal* during 1978 and 1979. Of the 332 articles, 80 (24%) apparently met the definition of a series used here.

INTERPRETING A SERIES

A number of factors bear on the interpretation of a report of a series. Several of the most important are discussed on the following pages.

The Integrity of Counting

My definition of a series includes the word "all," and the word is essential. Conclusions based on "selected cases" are notoriously treacherous because selection can grossly affect the data. At the extreme, only the successes or only the failures might be reported. Presumably, the limitations of selected cases underlie the skepticism sometimes voiced about the usefulness of voluntary disease registries.

At minimum, the reader needs to know what criteria were used to determine the inclusion and exclusion of subjects, how many subjects were included, and what happened to each of them. Here is where the concept "all" enters as essential to the study's value. Two kinds of problems lurk here. The first is operational: it may be difficult or impossible to learn some of the essential information in retrospect. The outcomes for some patients who belong in the series may be unknown. Patients who cannot be followed often differ on average from those who can be followed; more of the former may be dead or cured. Without complete follow-up, the available figures lose much of their meaning.

The second type of counting problem is definitional. The series report, to avoid being a recital of selected cases, needs to describe what was done to all eligible patients and the outcome for each of them. Who is (or was) eligible may depend on diagnostic criteria that require judgment calls. What was done to the patients may involve judgment as well: if the intervention is a new surgical procedure that has changed somewhat with time, then determination of which patients did and which did not receive "the" new operation requires a decision by the author. Even identification of the outcome for a patient may demand a judgment call. If the patient dies on the operating table, for instance, there may be a question (and a decision) about whether death was due to anesthesia or to treatment failure.

The definitional and operational problems of counting are likely to loom larger if the series study is planned after the data have been collected.

Adjustment for Interfering Variables

In the United Kingdom a series report on 5174 births at home and 11,156 births in hospitals stated that perinatal mortality was 5.4 per 1000 home births and 27.8 per 1000 hospital births.[5] What use can be made of these numbers? A moment's thought fills the mind with questions about the comparability of the two series of mothers. How did they differ in age, parity, prenatal care, prenatal complications, home circumstances, general health, and disease status? Without answers to these questions, we must withhold any firm interpretation of the data. With information on all these variables—and doubtless some others—we are better off. But even with such information, we still face the hard question of how to adjust the raw results for differences in these other variables. They are likely to be relevant to perinatal mortality, but we do not know "the right way" to adjust numerically for these factors, even if we have the information.

The complexities of adjustment are nicely exemplified in a study of more than 15,000 consecutive (eligible) deliveries at Beth Israel Hospital in Boston, about half involving electronic fetal monitoring, which was the intervention being studied.[6] The authors identified many variables as risk factors; among them were gestational age, hydramnios, placental and cord abnormalities, multiple birth, breech delivery, and prolonged rupture of membranes. Their primary analysis used 18 variables in a multiple-regression–derived risk index, on which each delivery was scored. Each case was then assigned to one of five (ordered) strata, depending on the risk score. In addition to the primary analysis, the authors applied risk stratification in two other ways and also analyzed the data independently in terms of log-linear models. Clearly, the answer to the question of how to adjust the data is not always straightforward. The authors qualified their results with this observation: "Since we are applying our risk score to the set of data from which the weights for the score are computed, we may be overstating the concentration of benefit in the high-risk categories." This candid caveat further attests to the intrinsic difficulty of adjusting for relevant variables in the effort to interpret the results in a series.

The message here is that interpretation of even an apparently sharp difference in a series-based study may require additional information about the data in the series. Moreover, even with such additional information, the results may remain ambiguous.

Control of Interfering Variables by Matching

Another strategy for assessing treatment outcome after adjusting for interfering variables like patient mix, referral patterns, and so forth, is to use matching. The idea is to construct a second series consisting of patients "like" the ones who get the intervention under study, and then compare the outcomes. Cameron and Pauling[7] used this approach in a series-based assessment of supplemental ascorbate on extending survival in terminal cancer patients. The investigators selected from the files 100 patients who were judged to be no longer able to benefit from any conventional treatment and who were given ascorbate. (This is not readily perceivable as "all" of any well-defined group; the investigators regarded them as "represent[ing] a random selection of all the terminal patients in [the] hospital, even though no formal randomization process was used.") Then, for each of these patients, 10 comparison subjects were chosen from the files of the same hospital; matching variables were sex, age (within five years), cancer of the same primary organ, and histological tumor type. The response variable was the survival time past initiation of ascorbate for the treated subjects, and the response variable for the controls was length of survival past the judged date when disease became untreatable. In all, there were 100 cases and 1000 controls. The authors reported a marked prolongation of survival with ascorbate. Later, Moertel et al.[8] reported a randomized clinical trial of the same question. The results of that trial slightly favored the placebo; the authors' analysis concluded, "There is no reasonable likelihood that vitamin C produces even a 25% increase in (terminal) survival times over placebo ($p = 0.017$)." The conflicting results suggest that effective matching—especially in retrospect—can be hard to accomplish. In particular here, the determination from records of just when a patient's disease became untreatable would be hard to equate with a determination of that same matter made face-to-face with the patient (i.e., when vitamin C treatment began).

The generic limitations of matching include: (1) some important variables may have gone unmeasured, and so cannot be used for matching; (2) though it may be possible to match on one or two variables, the difficulty of finding subjects who match on them all grows as the number of matching variables is increased; (3) the two groups of subjects may differ in ascertainment (of eligibility or outcome, as would seem to be the case in the ascorbate study). A full treatment of matching is given by Cochran.[9]

Necessary Information

At minimum, to interpret the findings of a series-based study accurately, we need to know answers to the cub reporter's legendary questions: *Who* were the subjects (i.e., what were their relevant characteristics)? *What* was done? (This calls for definitions of treatment, diagnosis, staging, adjuvant care, follow-up, and so forth.) By *whom* was it done? (By world-class experts? By teaching-hospital staff? By community-hospital staff?) *When* was it done? (Over a time span long enough to permit the appearance of large trends of various sorts?) *Why* was a certain treatment used? (Because other treatments had already failed? Because the patients were not strong enough to tolerate other treatments? For palliation? For cure?)

The randomized clinical trial is especially effective in addressing these questions for two reasons. First, since a protocol is prepared in advance, the key design questions have explicit answers that are unlikely to change. Second, randomization provides escape from the reality that differently constituted groups are hard to compare; this escape is effected by constructing a *single* group of patients eligible for and willing to receive either intervention and by then applying the different interventions to random subsets of this one group.

Effects of the Absence of a Protocol

The absence of a protocol prepared before data are acquired may give rise to certain kinds of defects in the study. Exactly what interventions were performed on what kinds of patients for what indications may be unclear in hindsight. Decisions about which patients to count as eligible, and therefore to include, and which patients to omit may have been based on subjective judgment. Withdrawals may be poorly documented or even undocumented, with possibly major effects on results. The reader may wonder whether the reported results have been selected from among many possible endpoints and are therefore less likely to be reproducible than significance tests indicate. Increasing numbers of studies have been performed in which the research was planned after the data had been collected. Fletcher and Fletcher[10] studied articles in the *Lancet* and the *Journal of the American Medical Association* and found that 24% of those published in 1946 fit this description; for articles published in 1976, the corresponding figure was 56%. Of course, difficulties of this type can be mitigated by careful reporting, but they can be eliminated only if the data have been gathered so systematically as to conform to an implicit protocol in all important respects.

Effects of Nonrandomization

The series-based study is vulnerable to the many dangers that randomization forestalls. The key considerations are the comparability of patients receiving different interventions and the equivalence of outcome evaluations. In the absence of randomization, doubts about interpretation can, and should, nag the reader. The effects of crossing over illustrate the difficulties.

Suppose that a serious disease can be treated effectively by surgery, but operative mortality and postsurgical sequelae are drawbacks. A medical therapy is therefore an attractive alternative. If there is a class of patients for whom the two treatments appear to be equally reasonable, then a suitably designed and executed randomized controlled trial should indicate which treatment is actually superior in that class of patients. Now, it may happen that some medically treated patients do not respond, and the gravity of the disease may require that they receive the surgical treatment after initial assignment to the medically treated group. This change is called *crossing over*.

In a randomized controlled trial, the effect of crossing over is simply to change the research question to a new form: For patients of the class originally defined, is the superior policy to perform surgery immediately or to give medical treatment and avoid surgery unless it becomes indicated? This is very likely to be a better—i.e., a more realistic and practical—question than the original one, so no harm is done.

In nonrandomized studies, crossing over is more likely to cause serious problems of interpretation. The two policies—surgery immediately or a medical therapy until surgery may be necessary—can be difficult to compare, because in retrospect it may not be clear which policy has been applied to a patient treated surgically.

Assessing Individual Studies

A summary of the discussion to this point would suggest that series-based studies are liable to grave difficulties, although of course not every study comes to a false conclusion. Determining the evidential value of the individual study under consideration amounts to assessing whether the selection of patients has biased the results, whether the evaluation of treatment outcomes has differed according to the treatment, and whether the withdrawal of patients from the study has biased the results. The reader may recognize the questions but be powerless to answer them with the information published. The investigator may be unable to answer them on the basis of the records. These difficulties are more formidable when the research plan is established after the data have already been recorded.

The timing of observations also affects a series in another way. The cases can be defined as all those present at one of several points in time. Thus, the series-based study (1) may take up each patient with a certain disease as he or she presents in a given setting during a stated time interval; (2) may first take cognizance of a patient at the time of initiating treatment A or treatment B; or (3) may look backward and capture all subjects who began treatment A or B during that stated interval. Difficulties of interpretation grow as the series originates at later stages in the sequence above. Starting at (2) rather than (1) blurs information about the inclusion and exclusion criteria that were applied. Starting instead at (3) further adds problems of data availability and quality. It is essential also that the starting and ending times for the series be representative in some sense; they must not be chosen to include or exclude "runs" of success or failure.

THE "CLEAR-CUT" SERIES

The reader may think that the picture of series has been presented too negatively and may reason, "If a small series is studied, clear differences may be observed at once, and the complexities described may not need to be unraveled. If a new approach is so good that it has an explosive impact, then an acceptable study can be devised readily enough." This objection raises fair questions. Isn't a large fraction of medical practice based on the results of series-based studies? Aren't there many instances in which such studies—e.g., those of penicillin and ether anesthesia—have unambiguously demonstrated the truth? Certainly, medical practice has evolved largely from series-based information. But we also know that much of today's accepted doctrine will be discarded when more and more-careful evaluations are performed. The problem is to ascertain which series (i.e., which uncontrolled studies) point to the right answers and which do not.

What about penicillin for syphilis, sulfa drugs against pneumococcus, and similar examples? These have been called "slam-bang" effects. When they occur, they are dramatic. The very fact that they are so dramatic should remind us that they are also rare. An effort to enumerate brings to mind the use of vitamin B12 against pernicious anemia, penicillin for subacute bacterial endocarditis, x-ray films for setting fractures, cortisone for adrenal insufficiency, insulin for severe diabetes, propranolol for hypertrophic aortic stenosis, methotrexate for choriocarcinoma, indomethacin for patent ductus arteriosus, and perhaps two or three times as many. But have there been more than one or two such cases per year in the last half century? Perhaps not.

Slam-bang effects are uncommon. They account for only a small number of the thousands of studies published each year. Furthermore, they are not always open-and-shut cases. In 1847, the year that Snow published his report on the ether series, J.Y. Simpson reported his results lauding chloroform anesthesia. Controversy about the comparative merits of the two anesthetics persisted at least until the Lancet Commission examined the matter in 1893. Between 1848 and 1893, a total of 64,693 administrations of chloroform and only 9380 administrations of ether had been identified. The commission recommended ether as safer than chloroform in general surgery "in temperate climes."[11] Similarly, x-ray films for diagnosing fractures clearly work, but how long did it take to discard x-ray therapy for the treatment of acne? Prefrontal lobotomy for schizophrenia stands as a reminder that a treatment may come to be widely used on the basis of inadequate evidence—only to be discarded later. The occasional slam-bang effect, clearly detectable from an uncontrolled study, is at the favorable end of a spectrum; at the other end lie series-based studies that defy interpretation.

The Office of Health and Technology Assessment (OHTA)[12] reviewed the nine published series that report at least 10 cases of transsexual surgery. Its assessment report states:

> These studies represent the major clinical reports thus far published on the outcome of transsexual surgery. None of these studies meets the ideal criteria of a valid scientific assessment of a clinical procedure, and they share many of the following deficiencies:
>
> a. There is often a lack of clearly specified goals and objectives of the intervention, making it difficult to evaluate the outcomes;
>
> b. The patients represent heterogeneous groups because diagnostic criteria have varied from center to center and over time;

  c. The therapeutic techniques are not standardized, with varying surgical techniques being combined with various other therapies;

  d. None has had adequate (if any) control groups (perhaps this is impossible);

  e. There is no blinding, with the observers usually being part of the therapeutic team;

  f. Systematically collected baseline data are usually missing, making comparison of pre- and post-surgery status difficult;

  g. There is a lack of valid and reliable instruments for assessing pre- and post-surgery status and the selection of scoring of outcome criteria usually involve arbitrary value judgments;

  h. A large number of patients are lost to follow-up, apparently due in great part to the desire of transsexuals to leave their pasts behind; and,

  i. None of the studies are presented in sufficient detail to permit replication.

Although the procedure under consideration is quite unusual, most of the difficulties listed are threats to the majority of assessments using series of patients receiving a new treatment or procedure. They also amount to a list of most of the problems that the protocol of a randomized clinical trial is intended to forestall.

ADDITIONAL ISSUES IN INTERPRETATION

A number of other issues also affect the usefulness of a series in providing information on the value of an intervention or procedure.

Subgroups

The difficulties associated with direct reliance on data in a whole series are exacerbated if one attempts to pick out subclasses marked by strikingly good or bad results. The idea seems reasonable enough, but it ignores a somewhat subtle, inescapable fact: one can always expect to find some good-looking and some bad-looking subsets in any body of data, even when no bias has influenced any part of it. Furthermore, such differences among subsets can easily be large enough to look quite convincing to the unsophisticated analyst (as discussed in Chapter 15).

Suppose that n subjects, a random sample from some population with standard deviation σ, are further divided at random into k equal-sized subgroups. Then the standard error for the mean of the undivided sample is S.E. = $\sigma/\sqrt{n}$. Now, of course, the largest of the subgroup means must exceed the mean for the whole group, but it can be surprising how large this excess must be. If $k = 4$, the average excess of the largest subgroup mean over the whole-group mean to be expected from random division is 2.06 S.E.; if $k = 7$, it is 3.56 S.E.; and if $k = 10$, it is 4.87 S.E. Comparison of the best and the worst subgroups can produce differences that appear even more vivid but are meaningless. The following rule of thumb demonstrates this point: If a group of n subjects is divided at random into k equal-sized subgroups, then the difference between the largest and the smallest subgroup means has an expected value that is approximately k times the standard error of the mean of the whole group (when k is not more than 15).

With such large subgroup differences to be expected by random division, we must temper our enthusiasm when we identify a series subset that differs strikingly from the whole group. We should face the question, Is this difference large enough to accept as meaningful, considering what chance alone would produce? There are methods for answering the question, which also arises with randomized controlled trials.[13]

Temporal Drift

If a series has been accumulated over a long time (as happened with Louis's study, but not with Snow's), additional problems are likely. Over a long period, shifts can occur—indeed, they are to be expected. The patient population may change as referral patterns alter; thus, the demographic composition of the sample may drift. Supportive care, diagnostic criteria, and exposure to pathogenic agents may change over time; even the treatments themselves may change. It follows that information about the sequence and timing of the cases in the series may be essential to a realistic analysis. The issue here is not hypothetical; Schneiderman[14] gives examples of clinical trials in which a second control group was initiated because treatments were modified during the trial. Analysis then showed that the two successive control groups, although seen in the same setting and meeting the same criteria, differed importantly with respect to survival.

Grab Samples

Statistical inference is a powerful tool for learning from experience. It is at its best when data are obtained in ways that permit the correct application of probability theory—e.g., with random sampling from a population or with data from a randomized clinical trial. When the probabilistic structure is chaotic or unknown, the data constitute what is often called a "grab sample." Inference from such samples, whether by application of formal statistical methods or by other means, is treacherous. The experience of a single physician is in some sense a grab sample; so are the case study and the series of successive cases. The fact that we can learn from experience shows that it is not impossible to reach valid conclusions from grab samples, but the process is fraught with difficulty, uncertainty, and error.

Data from a grab sample are more likely to be useful when two conditions obtain: first, when the data come from a well-defined setting that is relatively stable over time, and second, when the data are taken from this setup at regular intervals over a protracted period.

Two examples help explain this point. First, statistical reports from the Metropolitan Life Insurance Company have long given useful indications of trends in longevity and disease attack rates despite the fact that, because of selective factors that apply to insurance policyholders, its statistics could not wisely be used to estimate the average longevity and the attack rates of diseases for the U.S. population. Similarly, cross-sectional information from the populations covered by particular healthcare facilities such as the Kaiser Health Plan, the Mayo Clinic, and Professional Activities Study (PAS) hospitals would not be expected to apply directly to larger or different groups, although changes in such series over time might so apply.

Second, air pollutants are monitored at stations situated in particular locations; the relation of pollutant levels at such stations to the levels experienced by people in the schools, homes, and factories or on the roads near the monitoring stations is in general poorly known. Nonetheless, when those monitored levels rise or fall, we feel justified in thinking that the pollution levels experienced by the nearby population rise or fall as well. The monitored pollutant levels would serve less well, or even not at all, as measures of the absolute dose to the population nearby.

Even such restricted use, to indicate trends, depends strongly on the assumption of stability in the system. For example, a change in membership, fee structure, or reporting methods could affect the interpretation of trends observed in the statistics of a health plan. Similarly, a seasonal change in the prevailing wind direction might cause some areas to receive higher levels of pollution, even though every monitoring station showed lower levels. Consider, for instance, a location near a major pollution source that is upwind of that source during the region's high-pollution season but is downwind from it during the region's low-pollution season.

So the message here, again, is that the meaning and reliability of the data in a series are generally obscure until clarified by detailed study. It is possible that detailed study will reveal essential flaws that bar trustworthy interpretation of the kind that one might initially hope would be feasible.

CONCLUSIONS

A series study is a record of experience; as such, it has prima facie value. It may provide useful information about how to apply a new technique and about what kinds of difficulties and complications are encountered in its application. This is the case with Snow's book. Postmarketing surveillance produces what might be called partial series, in which the total number of cases under observation can only be estimated. It is a method of study that has its just role in medical investigation. The series is most liable to be inadequate as an indicator of the effectiveness of treatments. The two principal threats to its validity in such cases are vagueness and bias.

Advance planning and full, careful reporting can do much to mitigate problems of interpretation. The planning should be done while the investigators contemplate the way in which they would study the problem if they could use a randomized controlled trial; they can identify probable disturbing variables and can measure and report them. It is impossible to make two differently constituted groups reliably comparable by means of statistical adjustments, so doubts about selection and assessment bias ordinarily cannot be removed entirely. Nevertheless, fuller information helps with the difficult task of interpretation.

The description of a series of successive cases provides readers with vicarious experience, acquired with little outlay of effort. Often, collating and reporting the experience has cost the investigator relatively little effort as well. Thus, in terms of effort, the series may be regarded as an efficient information source.

Useful interpretation of this vicarious information, however, is likely to involve considerable difficulty. A thorough knowledge of surrounding circumstances is ordinarily necessary, but the series study may not adequately report these facts. Even if the necessary supplementary information is reported, quantitative methods for taking accurate account of it may be hard, or even impossible, to devise.

Acceptance of the results of a series study at face value is almost never justified. Any statistic is simply the reported outcome of some process; until the details of the process are known, one cannot know what the statistic means, however it may be labeled. Thus, the interpretation and use of results from a series-based study typically call for analysis, which will prove to be feasible in some instances but infeasible in others.

REFERENCES

1. Snow J. On the inhalation of the vapour of ether in surgical operations. London: John Churchill, 1847.

2. Louis P. Researches on the effects of bloodletting in some inflammatory diseases, and on the influence of tartarized antimony and vesication in pneumonia. Boston: Hilliard Gray, 1836.

3. Feinstein AR. Clinical biostatistics. XLIV. A survey of the research architecture used for publications in general medical journals. Clin Pharmacol Ther 1978; 24:117–25.

4. Bailar JC III, Louis TA, Lavori PW, Polansky M. A classification for biomedical research reports. N Engl J Med 1984; 311:1482–7. [Updated in Chapter 8 of the second edition of this book.]

5. Is home a safer place? Health Soc Serv J 1980; 90:702–5.

6. Neutra RR, Fienberg SE, Greenland S, Friedman EA. Effect of fetal monitoring on neonatal death rates. N Engl J Med 1978; 299:324–6.

7. Cameron E, Pauling L. Supplemental ascorbate in the supportive treatment of cancer: prolongation of survival times in terminal human cancer. Proc Natl Acad Sci USA 1976; 73:3685–9.

8. Moertel CG, Fleming TR, Creagan ET, et al. High-dose vitamin C versus placebo in the treatment of patients with advanced cancer who have had no prior chemotherapy: a randomized double-blind comparison. N Engl J Med 1985; 312:137–41.

9. Cochran WG. Planning and analysis of observational studies. New York: John Wiley, 1983.

10. Fletcher RH, Fletcher SW. Clinical research in general medical journals: a 30-year perspective. N Engl J Med 1979; 301:180–3.

11. Report of the Lancet Commission appointed to investigate the subject of the administration of chloroform and other anaesthetics from a clinical standpoint. Lancet 1893; 1:629–38, 693–708, 761–76, 899–914, 971–8, 1111–8, 1236–40, 1479–98.

12. Office of Health Research Statistics and Technology. Transsexual surgery. Washington, D.C.: Department of Health and Human Services, 1981 (Assessment report series. Vol. 1. No. 4).

13. Ingelfinger JA, Mosteller F, Thibodeau LA, Ware JH. Biostatistics in clinical medicine. 2nd ed. New York: Macmillan, 1987:280–2.

14. Schneiderman MA. Looking backward: is it worth the crick in the neck? or: pitfalls in using retrospective data. Am J Roentgenol Radium Ther Nucl Med 1966; 96:230–5.

CHAPTER 7
CZ

Biostatistics in Epidemiology: Design and Basic Analysis

MARK S. GOLDBERG, PH.D.

ABSTRACT   This chapter surveys the designs used in epidemiological studies to investigate health states. These designs do not stand alone: They are tools
to address specific scientific questions related to populations, broadly defined,
including disease etiology. The chapter stresses the importance of defining objectives in a clear and operational way so that an epidemiologic study can identify
the relevant target population, select the appropriate design that leads to the identification of the source and study populations, and analyze appropriate health
outcome variables, exposure variables, and covariates.

E pidemiology has been defined as "the study of the distribution and determinants of health-related states or events in specified populations, and
the application of this study to the control of health problems."[1] Historically the focus has been on etiology; some classic studies include a survey of
British physicians to determine the health effects of smoking,[2] the Framingham
study to identify risk factors for cardiovascular disease,[3] and studies of the
effects of ionizing radiation on victims of the atomic bomb explosions at Hiroshima and Nagasaki.[4]

Epidemiology still includes studies of etiology,[5–9] but has expanded to cover
such questions as those listed in Box 1. Thus, knowledge of epidemiologic
methods and findings is critical for the full range of health practitioners.

The epidemiologic methods, including statistics, that can be used to answer
these research questions depend mainly on the type of study design (e.g., cohort,
longitudinal, case-control, cross-sectional), how the outcome is measured (e.g.,
binary, continuous, failure-time), and whether the outcome can occur only once
for each subject (e.g., a first myocardial infarction) or whether it can recur
and be measured periodically during the study period (e.g., number of asthma
attacks). The specific analyses that need to be carried out, such as what variables are included in a statistical regression model, depend on the objectives of
the study as well as on the type of information collected.

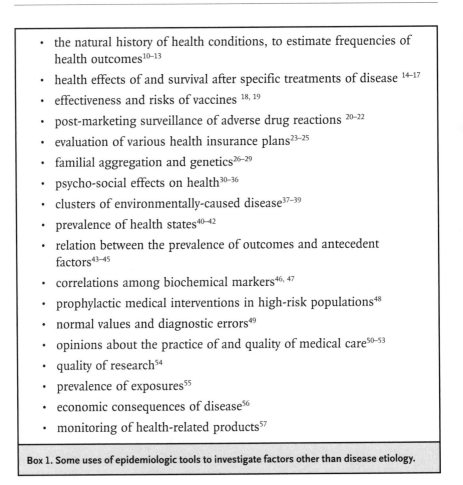

- the natural history of health conditions, to estimate frequencies of health outcomes[10-13]
- health effects of and survival after specific treatments of disease [14-17]
- effectiveness and risks of vaccines [18, 19]
- post-marketing surveillance of adverse drug reactions [20-22]
- evaluation of various health insurance plans[23-25]
- familial aggregation and genetics[26-29]
- psycho-social effects on health[30-36]
- clusters of environmentally-caused disease[37-39]
- prevalence of health states[40-42]
- relation between the prevalence of outcomes and antecedent factors[43-45]
- correlations among biochemical markers[46, 47]
- prophylactic medical interventions in high-risk populations[48]
- normal values and diagnostic errors[49]
- opinions about the practice of and quality of medical care[50-53]
- quality of research[54]
- prevalence of exposures[55]
- economic consequences of disease[56]
- monitoring of health-related products[57]

Box 1. Some uses of epidemiologic tools to investigate factors other than disease etiology.

In conducting epidemiologic studies and evaluating research papers on any of these topics, several principles of research design and conduct are important in evaluating the data and the analysis. Critical questions include:

1. Are the objectives of the study stated precisely and clearly?

2. Is the study design appropriate for the purpose?

3. Does the study population represent the target population without appreciable biases in study enrollment, including sampling of subjects and response rates?

4. Were enough subjects enrolled to meet the objectives (i.e., is there sufficient statistical power to study the problems and assess the primary questions with adequate precision)?

5. Were the measures of outcome and exposure reliable and valid?

6. Are the (possibly implicit) statistical models appropriate? Namely:

    • Do they match the design and the type of outcome variable used, and are the underlying assumptions at least approximately true?

    • Are known risk factors for the outcome(s) included as potential confounding variables, and does the research strategy adequately deal with confounding?

    • Were associations among covariates assessed?

    • Was effect-modification evaluated?

    • Are the data used to their fullest extent; could the method of analysis have caused a loss of information and possibly distorted the findings (e.g., transforming a continuous variable into a binary one; use of logistic regression instead of ordinal regression for ordinal outcomes)?

    • Are missing data dealt with adequately, so that losses of subjects or missing data elements do not bias the findings?

    • Did the reported analysis follow the stated procedures?

The present chapter deals with the first two of these questions, and Chapter 18 deals with some of the remaining questions. Much of the discussion here is based on a survey of four leading clinical journals (*New England Journal of Medicine, British Medical Journal, Journal of the American Medical Association*, and *Lancet*) using the PubMed database, 2000–2003 with the keywords "cohort study" (which identified 125 papers, including 27 nested case-control studies and 19 follow-up studies), "case-control study" (84 papers), and "cross-sectional study" (75 prevalence studies, 2 cross-over studies of acute effects on health, and 2 time-series studies).

Key to answering each of these questions is the concept of *incidence*; that is, the number of new occurrences of an outcome over a period of time (such as new cancers of the lung in a year). Essential concepts are:

1. The *cumulative incidence proportion* (or *risk*), defined as the number of events occurring in a specified time period divided by the number of persons at risk at the beginning of follow-up. For studies that are of short duration and those that have no appreciable losses to follow-up, the cumulative incidence proportion is a good estimator of incidence rates.

2. The *incidence rate* (the incidence per unit population, such as new lung cancers per year per 100,000 person-years). Unlike the cumulative incidence proportion, an incidence rate can reflect the changing number of persons at risk because it accounts explicitly for such events as loss to follow-up and mortality.

3. The *prevalence proportion* (the number of persons per unit population who have some condition at any given time, such as the number of asthmatics per 100,000 population on a given date).

4. The *incidence rate ratio*—the ratio of incidence rates for the same outcome in two different populations or at different times.

A wealth of approaches exist. For example, in chronic disease epidemiology, where health outcomes are usually defined in terms of binary, non-recurrent health states (e.g., death or incidence of cancer), rare outcomes would usually imply that a case-control study is needed, whereas rare exposures may call for a cohort design. In studies of acute effects, such as investigating triggers for myocardial infarction, time series analyses and case-crossover designs may be used. Cohort studies and case-control studies are often used to investigate etiology.

Two general lessons from this chapter are that 1) the investigator usually has a choice of methods to use in a given setting, but the methods are not in general equally appropriate for each circumstance; and 2) a good protocol is not enough—it must be followed, with any deviations recorded and examined for their possible effects on findings and interpretations.

ARE THE OBJECTIVES OF THE STUDY STATED PRECISELY AND CLEARLY?

The crafting of clear and cogent objectives is critically important, not only in designing and conducting studies, but also in allowing readers to determine whether the study design and methods answer the research question. In writing objectives, the study population, the exposures, and the outcome should all be stated clearly, explicitly, and in enough detail for the reader to understand what was intended. One popular approach is the "PICO" model (Population, Intervention [including exposures to agents], Comparison of interventions [including comparisons between exposure groups], and Outcome) (see http://www.uic.edu/depts/lib/lhsp/resources/pico.shtml[58]) (Table 1).

For example, one may want to know whether past use of oral contraceptives increases the risk of developing a myocardial infarction.[59] A clear research question could be framed as: "Among women 18–49 years old living in the Netherlands, is the incidence rate of myocardial infarctions related to past use of oral contraceptives." An essential aspect here is the need to "estimate," to compute a value for the parameter of interest (e.g., ratio of incidence rates) from a sample of subjects. As well, the issue of stating that exposures will be evaluated in the past, though not described perfectly here, implies a historical focus for gathering information and suggests the need for specific types of instruments that can be used to collect accurate information about past exposures. Questions

---

TABLE 1. P.I.C.O. Model for Clinical and Epidemiological Questions.*

Patient, Population, or Problem	How would I describe a group of patients similar to mine?
Intervention, Prognostic Factor, or Exposure	Which main intervention, prognostic factor, or exposure am I considering?
Comparison or Intervention (if appropriate)	What is the main alternative to compare with the intervention?
Outcome you would like to measure or achieve	What can I hope to accomplish, measure, improve, or affect?
What type of question are you asking?	Diagnosis, Etiology, Therapy, Prognosis, Prevention, Harm
Type of study you want to find	What would be the best study design / methodology?

Template for P.I.C.O. Questions

In people with _____

Does (intervention, characteristic, exposure)_____

In comparison to (another intervention, characteristic, no treatment, exposure) _____

Affect (outcomes) _____

---

*Adapted from http://www.uic.edu/depts/lib/lhsp/resources/pico.shtml[58]

that the investigator could pose to members of the study population to meet this objective include: "Have you ever taken birth control pills?"; "If yes, did you take birth control pills for at least 12 consecutive months?"; "How old were you when you took birth control pills? [list all dates]" Estimates of risk are subject to various kinds of uncertainties, such as sampling variability (commonly expressed as confidence intervals), and selection, confounding, and misclassification biases (see below). The art and science of epidemiology focus largely on understanding and controlling such uncertainties.

The eventual selection of a research design will depend on many factors, including the prevalence and incidence of the health condition, costs, availability of subjects, feasibility of assessing exposure information, and issues related to sample size and statistical power. The PICO framework gives researchers and readers a basis for thinking critically about these matters.

Table 2 illustrates the objectives and principal findings of selected papers from the search of the literature described above. The studies are classified under five headings: cohort studies; case-control studies; time-series, case-crossover, other

Table 2. Design, Objectives, and Principal Findings of Selected Observational Studies in the Literature.*

Design and Objectives	Principal Findings
1. Cohort studies	
"To assess possible associations between smoking and [mortality from] dementia in the British doctors prospective cohort study"[119]	No strong association
"To examine simultaneous effects of [exposure to ambient] ozone and PM2.5 at levels below EPA standards on daily respiratory symptoms and rescue medication use among children with asthma"[120]	"Asthmatic children using maintenance medication are particularly vulnerable to ozone . . . at levels below EPA standards"
"To assess the associations between birth weight and gestational age and risk of type 1 diabetes" [in a birth cohort][121]	". . . weak but significant association between birth weight and increased risk of type I diabetes . . ."
"To evaluate [in a population-based cohort] the incidence of chronic renal failure, risk factors for it, and the associated hazard of death in recipients of non-renal transplants"[122]	"The occurrence of renal failure [in this population] is associated with" a four-fold increased risk of death
"[Among children born to parents with type 1 diabetes mellitus], to determine whether breastfeeding duration, food supplementation, or age at introduction of gluten-containing foods influences the risk of developing islet autoantibodies"[123]	"Ensuring compliance to infant feeding guidelines is a possible way to reduce the risk of development of type 1 autoantibodies"
"[To determine] the relation between the dose of inhaled glucocorticoids and the rate of bone loss in premenopausal women with asthma"[124]	"Inhaled glucocorticoids lead to a dose-related loss of bone at the hip"
2. Case-control studies	
To determine whether use of oral contraceptives is associated with subsequent increased incidence rates of myocardial infarction among women 18–49 years old living in the Netherlands[59]	"The risk of myocardial infarction was increased among women who used second-generation oral contraceptives"
To identify risk factors for the incidence of common acute lymphoblastic leukemia in childhood[125]	Folate supplementation in pregnancy appears to reduce the risk of common acute lymphoblastic leukemia in childhood
"To determine whether crosswalk markings at urban intersections influence the risk of injury to older pedestrians"[126]	"Crosswalk markings appear [to be] associated with increased risk of motor vehicle collision to older pedestrians at sites where no signal or stop sign is present"
To determine whether a polymorphism in a genotype for ATP-binding cassette sub-family B is associated with resistance to multi-antiepileptic drugs[127]	"These pharmacogenomic results identify a genetic factor associated with resistance to antiepileptic drugs"

To determine whether duration and patterns of use of combined estrogen and progestin hormone replacement therapy are associated with postmenopausal invasive breast cancer[228]	Combined estrogen and progestin hormone replacement therapy is associated with increased risk of breast cancer
"To assess the quality of care given to elderly people. . . ."[129]	"The quality of medical care that elderly patients receive in one UK city . . . is inadequate"

3. Time series, case-crossover, other self-controlled designs

Time series:

"To determine the impact of introducing prescription drug cost-sharing on use of essential and less essential drugs among elderly persons"[23]	". . . increased cost-sharing for prescription drugs . . . was followed by reductions in essential drugs and a higher rate of serious adverse events and Emergency Department visits . . ."

Case-crossover:

To determine the risk of sudden cardiac death associated with vigorous exertion 30 minutes before the attack[130]	". . . habitual exercise diminishes the risk of sudden death during vigorous exertion"
". . . to assess whether vaccinations increase the risk of relapse in multiple sclerosis"[131]	"Vaccination does not appear to increase short-term risk of relapse . . ."

4. Longitudinal studies with outcomes measured more than once

"To determine whether the priority given to [Scottish] patients referred for cardiac surgery [and on National Health Service waiting lists] is associated with socioeconomic status"[132]	"Socioeconomically deprived patients . . . [have] to wait longer for surgery because of being given lower priority"
"To examine the combined effect of social class and weight at birth on cognitive trajectories during school age. . . ."[133]	"The postnatal environment has an overwhelming influence on cognitive function . . . but these strong effects do not explain the weaker but independent association with birth weight"

5. Natural experiments (deliberate but uncontrolled experiments)

To determine the effect of air pollution controls on particulate air pollution and death rates[134]	"The net benefit of the reduced death rate was greater than predicted from results of previous time-series studies"
"To determine whether the more intensive screening and treatment for prostate cancer in the Seattle-Puget Sound area . . . led to lower mortality . . . than in Connecticut"[135]	There was no association between intensive screening and mortality

* From a search of the bibliographic PubMed database, 2000–2003, in *British Medical Journal, Journal of the American Medical Association, New England Journal of Medicine,* and *The Lancet.*

[. . .] indicates text added by the author to clarify the context.

self-controlled designs; longitudinal studies with outcomes measured more than once; and natural experiments. (This classification builds on a taxonomy developed for biomedical research reports.[60]) Not all examples contained in the table were precisely described, and often the study population and its characteristics (e.g., age or racial distribution) were not specified.

IS THE STUDY DESIGN APPROPRIATE
FOR THE PURPOSE?

With objectives clearly described, often in terms of PICO, the stage is set to ask questions about the study design, including the methods of identifying and recruiting subjects, specifying the principal exposures and outcomes, delineating potential confounding variables, estimating sample size, and other components of design and fieldwork.

Figure 1 is a schematic of the populations involved in most epidemiological studies. An essential element is the target population, from which a specific source population is established (sampling frame), and from which potential participants are selected (study population). Inferences from the study population are made to the target population (internal validity), and the results may be generalized to some "overarching population" or "universe" (external validity).

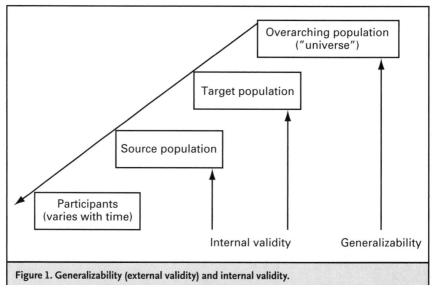

Figure 1. Generalizability (external validity) and internal validity.

A study would be valid internally if subjects are selected from the target population without bias (no selection bias) and if there are no biases inherent in the study population (no confounding, no serious information bias, reasonable specification of the statistical model to summarize the data).

For example, the universe might be all persons in some city who have asthma, the target population might be those who have been treated in any hospital in the city, the source population may comprise those who can be identified and found from records in the hospitals, and the participants are the subset who are invited and eventually participate in the study.

Internal validity refers to whether the conclusions of the study would be similar to those that would have been obtained had the entire target population been investigated. It is enhanced by such features as unbiased selection of subjects into the study, few losses to follow-up, accuracy of the measurement processes used to define the outcomes, exposures, and other variables, and absence of bias from confounding. The population to which we would like to make inferences is often different and much larger than the target population of the study, and the validity of such inferences to the larger population is usually referred to as generalizability or "external validity."

Bias is generally the biggest threat to drawing sound conclusions from an epidemiologic study. Biased selection of subjects into a study generally arises from two sources: 1) the selection of a study population that is not representative of the target population, or 2) the subjects who actually participate do not fairly represent the target population even though the process of selection was unbiased. Bias is present when the study population's distributions of exposure and health outcomes are such that the estimated parameter comparing the populations (e.g., odds ratio, incidence rate ratio) differs from the value that would be obtained from the entire target population.

Study design and appropriate fieldwork methods are critical to internal validity, which requires that "the index and comparison groups are selected in such a manner that the observed differences between them on the dependent variables under study (i.e., the health outcome variables) may, apart from sampling variation, be attributed only to the hypothesized effect under investigation."[1] Four important types of bias must be considered (e.g.,[1, 61, 62]):

1. Selection bias: The constitution of the study population leads to incorrect estimates of effect because of systematic differences in characteristics between those who take part in the study and the larger population ("target") for which inferences are to be drawn. Losses to follow-up may also lead to bias.

2. Confounding bias: A variable that is associated with both the health outcome and the exposure (very broadly defined) is not considered adequately in the design stage (e.g., matching), the analysis stage (e.g., regression analysis), or both.

3. Information bias: Errors in the measurement of outcomes, exposures, and confounding variables affect findings and conclusions.

4. Model mis-specification bias: Incorrect analytic methods are used, or the models do not account adequately for any relevant differences between the index and comparison groups (related to confounding or to the relation of response to the exposures).

The example above of a study of myocardial infarction and past use of oral contraceptives was designed and conducted as a population-based case-control study.[59] The target population from which study subjects were drawn and for which inferences were made included all women 18–49 years old living in the Netherlands, 1990–1995, who were at risk of developing a first myocardial infarction. Although rates of myocardial infarction are low in this age range, the prevalence of concurrent exposure should have been maximized. The source population consisted of case subjects identified from 16 medical centers and control subjects drawn randomly from the general population through random-digit (telephone) dialing.

"Random" means that the method of selection gave every subject the same, statistically independent probability of being selected. Tossing a fair coin means that the probability of selection is $\frac{1}{2}$. Computer programs that have a random number generator can also be used. In the case of simple random-digit dialing, for example, a computer program could select a predetermined number of telephone numbers, such that each telephone number has exactly the same probability of selection. (Techniques exist to handle non-independent samples [e.g., members of the same family] and to handle unequal probabilities of selection; use of these techniques generally requires special expertise in sampling methods.)

Considering the study of oral contraceptive pills, one overarching population to which one would like to make inferences is all women of reproductive age living anywhere in the world. The generalization to all age groups will depend on whether the effects, if any, would occur before the age of 18 years. The generalization to all women in the world (or, perhaps, of European descent) will rest on whether the sample from the Netherlands is representative for the purpose, and the validity of the latter generalization may depend on many factors, such as relationships with socio-demographic and genetic characteristics.

More crucial than generalizability, however, is that the results should be valid internally (i.e., no substantial biases from measurement error, confounding, and selection of subjects who represent the exposure experience of the target population). *Confounding* of the association between exposure and outcome is the distortion of the apparent effect of an exposure on an outcome that arises from the association of both exposure and outcome with other factors that can influence risk ("risk factors"). These factors need to be causal or represent a process that causes such a distortion. Thus, a confounding factor is a variable that is associated with both exposure and a risk factor for the health outcome and, if not accounted for adequately, may distort (or confound) the true association (Figure 2). An example is the comparison of cancer mortality rates in two countries with different age structures. Age differs between the countries, and age affects cancer rates, so that even if rates in the two countries are identical for each age group, the overall rate in the country with the older age distribution will be higher than in the comparison country. That is, age would "confound" a direct comparison. The extent of confounding bias depends on the strength of associations among any confounding variables, the health outcome, and the exposure (Figure 2). The direction of bias can be either away from or toward the null value, depending on the specific distributions. Later, the chapter discusses ways to reduce or eliminate confounding by statistical methods (adjustment, modeling, matching, stratification).

Information bias refers to flaws in measuring exposure or health outcomes that result in inaccurate information. Almost all measures are inaccurate to some degree. The extent of the bias depends on the degree of misclassification and on whether the variable being misclassified is the health outcome, the exposure, or the confounding variable. In general, if the errors in measurement do not depend on the health outcome (cohort studies) or exposure status (case-control studies), the direction of the bias will be toward the null value (referred to as non-differential misclassification).

Types of Study Designs

The manner in which subjects are selected ("sampled") from a target population is an essential element for distinguishing and classifying epidemiologic studies. The fundamental design is the *cohort study*, in which groups of individuals having some element in common are sampled and followed through time to identify occurrences of health events or to measure states of health. The two

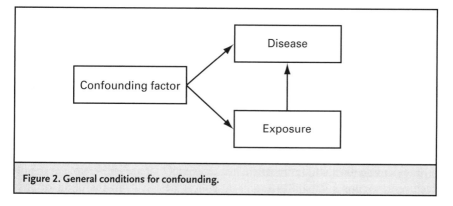

Figure 2. General conditions for confounding.

other principal designs used commonly in analytical epidemiology are the case-control study and the cross-sectional study. These designs are based on the cohort study, either implicitly or explicitly,[61–64] and they differ from it in the procedures used to sample subjects from the target population.

Case-control studies sample subjects according to health status, usually over a short period of time in well-defined geographic regions (e.g., the general population of one or more metropolitan areas); the target population is defined by a cohort that represents the general population but whose members are not enumerated explicitly. *Cross-sectional studies* (a synonym for surveys) sample from a cohort at one point in time, independent of exposure status and independent of disease status. These studies can also be nested within a well-defined cohort or can be a sample from a more general population.

A second axis for classifying epidemiological studies is the way in which health states are defined and determined, and their use will distinguish between the types of statistical procedures that should be used:

- A health state that is irreversible and non-recurrent (also referred to as an "absorbing health state" or "failure"). This is represented by a binary outcome variable (e.g., incidence of histologically confirmed lung cancer) whose time of diagnosis is recorded and, thus, incidence is measured. Examples are death from cancer and first myocardial infarct (because one cannot have the first event a second time).

- Health states that are defined on interval, nominal, or ordinal scales that may recur and may be reversible. Clear operational definitions are required. Depending on the design, these health states may be measured more than once during the follow-up period. Examples include hypertension, degree of back pain, and exacerbations of asthma. These types of outcomes may be used in cohort, longitudinal, or cross-sectional studies but would need to be modified for case-control studies so as to fit into the failure-type framework.

Cohort Studies

Incidence Cohort Studies
All cohort studies (incidence, longitudinal) require follow-up of individuals through time to determine each health outcome of interest and the time when it occurs, identify censored subjects (that is, those who have been lost to follow-up before the study ends), and assess confounding variables (which may change during follow-up).

Incidence cohort studies measure health events that are irreversible and non-recurrent. Figure 3 illustrates the basic cohort design from the point of view

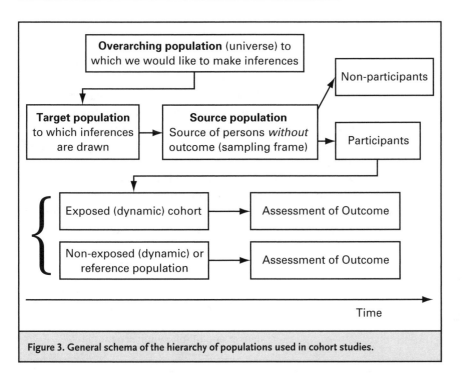

Figure 3. General schema of the hierarchy of populations used in cohort studies.

of the populations involved. Once the objectives of the study have been established, and the cohort study has been chosen as the optimal design, the populations from which the sample is to be drawn must be identified. The target population, or primary study base, is the population from which subjects are to be selected, either randomly or systematically. The source population represents the sub-population that is drawn from the target; the study population, which is shown simply as two groups of exposed and unexposed subjects, comprises individuals who participate. Exposure can change with time (dynamic), and subjects can therefore move between exposure groups during the follow-up period. Some subjects may be censored during the follow-up period (i.e., from death, loss to follow-up, or withdrawal at the end of the study), but they are not shown here.

Incidence cohort studies compare incidence rates in the study group, either with an external reference population (e.g., rates from the general population) or between sub-cohorts (e.g., defined by differing levels of exposure). These sub-cohorts are often defined by their status at the beginning of follow-up, in which case it is assumed that early exposure is what matters or that exposure is constant throughout the follow-up; special analysis is needed to account for changes in exposure status through the follow-up. The specification of the appropriate reference population in the objectives is crucial to the analysis and interpretation of the study. For example, if the cohort is exposed uniformly, or the measurements cannot distinguish among cohort members with different levels of exposure, then a reference population external to the cohort must be used. Sometimes a critical health issue cannot be investigated with internal controls. A typical external population is the general population from which the study population is a subset, but the analysis should deal with any relevant differences in age, sex, racial, or other characteristics of the study group and the reference population.

Figure 4 shows the general layout of an incidence cohort study. The risk period for the entire study is the period of time from start to end of follow-up. The actual risk period for a particular subject is defined as the period of time between entering and leaving the cohort. The exposure period can start during

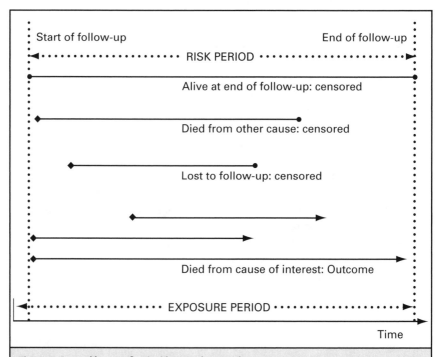

Figure 4. General layout of an incidence cohort study.

A line ending in an arrow represents a subject who had an event, and a line ending in a small circle represents a subject who was censored. The risk period for the entire study is defined as the period of time from start to end of follow-up. The actual risk period for a particular subject is defined as the period of time between entering and leaving the cohort. The exposure period can occur during the risk period and may end before the last date of follow-up, but it can also be defined as occurring before entry into the cohort.

the risk period and may end before the last date of follow-up, but it can also be defined as starting before entry into the cohort. For example, in the Harvard Nurses' Health Study,[65] one could have inquired about age at menarche (a risk factor for breast cancer), which would occur well before becoming a nurse and entering the study. Subjects who are censored are still at risk until the time they are censored; thus, in counting incidence time, one must include the person-time experience of these subjects.

Subjects in cohort studies generally have one or more characteristics in common, such as being army conscripts,[66] women who attended family planning centers,[67] or sibs,[68] or having atrial fibrillation.[14] Alternatively, cohorts may represent samples from the general population, such as birth cohorts,[69] or from participants in a cohort from the general population, such as the Honolulu Heart Program[70] or the American Cancer Society Cancer Prevention Study-II (ACS CPS-II).[71] The period of follow-up can be short or long, and the data collection may use either a prospective or a retrospective method, depending on whether subjects are followed from the present time forward, or records are used to determine what has happened in the past.

Incidence rates of one or more health outcomes will be estimated, and these will be compared between subgroups defining different levels of exposure, most often as an incidence rate ratio. When the health outcome is reversible and may recur during the follow-up period, the comparison of health outcomes between subjects on levels of exposure becomes more complicated, and special methods are required (see longitudinal studies below).

Cohort studies can be quite complex, and the reader may sometimes find that it is useful to draw a timeline of the essential features. For example, Figure 5 shows a timeline of the Western Electric cohort study[72] that was used to determine whether cancer mortality is associated with dietary vitamin C or beta-carotene. Because mortality is being considered, the study is regarded as an incidence (i.e., the incidence of death) study. A random sample of 3102 workers (from 5397 employed at a plant in Chicago, Illinois between 1957 and 1958) defined the cohort. Examinations and questionnaires were administered at baseline, followed by periodic medical examinations until 1969. Mortality was assessed between 1957 and 1982 in relation to levels of beta-carotene and vitamin C at baseline. Mortality from all causes of death, from cancer, and from cardiovascular disease was found to decrease with increasing levels of consumption of these vitamins.

The Bronx Aging Study followed 488 individuals, ages 75–85 years, over a 21-year period to estimate the incidence of dementia, which was assessed every 12–18 months using neuropathological tests.[12] The incidence of dementia was then related to leisure activities measured at the time of enrollment, and it was found that increased levels of leisure activities were correlated with a reduced

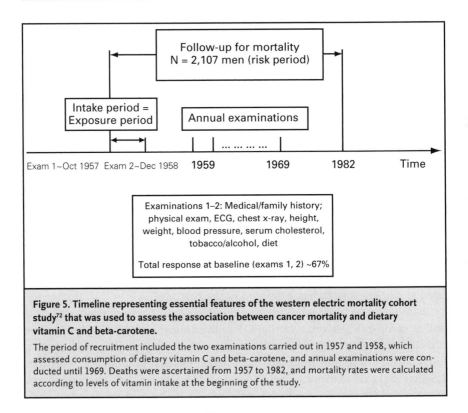

Figure 5. Timeline representing essential features of the western electric mortality cohort study[72] that was used to assess the association between cancer mortality and dietary vitamin C and beta-carotene.

The period of recruitment included the two examinations carried out in 1957 and 1958, which assessed consumption of dietary vitamin C and beta-carotene, and annual examinations were conducted until 1969. Deaths were ascertained from 1957 to 1982, and mortality rates were calculated according to levels of vitamin intake at the beginning of the study.

risk of developing dementia. It is likely that the pitfall of reverse causality was eliminated or reduced: if dementia leads to decreased activity, then the simultaneous measurement of both exposure and dementia would be difficult to interpret, whereas in this study the authors were careful to measure activity at baseline and then assess dementia.

The cohort must consist of only incident cases (i.e., new cases), because persons with prevalent disease cannot develop a new instance of the disease. What is considered prevalent must be defined by the investigator; for example, some researchers might exclude all patients with a history of any cancer, whereas others would exclude only those with cancer at the site of interest. This exclusion can be either at the time subjects enter the study or at the time of analysis. For example, subjects in the Framingham study[73] were examined at baseline, and those who already had coronary heart disease were excluded from the cohort. In the ACS CPS-II mortality study,[71] subjects who said that they had a diagnosis of any type of cancer before entering the study were excluded at the time of analyses. Subjects were also excluded if they had recently lost 2.5 kg or more, because such weight loss may have indicated undiagnosed cancer. Another study used computerized hospital discharge records to exclude patients known to have had a myocardial infarction during the eight years before the study started.[74]

The Framingham and the ACS CPS-II studies excluded subjects with existing cardiovascular disease and cancer, respectively, because the main objectives were to identify risk factors for developing new cases of these diseases. However, secondary analyses of other outcomes are conducted frequently, and subjects having these diseases are likely to be included at baseline. If existing disease cannot always be identified at the time of entry, one strategy is to assume that the condition, if present, will become overt during some specified interval after start-up, such as within the first three years. That part of the follow-up would be set aside, and only after that time would subjects become at-risk for incidence, and the critical follow-up interval for estimating incidence would begin. (Thus, all events and person-time in the exclusion interval would be discarded.) For example, in a cohort study to determine whether appendectomy reduced the risk of ulcerative colitis, subjects diagnosed with ulcerative colitis during the year after the appendectomy were excluded.[75]

Cohort studies also use other types of sub-designs. Nested case-control (and case-cohort) studies select sub-samples of subjects from an explicitly defined cohort. (Chapter 18 discusses nested case-control studies in more detail.) The statistical power (i.e., the probability of detecting an excess risk, should it exist) in cohort analyses derives mostly from the number of subjects who develop the outcome of interest. Thus, if one requires additional information that is not readily available for all members of the cohort, it wastes resources to obtain this information for each control subject. Usually, all cases are included in these studies, but only a random subset of the identified control group is studied.

An example is a case-control study of multiple sclerosis nested within the Nurses' Health Study.[65] Instead of collecting detailed information for every potential control subject, a subset of the at-risk population was defined by selecting nurses who did not have a diagnosis of multiple sclerosis at the time the case was diagnosed. Thus, controls were matched to each case by date of diagnosis. An important feature of this design is that controls could develop the disease after this date, and this is consistent with the underlying statistical theory. Auxiliary information about hepatitis B vaccination was obtained by means of a postal questionnaire, but only from the selected controls.

An example of a nested case-cohort study is a Dutch dietary study that assessed the effects of ambient air pollution on cause-specific mortality: The analysis consisted of a sub-cohort that included all deaths in the risk period (the "case" component) and a randomly selected sub-cohort.[76] Both sub-cohorts are selected independent of exposure, and the "control" sub-cohort can actually contain cases.

It is unusual to ignore censoring in long-term studies because it can be important, and accurate calculation of incidence rates requires that the denominators account for subjects lost to follow-up. Time was ignored, for example, in a study of cannabis use and subsequent development of schizophrenia among men who were conscripted into the Swedish army between the ages of 18 and 20 years.[66] Cannabis use was assessed by questionnaire at time of conscription, and this large cohort was followed for psychiatric admissions from 1969–1970 until 1996 using record linkage to the Swedish hospital discharge registry. Logistic regression, a regression method for binary outcomes (see Chapter 12), was used to estimate odds ratios (which approximate risk ratios when the disease is rare). This is an unusual approach for a long-term study because censoring was ignored, and person-time was not calculated. If death rates and losses to follow-up were low, and if the entire cohort was covered by the hospital registry, then the results would be similar to a proper full-cohort analysis, as the authors indicated. On the other hand, if deaths are not fully identified from a vital statistics or hospital registry, or if there was "substantial" loss to follow-up, then these analyses would be biased, so that the finding of twice the risk of being admitted for a psychiatric diagnosis among users of cannabis (odds ratio = 2.1, 95% confidence interval [CI]: 1.2–3.7) may not have been valid.

Cumulative Incidence Studies

Cumulative incidence sampling, in which the time of the event during the course of the study is ignored and the comparison population comprises subjects without the outcome, is illustrated in a study of uterine ruptures during labor among women who had a previous cesarean delivery.[77] The cohort comprised primiparous women who gave birth to their first baby by cesarean section and were followed through a database (Washington State Birth Events Record Database) to identify a second delivery. The outcome was defined as having a uterine rupture during their second delivery, classified by whether the second delivery was a cesarean section without labor, spontaneous onset of labor, or induction of labor with or without prostaglandins. The calculation of rates depended on women who were actually at risk of having a uterine rupture, which can happen only when they are pregnant and deliver. Thus, counting person-time at risk from time of entry does not apply. However, risks can be calculated as the number of events occurring during delivery divided by the number of women delivering during the study period. If conditions change during the study period, event rates can be calculated for separate periods.

In cohort studies for which the follow-up is short, time will have little effect on the rates, so person-time need not be calculated and, thus, risk will approximate the incidence rate. However, differences in covariates at baseline (e.g., age structure) would need to be assessed using either the stratified methods described below (replacing person-time by number of persons at risk) or by logistic regression. An example is a one-year study of deaths of children living in North Carolina after a traumatic brain injury.[78] Cohorts of children with injuries inflicted by others (usually from child abuse; referred to as the "inflicted cohort") and with non-inflicted injuries (mostly accidents) were established, and mortality rates in the inflicted cohort were compared to the non-inflicted cohort, the general population (from general statistics), and a random sample of 300 births. The latter comparison group was needed to identify factors not available from the aggregated data, and multivariable logistic regression was used to adjust for potential confounding.

Longitudinal Studies

Longitudinal studies are cohort studies but distinguished from incidence studies because outcomes are reversible or can recur, and each subject may experience an outcome more than once during the follow-up period. As with incidence cohort studies, exposures and confounding variables can also be assessed periodically. Incidence can be assessed in longitudinal studies if an outcome is considered a failure.

The health states can be defined on categorical (nominal, ordinal) or on interval scales. An example of a binary, recurrent outcome is relapse of moderate symptoms of multiple sclerosis, and an example of an interval scale is blood pressure. Incidence (and prevalence) rates are not defined for outcomes measured on interval scales. Incidence can, however, be estimated by transforming the outcome to a binary scale and by including the dimension of time (e.g., first time that lung function was less than 80% of predicted). Such transformations, however, may entail serious losses of information.

Some recurrent events can be converted to binary scales. For example, asthma attacks (e.g., wheezing lasting two or more days) are not failure-type events because exacerbations are transient and recurring (a clear definition of an asthma attack is required). If the time of the first occurrence can be measured accurately, then incidence rates for the first attack of asthma can be estimated. As another example, second falls in an elderly population can be considered as incidence, but only persons who have fallen once before are at risk of falling again.[79]

In the British Doctors Study, assessments of cigarette smoking were made throughout the study period, but this is not considered a longitudinal study because the outcome was defined exclusively as a failure (namely, cause-specific mortality). In the Framingham study, examinations and questionnaires were administered periodically through the follow-up period, so it can be considered a failure-time study for outcomes that do not recur (e.g., breast cancer),[80] but longitudinal for outcomes that are measured continuously (e.g., changes in lung function).[81]

Statistical methods become more complicated when outcomes are measured repeatedly. Measurements of outcomes through time can provide a great deal of information on health and how it changes with time, as well as how exposures affect changes in health. However, the use of repeated measurements presents challenges to the statistical analysis because the assumption of independence of the observations is not satisfied. One consequence is that the effective sample size will generally be greater than if each subject contributed a single observation, but less than the total number of observations, because correlated observations do not bring as much new information as independent ones. Thus, estimates of variances are greater than if the observations came from different subjects. Lack of independence can be handled effectively using random-effects regression methods. Another important issue is that some measures may not show a great deal of intra-subject variability, which means that one event in a subject will predict future ones (i.e., autocorrelation is large). For example, in a daily diary study of congestive heart failure that the author conducted[82] over a two-month period in 31 subjects, individual values of oxygen saturation (measured using a pulse oximeter) were correlated within themselves to about 8%, but consecutive values of pulse rate had a correlation of about 17%. This occurred because past health status reflected current health status. The additional serial correlation in pulse rate clouded the interpretation of the analysis by increasing estimated variances.

Assessment of Exposure and Outcomes

Validated and reliable methods must be used to assess outcomes. Despite any differences in method of analysis, outcomes must be determined with the same accuracy and completeness in both the study and comparison groups. This requires that appropriate criteria be established and used in the same way in the two groups, both to identify the study groups for possible instances of the end-point of interest and to confirm the diagnosis where it is suspected. For example, there can be substantial misclassification of causes of death, particularly for cardio-respiratory illnesses. If misclassification of outcome is independent of exposure (non-differential misclassification), the direction of the association between exposure and outcome will probably be preserved, but rate ratios will be underestimated. Problems are increased if the likelihood of misclassification is not constant. For example, cancer studies often require histological confirmation of tumors at specific anatomical sites. Non-uniform use of technologies that detect very small or early lesions may introduce a bias because the investigator is studying, in part, who has a certain result on a test rather than who actually has the disease. Examples include mammography for breast cancer and PSA testing in prostate cancer, each of which identifies a state that may be an early indicator of a serious problem, though some lesions may resolve or not progress to invasive cancer if just left to themselves. Such biases may be reduced by defining outcome in ways that exclude some cases (e.g., by size or other characteristics). This strategy reduces sample sizes, but may pay dividends in increased statistical power and reduced bias from misclassification.

Calculation of Incidence Rates

A long follow-up period may result in important losses of subjects from the cohort as well as gains as new subjects are enrolled. These changes in the structure of the cohort are accounted for in the calculation of incidence rates by accumulating person-time at risk for each subject, which is the time that a subject is under study and at risk of the outcome studied, and summing over all subjects. Health events are then tallied and are allocated to levels of variables (referred to as strata) that are accepted or suspected risk factors. Thus, the investigator needs precise criteria to determine the dates of critical events—when subjects entered observation for the study, had the health event of interest, were lost to follow-up because of migration, died of other causes, or were still alive at the end of the study.

Person-time is easy to calculate when potentially confounding variables are independent of time (e.g., gender);[83] in each separate stratum, incidence rates are calculated by dividing the number of events by the accumulated person-time. However, the calculation of person-time is more complex when rates vary

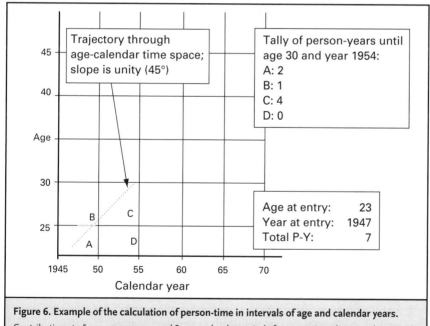

Figure 6. Example of the calculation of person-time in intervals of age and calendar years.

Contributions to 5-year age groups and 5-year calendar periods from a patient diagnosed at age 23 in 1947 and followed until age 30 in 1954: 2 person-years to age 20–25, 5 P-Y to age 25–30, 3 P-Y to 1945–50, and 4 P-Y to 1950–55.

by calendar year as well as age, or by other temporal factors that differ among subjects (see the diagram in Figure 6). Person-time is usually partitioned so that the experience of each subject through time is allocated according to age and calendar year strata, and these are then summed to form the denominators of stratum-specific incidence rates. Standard methods for calculating person-time have been developed,[83, 84] and computer programs can be used for this purpose (e.g., an elegant SAS program developed by Pearce and Checkoway,[84] the NIOSH LTAS system (http://www.cdc.gov/niosh/LTAS/), OCMAP (http://ocmap.biostat.pitt.edu), or EPICURE (http://www.hirosoft.com/).

Stratified Methods for Adjusting for Confounding
As defined previously, a confounding factor is a variable that is both associated with exposure and a risk factor for the disease. Both of these conditions must be present for a variable to distort (or confound) the true association (Figure 2). Other situations in which a variable is within a causal pathway (Figure 7a) or is a correlate of exposure (Figure 7b,c) (referred to as overmatching) are not confounding, and adjusting for such a variable, either in the design stage through matching or in the analysis stage, can remove part or all of the effect.

The primary tool to account for confounding in the design stage is matching, whereby at the time of enrollment subjects are made equivalent on certain strong potential confounding factors. In cohort studies, matching is inefficient,

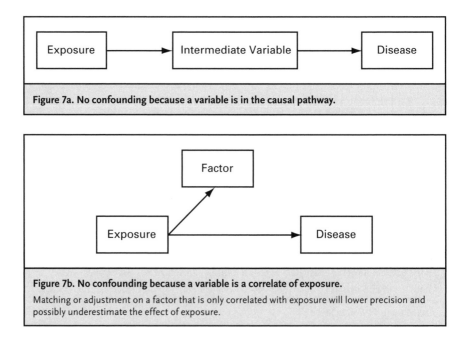

Figure 7a. No confounding because a variable is in the causal pathway.

Figure 7b. No confounding because a variable is a correlate of exposure.
Matching or adjustment on a factor that is only correlated with exposure will lower precision and possibly underestimate the effect of exposure.

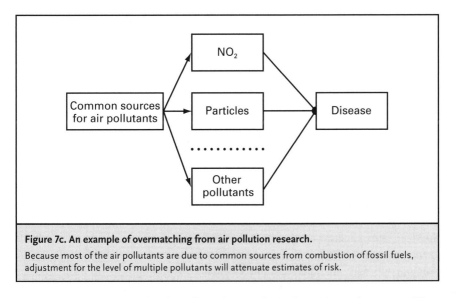

Figure 7c. An example of overmatching from air pollution research.
Because most of the air pollutants are due to common sources from combustion of fossil fuels, adjustment for the level of multiple pollutants will attenuate estimates of risk.

although it does not lead to bias.[85] During analysis the main tools are stratification techniques and regression modeling. Stratification refers to the division of the study and control groups into categories defined by the potential confounding variable. (Chapter 18 discusses regression modeling.) For example, the confounding effect of age in comparisons of cancer mortality rates may be nearly eliminated by studying rates within narrow age ranges, such as 0–10 years, 11–20, etc. Rates are then estimated and compared within strata (e.g., by taking ratios), and a weighted average ratio is computed across the strata.

One important consideration in the use of stratification techniques for variables that are measured on interval scales is the concern that additional errors can be introduced if the rate ratios, for example, are not homogeneous within strata. For example, in analysis of cancer rates in adults, the stratification of age into five-year rather than one-year intervals is unlikely to lead to appreciable bias, but in a study of childhood leukemia five-year intervals may be too long because rates change rapidly during the first five years of life.

Empirically, confounding is apparent when stratum-specific rate ratios vary appreciably from the crude ratio obtained by ignoring the strata. The partitioning of person-time and the assignment of events to the appropriate strata mean that incidence rates are estimated within each stratum.[83] This stratification produces many more rates than a crude analysis, with the result that they may be confusing and will each have larger standard errors than the crude rate. Adjustment refers to a set of techniques that summarize the stratum-specific rates into a summary estimate. A key assumption in adjustment is that the rate ratios do not vary substantially among the strata (homogeneity); otherwise the average may be difficult to interpret or may obscure important trends. (Departures from homogeneity produce heterogeneity, often in the form of statistical interaction: the effect of the exposure on the outcome varies among levels of a covariate.) Specific statistical tests are available to test for interactions, and they should be conducted routinely. As with all statistical tests, small sample sizes may imply that there is insufficient power to detect an interaction; if the sample sizes are very large, then non-meaningful interactions may be detected.

Direct adjustment produces a weighted average of the stratum-specific rates, with weights derived from some suitable population. This may be a national population, the total of subjects in the study itself, or something else. When comparing two or more cohorts, the ratio of directly standardized rates represents a weighted average of the rate ratio (referred to as the *cumulative mortality figure*, CMF). (The weighted average will lie within the range of the stratum-specific rates.) *Indirect adjustment* "reverses" the process used in direct adjustment; it compares the overall (not stratified) observed number of events in the study group with an expected value calculated by multiplying, in each separate stratum, the rates in the standard population by the number of person-years accumulated. The expected number of events is based on the null hypothesis that the stratum-specific rates in the standard population should apply in the cohort. The *standardized mortality ratio* (SMR) is such an estimator. Like the CMF, it represents a weighted average of stratum-specific rate ratios. Another weighted average, a stratification method, is the *Mantel-Haenszel estimator*, whose weights are the inverse of the variances in each stratum.

Basically, these three estimators differ only according to what weights are used. SMRs generally have lower variances than CMFs, and it is for this reason, especially when dealing with rare outcomes, that the SMR has often been preferred over the CMF. However, the SMR can, in some instances, give biased estimates of effect. The Mantel-Haenszel estimator is unbiased, has the smallest variance of all three stratified estimators, and is thus the one preferred today.

Examples of Cohort Studies That Illustrate Stratified Methods of Comparison and Adjustment for Confounding

As an illustration of stratified analysis to adjust for confounding, Table 3 shows the data from a retrospective cohort study of mortality among young persons in Australia[86] who had been convicted of legal offenses. This study was motivated by the need to appreciate whether socially disadvantaged youth, who generally have many more health problems than expected, are also at higher risk of early death. Consider first the comparison of rates in the full population between women and men, where mortality rates among women were much lower than among men (crude rate ratio = 0.43). The stratum-specific rate ratios varied from 0.33 to 0.85, and the age-adjusted Mantel-Haenszel estimate of the rate

	Men			Women			Age-specific mortality rate ratio (B ÷ A)
Age	Person-Years	No. of Deaths	Mortality Rate (A)	Person-years	No. of Deaths	Mortality Rate (B)	
Young offender cohort							
≤14	71.7	1	0.013947	7.0	0	0	0
15–19	4840.7	33	0.006817	311.7	7	0.022457	3.29
20–24	5282.5	52	0.009844	275.5	1	0.003630	0.37
≥25	518.8	2	0.003855	25.0	0	0	0
Total	10713.7	88	0.008214	619.2	8	0.012920	1.57
Population rates							
≤14	670,718	146	0.000218	274,589	51	0.000186	0.85
15–19	1,667,791	1080	0.000648	1,584,927	428	0.000270	0.42
20–24	873,365	878	0.001005	845,754	294	0.000348	0.35
≥25	109,413	131	0.001197	107,117	43	0.000401	0.34
Total	3,321,287	2235	0.000673	2,812,387	816	0.000290	0.43

Table 3. Mortality Rates in Victoria, Australia, and among Young Offenders.*

*Adapted from[86].

ratio was 0.40 (95% CI: 0.37–0.43), close to the crude rate ratio in the table. However, the stratum-specific rates differed significantly from each other (Mantel-Haenszel test of heterogeneity X^2 = 29.0, p = 0.000002). Thus, two summary estimates of the rate ratio were needed to describe in the general population the comparison of women to men: in children under the age of 14 years, the rate ratio was 0.85, whereas for the other age groups the rate ratio was about 0.40.

The person-years distribution in the young offender cohort implies many more young offenders among men than among women. Age by age, the risk of death was higher for male offenders than in the general population, and the same pattern holds for females except in the two age groups with the smallest numbers of person-years. Because of the small numbers of person-years, especially in women, rates in the cohort of young offenders were highly uncertain, with females having a higher rate than males in one age group (15–19 years) and lower rates in the other three age groups. The crude rate ratio comparing rates in women to those in men was 1.57, and the Mantel-Haenszel estimator was 1.58 (95% CI: 0.77–3.26), opposite to what was found in the general population, where men had higher rates. Although the stratum-specific rate ratios appeared to be variable, the test for heterogeneity was not significant (X^2 = 6.0, p = 0.11), suggesting that one summary estimate was sufficient to characterize the association. Another estimate of the rate ratio is obtained by calculating the ratio of SMRs between women and men using the rates in the total cohort as the reference population: SMR_{men} = 0.97 (95% CI:

0.78–1.19) and SMR_{women} = 1.53 (95% CI: 0.66–3.01), and the ratio of SMRs was RR = 1.58 (95% CI: 0.66–3.25), almost identical to the Mantel-Haenszel estimator but with a larger confidence interval.

As indicated above, rates in men and women in the cohort were much higher than in the general population: the SMR for women was 41.8 (95% CI: 18.03–82.36) and for men it was 9.69 (95% CI: 7.77–11.94). The ratio of these SMRs, which is another estimate of the internal rate ratio comparing the gender-based sub-cohorts, was 4.31 (95% CI: 1.81–8.88). Although these sex-specific SMRs are computationally correct, they are hard to interpret because the estimated rate ratios of the sex-specific age distributions within the cohort differed dramatically from those in the general population. Thus age is a potential confounder for these analyses. This well-known problem in comparing SMRs using an external population occurs only in such extreme examples; if the age distributions do not differ considerably, then the ratio will provide estimates similar to the internal analyses.

Sometimes stratification and adjustment fail to remove enough of the bias introduced by confounding variables. A study in Toronto, Ontario[30] compared age-specific mortality rates in a cohort of homeless men using shelters to rates in the general population, but the age groups were broad. The rate ratio for all-cause mortality among men at ages 18–24 years was 8.3 (95% CI 4.4–15.6), and among men age 45–64 years it was 2.3 (95% CI: 1.8–3.0). Although it appeared that homeless men, especially younger ones, are at much higher risk of death than the general population, residual confounding effects within each age category may have occurred, so that the reported risk ratio may not well represent the actual one. (This may have occurred if the distribution of cohort subjects within each age category was not similar to that of the general population.) For example, in the general population, mortality rates increase dramatically from age 45 to age 64, but it is not known whether or how much this trend holds in homeless men. A simple solution to this problem would have been to adjust for age within each category, as was done by Doll and collaborators in the British Doctors Study cohort.[87] Another component of this study compared the cohort of homeless men to cohorts in three U.S. cities. After adjusting for race, mortality rates in Toronto were lower than in these U.S. cities. The discussion of these calculations did not indicate whether adjustments by age were undertaken; presumably, the age distributions of the various cohorts were similar. If the Canadian and American cohorts differed in age structure, results may have been biased.

Comparison of Cohorts to Reference Populations
Separate exposure groups can be defined in studies that have variability in measured exposures within the cohort. In the simplest situation, exposure groups are defined at the beginning of follow-up and do not change through time.

Incidence rates can therefore be compared: 1) between each exposure group and the general population (external comparisons); 2) between each exposure group and the total cohort population; and 3) between exposure groups using one group as the reference.

For example, the Oxford Family Planning Association contraceptive study involved a cohort of 17,032 women who were 25–39 years of age during the years 1968–1974.[67] When women reached the age of 45 years, they were classified into groups of oral contraception users according to number of years of use. The analysis involved classifying women according to their cumulative exposure ("never used," "used for 48 months or less," "used for 49 to 96 months," "used for more than 96 months"). Only those who were never users or those who had more than eight years of non-contiguous use were then followed until mid-1994 (the authors argued that this would maximize the contrast between exposed and non-exposed). Subjects were also classified into one of four categories of average daily intensity of cigarette smoking as assessed at time of enrollment. The authors used indirect standardization: rates in the entire cohort served as the reference, and the rates in the various sub-cohorts were compared to those in the total cohort. This method of analysis has the advantage that adjustments can be made for all potential confounding factors measured in the cohort. Indirect standardization is preferred here because the standard errors are smaller than for direct standardization, especially important when the number of deaths is small,[83] but the Mantel-Haenszel technique will lead to unbiased estimates having minimum variances. (Regression methods, such as the Cox model, will yield similar answers and are able to account for continuously measured covariates without resorting to categorization, among other advantages.) In this study, incidence rates in the categories of oral contraceptive use and smoking were compared to rates in the unexposed cohorts, after

Table 4. Results for Breast Cancer from the Oxford Family Planning Association Mortality Study.[67]							
Duration of use of oral contraceptives[1]				Smoking status[2]			
Total duration of oral contraceptive use before age 45 years (months)	No. of deaths	Rate ratio	95% CI	Determined at time of recruitment	No. of deaths	Rate ratio	95% CI
Never used	83	1		Non-smoker	118	1	
<48	29	0.8	0.5–1.2	Ex-smoker	27	1.1	0.7–1.7
49–96	40	0.8	0.6–1.2	1–14 cigarettes/day	24	0.6	0.4–1.0
≥97	42	0.8	0.5–1.2	≥15 cigarettes/day	25	1.0	0.6–1.5

[1]Adjusted for age, parity, social class, and smoking.

[2]Adjusted for age, parity, and social class.

adjusting for age, parity, social class at entry, and other risk factors. Smoking was assessed at baseline (constant sub-cohorts), but duration of use of oral contraceptives was accumulated over follow-up, making it a time-dependent variable. Table 4 shows adjusted rate ratios for breast cancer: these ratios are interpreted as representing rates of mortality for breast cancer among oral contraceptive users and smokers compared to the rates among unexposed women, after adjusting for other covariates. No excess risks were observed. This method of analysis was also used in the British Doctors Study.[87]

This study illustrates another feature common to many cohort studies. Although the study population was relatively large and the average period of follow-up was relatively long (~25 years), there were only 889 deaths. The reason for the small number of deaths was that the population was relatively young (age 25–39 years at recruitment in 1968–1974). This low number of deaths implies an even lower number of cause-specific deaths:

Cause of death	Number of deaths
Total	889
Breast cancer	194
Ovarian cancer	61
Melanoma	11
Ischemic heart disease	72

In addition, breast cancer has 10-year survival rates on the order of 75%, so the number of deaths would be substantially less than the number of incident cases, and the focus on mortality reduces statistical power. Cause of death is well known to be subject to misclassification, especially for cardio-respiratory outcomes, and misclassification will usually lead to underestimates of rate ratios. Consequently, the study may have lacked the statistical power needed to uncover modest associations for specific causes of death. However, as the number of deaths increases with time, future study of this group may provide valuable information on a variety of risk factors that were measured when the women were young.

Case-Control Studies

In case-control studies, incident (new) cases are sampled over a specified period of time in a well-defined geographic region (e.g., the general population of a large metropolitan area), and their "exposure profiles" are compared to a series of control subjects who do not have the disease. Case-control studies are usually used when the outcome is rare. Cohort studies, unless they are sufficiently large and/or have long follow-up periods, will not have enough events for effective study of rare outcomes.

An essential difference from cohort studies is that subjects in case-control studies are selected to represent persons with and without the outcome of interest, rather than those with and without the exposure of interest. Thus, a case-control study might compare smoking histories in persons who do or do not have lung cancer, rather than compare lung cancer incidence in smokers to non-smokers. Nevertheless, inferences in case-control studies are still to the target population that represents some defined cohort of persons. Thus, a critical element in the design of any case-control study is whether case and control subjects are indeed representative of the target population. Figure 8 shows a schematic of the populations inherent in a case-control study and is similar to that of the cohort study (Figure 3) except for the manner in which subjects are sampled from the source population.

Proper sampling—the means of selecting cases and controls, with analysis appropriate to the sampling—is fundamental to good epidemiology. It is common to assume that the target population (primary study base) is in a steady state (size and age structure are approximately constant during the course of the study)[63] and that it is the population from which subjects are to be selected. This assumption may not hold when cases accumulate over a long period of time, as in some cancer incidence studies. In practice, however, especially for rare diseases,

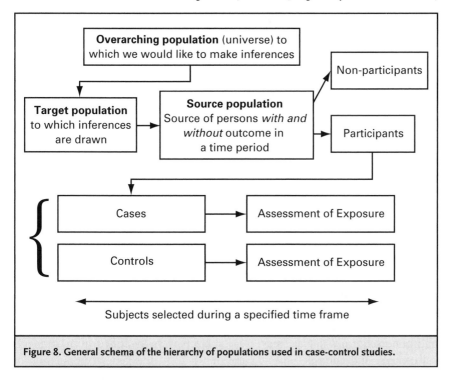

Figure 8. General schema of the hierarchy of populations used in case-control studies.

potential control subjects are accrued over short intervals of time (1–2 years) and then selected and interviewed. The members of the target population are not usually enumerated explicitly. The source population includes the sub-population that is drawn from the target and will include both cases identified during the course of the study and non-cases. Exposure is assessed retrospectively at the time of recruitment. The overarching population is the much larger population for which inferences will be made (generalizability). The main challenges of case-control studies are the selection of control subjects who represent the target population in all relevant ways except exposure and outcome (Figure 8), accurate measurement of exposures that reflect the etiological time period (before the outcome), and recruitment of subjects with sufficiently high response rates.

Both case and control subjects are selected from the source population using incidence density sampling; that is, at the time that each case is identified, potential control subjects include all persons who do not have the disease of interest at that time and are therefore at risk of developing it.[88–90] (This is the same method of sampling used in nested case-control studies, described in Chapter 18.) Constraints on eligibility applied to the case subjects must also be applied to the control subjects. Odds ratios based on incidence density sampling are estimates of incidence rate ratios. However, waiting until all cases have been accrued, which may take several years, is equivalent to cumulative incidence studies; then the odds ratio may not estimate the rate ratio, but, for rare diseases, it will estimate the relative risk.

Sampling defines two main types of case-control studies, according to whether cases and controls are 1) representative of the entire target population (referred to as population-based studies) and 2) selected from subsets of the primary base (referred to as secondary base studies).

Primary Base Studies
The goal of primary base studies is to ensure that subjects, though possibly not randomly selected, appropriately represent the target population. More often than not, all identified cases are selected (selection probability of 100%) so as to increase statistical power, whereas only a small fraction of potential controls are selected.

In the population-based, case-control study of oral contraceptive use and myocardial infarction,[59] the target population included all women 18–49 years old living in the Netherlands in 1990–1995 who were at risk of developing a first myocardial infarction. Although myocardial infarction is uncommon in this age range, many women in the target population use oral contraceptives, so that a national population could be expected to include enough cases in both users and non-users for a useful study. Case subjects were identified from 16 medical centers, and control subjects were drawn from the general population of the Netherlands through random-digit dialing, a technique that gives the same probability of selection to each telephone number in the dialing area, including those that are unlisted. Though the universe here was, initially, women in the Netherlands, one could also define the universe to include all women of reproductive age living in other countries. The generalization to all age groups will depend largely on whether the effects, if any, would occur before the age of 18 years, since very few women over 50 take oral contraceptives. The generalization to women elsewhere (or, perhaps, just women of European descent) assumes that the sample from the Netherlands is representative of the larger group in all relevant ways, and the validity of this assumption may depend on many factors, including socio-demographic and genetic characteristics.

Risk factors for myocardial infarction were ascertained in both groups, as they may also be associated with oral contraceptive use and therefore may confound the observed association; that is, extraneous factors correlated with both the exposure and outcome of interest may create or obscure an association that does not reflect cause and effect. Here, one might wonder whether oral contraceptive use might be correlated with myocardial infarction just because women with risk factors for myocardial infarction (such as smoking) are also more likely to take oral contraceptives. Where possible, investigators should choose study groups so as to minimize any serious confounding, but that is often difficult or impossible. An alternative is to measure and adjust for the effects of potential confounding variables. The Dutch investigators may not have had much information on how oral contraceptive use is correlated with other risk factors, so they prudently assessed a range of accepted and suspected risk factors that could be measured accurately, including smoking and biological markers (here, cholesterol levels and C-reactive protein). Almost 80% of subjects complied with a request for blood samples; these were used to assess certain genetic factors. In general, however, obtaining blood samples from subjects is difficult and expensive, and tends to reduce participation rates, so the relation between current levels of various biomarkers and past exposures may be complicated. (Non-invasive methods for obtaining DNA are now available, including collection of buccal cells and saliva.)

The meaning of questions related to exposure to oral contraceptives should not pose any specific difficulties, and quantitative estimates of exposure might be inferred from typical dosages used in each calendar period and access to computerized insurance claims for prescriptions. An important lesson from this study is the lack of specificity of the stated objectives—the authors were concerned, rightly, about changes in the composition of oral contraceptives, doses, and prothrombotic mutations during the course of their study. However, there seemed to be some ambiguity related to the timing of exposure to oral contraceptives; for example, one may postulate that long-term use affects the development of plaque, whereas exposures closer to the event may reflect other processes related to the development of thromboses. Although the authors stated that past and current use was assessed, the results did not refer to timing of exposure, so that the relation of the findings to possible biological mechanisms is obscure.

Another example of using a primary base is a Swedish study of acetaminophen use and chronic renal failure,[91] in which cases were identified from laboratory files of serum creatinine measurements above 250 μmol/liter (2.8 mg/dL) and eligibility was determined by the treating physicians. Population-based controls were selected from the universal Swedish Population Register and were frequency-matched to cases by age (10-year age groups) and gender. In a study of incident prostate cancer and vasectomy,[92] cases were identified through the New Zealand Cancer Registry, and control subjects, matched by 5-year age groups, were selected from the mandatory general electoral roll.

When national registers such as these are not available, investigators turn to other techniques to identify population controls. For example, a study of invasive pneumococcal disease and cigarette smoking[93] identified cases in three metropolitan areas of the U.S. and Canada through surveillance of laboratory findings. Control subjects from the general population were identified by random-digit telephone dialing and were frequency-matched to cases on month of positive culture (by month of enrollment), age group, and area of residence. To be included in the study, cases, like controls, must have had a telephone. The main issues with random-digit dialing are that response rates can be quite low, especially in the current era of intensive telemarketing, and they may be difficult to assess when the investigator cannot classify numbers that do not respond, although many business numbers can be identified.

A study from New Zealand[9] illustrates the use of a different type of sampling to estimate the population exposure distribution. Serious car injuries caused by driver drowsiness were investigated by including all accidents in the Auckland region, 1998–1999, that resulted in hospitalization or death. An estimate of the frequency of sleepiness in the primary base was obtained by sampling control subjects using a clustered approach in which 69 sites on the road network were selected and assigned randomly by day of week, time of day, and direction of travel. During a two-hour period, control drivers were selected in proportion to the volume of traffic to match case drivers, and interviews with drivers were conducted in hospitals or by telephone at home. The interviews were complex and included many factors, including two scales that measured drowsiness or alertness (Stanford and Epworth sleepiness scales).

Databases have also been used to conduct population-based case-control studies. For example, a study in New York State of women's own birth weights and their subsequent development of gestational diabetes at first pregnancy[94] used the hospital discharge file to determine all first births and thereby classify women according to whether they developed gestational diabetes. The data for these women were then linked to the state birth registry to obtain data on their own birth characteristics.

Secondary Base Studies

Secondary study bases refer to subsets of the target population from which subjects are selected. A common example is the use of controls identified from hospital records and matched to case subjects by hospital and other factors. The major challenge with such studies is to ensure that control subjects provide an accurate estimate of the exposure distribution of the target population from which the cases are selected. Advantages of this design include obtaining higher response rates than with general population controls, especially if biological samples are required, and minimizing differential information bias if control subjects are selected to have diseases that would lead to similar levels of recall as cases. Secondary bases include hospital controls, friend controls, and family controls. Wacholder and collaborators have discussed in detail the principles of selection of control subjects.[88-90]

Use of hospital controls is justified if "subjects who are admitted to the hospital for the case disease would have been admitted to the same hospital for the control disease" and if exposure is independent of admission.[88-90] An example is a study of brain cancer and cellular telephone use,[95] in which cases with well-defined types of brain cancers diagnosed in certain hospitals in Boston, Phoenix, and Pittsburgh were matched to hospital controls having a variety of nonmalignant conditions. Matching criteria included hospital center, age (10-year groups), sex, ethnic group, and proximity to hospital.

Not all studies that I reviewed used appropriate techniques for sampling subjects. In a small study investigating single nucleotide polymorphisms for adrenergic receptors in congestive heart failure, case subjects were enrolled from a major university hospital center, and control subjects were selected at voluntary blood draws and through newspaper advertisements.[29] This type of procedure violates the tenets of sound selection of controls: In a hospital-based study, unless the center covers the entire geographic area of the target population, controls must be drawn from the same secondary study base (e.g., the hospital center) to reduce possible referral biases that may be related to exposure. In this study, exposure refers to specific polymorphisms; it is possible that mechanisms related to ethnicity and associated with the polymorphisms could affect referral to this hospital, and not selecting controls from this hospital may have led to selection bias. (The authors indicated that allele frequencies varied considerably by race.) In addition, it is possible that the nonrandom controls may not represent the allele frequency distribution of the target population.

In another hospital-based case-control study of upper gastrointestinal bleeding and treatment with non-steroidal anti-inflammatory drugs (NSAIDs),[96] subjects were included if they were admitted to hospital for this disorder, thereby excluding individuals who were asymptomatic. Control subjects comprised hospital-based outpatients who did not have any conditions known to be associated with NSAIDs, frequency matched by age and sex. This is an appropriate strategy, as otherwise the prevalence of NSAID use will be overstated relative to the target population. All control subjects were appropriately tested to ensure that they were free from upper GI bleeds, but there was no screening for possible asymptomatic disease (e.g., excluding patients suffering from gastritis). The effect of including among the control series subjects with gastritis may attenuate the odds ratios, as this is associated with NSAID usage. This is a common problem in case-control studies; for example, in studies of prostate cancer, it is often unclear whether controls have undiagnosed prostate cancer. However, such health states are often unobservable, so the use of clinical diagnoses is the only appropriate practical strategy. Sensitivity analyses including only controls who had recent PSA tests (presumably negative) can be used to estimate the extent of this bias.

Clustered Case-Control Studies

Some studies are based not on the individual as the primary sampling unit but rather on an aggregation of subjects into groups (e.g., a family or a work location) that have common characteristics. This is referred to as *clustering*. When the unit of observation is a group, the study is referred to as a clustered case-control study. In one occupational study[97] designed to test whether robbery-prevention measures decreased the risk of homicides in the workplace, workplaces were selected as the unit of observation, rather than individuals. Thus, "cases" were those workplaces in which at least one employee was murdered, and the "controls" were those workplaces listed in a commercial business telephone list that did not meet the definition of a case. Control workplaces were then matched to a case workplace by month of the event and by broad occupational categories. An important finding was that having five or more control measures in the workplace showed a strong protective effect (OR = 0.5; 95% CI: 0.2–1.0).

Accuracy of Outcome and Exposure

Each endpoint must be defined clearly using valid, reproducible criteria. This may be difficult for health states that are diagnosed by complex criteria. The study of oral contraceptive use and the incidence of myocardial infarction[59] used elevated cardiac-enzyme levels and electrocardiographic changes to confirm the diagnosis of myocardial infarction. The report did not say whether these tests were used in the same way in cases and controls, but there is little reason to suspect that medical management would differ in this respect by use of oral contraceptives. A study of glaucoma[98] used specific criteria to define subjects who had losses of field of vision in advanced glaucoma (cases) and compared these individuals to those with early-stage glaucoma (controls) (Table 5). The study investigated possible socioeconomic differences between the presentation of new late (cases) and early (controls) glaucoma. This is not a study of incidence, and those subjects diagnosed previously were excluded, so it is also not a study of prevalence. Thus, the finding that lower social position was strongly associated with a worse state of glaucoma at the time of diagnosis is interpreted in terms of prognosis. (In general, the exclusion of prevalent cases of disease is crucial to the validity of an etiological study, as associations estimated from prevalent cases depend generally on duration of disease,[99] meaning that it is difficult to determine whether an identified factor was associated with incidence, prognosis, or both.)

In occupational case-control studies, Siemiatycki and his collaborators[100–103] used in-depth probing interviews to provide a portrait of a subject's workplace. This information was then passed on to a team of occupational hygienists and chemists to estimate intensity and frequency of exposure to hundreds of chemical and physical agents used in the workplace. The advantage of such a strategy

Table 5. Criteria for the Classification of Glaucoma in a Case-Control Study Identifying Socioeconomic Risk Factors.[98]

Cases (late presenters)

- Visual field loss consistent with a pattern of glaucomatous loss—for example, arcuate scotomas, residual temporal island—compatible with the patient's disc changes and in which there was no suggestion of other optic nerve pathology (for example, defects crossed the horizontal midline). For the late presenters, this field loss had to be within 5° of fixation and beyond 30° in one or both eyes.

- Glaucoma of any chronic type—that is, primary open angle, pseudoexfoliative, normal tension, chronic angle closure, aphakic, or pigment dispersion

- Two consecutive fields (threshold or suprathreshold) confirming the loss, except when field loss was so advanced that field testing was not possible

- Cup:disc ratio assessed as > 0.8 in the eye(s) with the field loss

Control group

- Visual field loss consistent with a pattern of glaucomatous loss, compatible with the patient's disc changes and in which there was no suggestion of other optic nerve pathology. No absolute scotomas within 20° of fixation in either eye

- Glaucoma of any chronic type (as above)

- Two consecutive fields (threshold or suprathreshold) confirming the loss

- Cup:disc ratio assessed as > 0.5 or difference of > 0.2 between the discs

Reproduced from Deprivation and late presentation of glaucoma: case-control study, Fraser S, Bunce C, Wormald R, Brunner E, BMJ 2001; 322(7287):639–43 with permission from BMJ Publishing Group Ltd.

is that most individuals do not know what they are exposed to, whereas trained experts can make reasonably accurate judgments.

One strategy to reduce recall bias is to choose controls who have diseases that will make their memory of past events similar to that of cases. For example, in a study of congenital birth defects,[104] controls were mothers of infants with defects other than the ones in the case series. Another illustrative example is a study in China to identify psychological characteristics that predispose individuals to suicide.[105] As information on subjects can only be obtained from next of kin, surrogate subjects were also selected as respondents. As well, controls were persons who died accidentally, as other diseases may affect quality of life and psychological profiles.

External data have been used to validate the distribution of exposure in the control series. For example, in a study of benzodiazepines and hip fractures in an elderly population,[106] matched hospital controls were used, and the distribution of exposure to benzodiazepines in the control series was shown to be similar to that in a survey conducted in the area. Another post-hoc validation method is to compare study results on known risk factors with findings from other studies. For example, my colleagues and I made use of cancer controls in an environmental study of postmenopausal breast cancer[107, 108]; we found that associations for the accepted risk factors were in the expected direction and magnitude.

Confounding in Case-Control Studies

The primary tools to deal with confounding in case-control studies are: matching, whereby at the time of enrollment both cases and controls are selected in ways that make them similar with respect to certain strong potential confounding factors; stratification; and regression modeling. Matching is the primary tool for dealing with confounding at the stage of study design, whereas stratification and modeling are used at the time of analysis. In general, matching has the defect that samples may be more difficult and time-consuming to gather, stratification leads to larger variances, and modeling requires that the chosen model be at least approximately correct, a matter that is often difficult or impossible to establish. (Of course, stratification also makes use of a model that is implicit in the method.) Thus, the choice of an approach requires educated judgment.

Stratification refers to the division of the study and control groups into categories defined by the potential confounding variable(s) and is similar to those methods used in cohort studies. For example, the confounding effect of age between case and control groups can be accounted for by estimating odds ratios within narrow age ranges, such as 0–10 years, 11–20 years, etc., and then use of the case-control version of the Mantel-Haenszel estimator to provide a weighted average.

Case-control studies usually employ some form of matching to eliminate confounding at the design stage by ensuring that case and control subjects have similar distributions of selected risk factors (e.g., age, sex).[61–64] An important criterion for matching is that the variable is recognized as a strong causal risk factor for the outcome; otherwise the improvement in data quality will be small and not worth the serious reductions in study size and flexibility. Also, the data must be analyzed using techniques that account for the matching; otherwise the summary odds ratios may be biased.

Frequency-matching refers to matching groups, rather than individuals, within strata. It is often used to ensure, for example, that the age distributions of cases and controls are similar. It entails setting in advance the strata, setting the control-to-case ratio, and then ensuring that the numbers of controls in each stratum are in this proportion. For example, a population-based study of breast cancer[109] identified cases from the provincial tumor registry and identified controls from the electoral roll of British Columbia. The recruitment strategy ensured that the number of controls was approximately equal to the number of cases in each five-year age group. An important inclusion criterion was that only Canadian citizens were enrolled and, because Canadian voter lists have almost 100% coverage, the case and control populations were representative of the target population (i.e., Canadian women, living in British Columbia 1988–1989, and under age 76 years). To account for the matching, conditional logistic regression was used to estimate the odds ratios, although ordinary logistic regression stratified by age would probably have sufficed.

Individual-level matching is used less often because cases may be excluded if no controls are found. For example, in the hospital-based study of benzodiazepines and the risk of hip fractures among persons aged 65 years and over,[106] control subjects were selected from other diseases not known to be related to benzodiazepine use. Up to four controls were sought for each case according to age (five-year groups), gender, and week of admission, but 74 cases (23%) had to be excluded because no controls were found. As well, the exclusion rate increased with increasing age of the case, which may have led to confounding by unmeasured factors associated with age. Although the authors indicated that the prevalence of exposure in the excluded cases was similar to the included cases, a considerable loss of statistical power occurred, and that may explain the essentially null findings.

In a study of estrogen replacement therapy and venous thromboembolism,[110] three hospital controls were individually matched to cases according to hospital center, date of admission, area of residence, and age within ±2 years (referred to as a caliper). Matching by area of residence would presumably have reduced possible referral biases to the institutions. Subjects from the secondary base who did not have diseases associated with estrogen use were selected, and this would have lessened attenuation of the odds ratios. The individual matching of cases to controls meant that a conditional logistic regression analysis was required.

The hospital-based study of benzodiazepines and hip fractures in the elderly[106] is instructive for interpreting associations when power is low. Although the study was designed to detect an odds ratio of 2, at 90% power, for exposures having prevalence of 20%, in one sub-analysis of specific drugs, as derived from measurements in blood samples, the largest prevalence of exposure (in controls) was 8.3%. Table 6 shows substantial variation in the odds ratios. The statistically significant association for lorazepam could have been due to chance (small numbers tending to produce more-extreme results with wider confidence bounds), and the predominant number of negative associations could have been due to low power.

Stratification Methods for Adjusting for Confounding
As with cohort studies, stratification methods of analysis have been developed for case-control studies to account for confounding. In the event that potential confounding variables (e.g., age, gender) can be classified accurately into strata

Table 6. Rate Ratios for Hip Fractures According to the Presence in Blood Samples of Specific Types of Benzodiazepines.[106]

	Exposed as % of total population		
	Controls (*n* = 817)	Cases (*n* = 245)	Odds ratio
Alprazolam	12 (1.5)	3 (1.2)	0.8 (0.2 to 2.7)
Bromazepam	64 (7.8)	21 (8.6)	1.02 (0.6 to 1.7)
Chlordiazepoxide	1 (0.1)	0	
Clobazam	3 (0.4)	3 (1.2)	3.1 (0.6 to 15.6)
Clorazepate	68 (8.3)	13 (5.3)	0.6 (0.3 to 1.1)
Clotiazepam	1 (0.1)	0	
Diazepam	1 (0.1)	0	
Flunitrazepam	12 (1.4)	5 (2.0)	1.4 (0.5 to 4.4)
Loflazepate	0	1 (0.4)	
Loprazolam	3 (0.4)	4 (1.6)	2.7 (0.5 to 13.6)
Lorazepam	44 (5.4)	25 (10.2)	1.8 (1.1 to 3.1)
Nitrazepam	3 (0.4)	2 (0.8)	2.2 (0.4 to 13.4)
Oxazepam	15 (1.8)	5 (2.0)	0.7 (0.2 to 2.2)
Prazepam	1 (0.1)	1 (0.4)	
Temazepam	4 (0.5)	4 (1.6)	2.7 (0.7 to 10.9)
Triazolam	0	0	
Zolpidem	35 (4.3)	15 (6.1)	1.3 (0.7 to 2.5)
Zopiclone	48 (5.9)	14 (5.7)	0.7 (0.4 to 1.4)

Reproduced from Benzodiazepines and hip fractures in elderly people: case-control study, Pierfitte C, Macouillard G, Thicoipe M, et al., BMJ 2001; 322(7288):704–8 with permission from BMJ Publishing Group Ltd.

and with a dichotomous metric for exposure (exposed vs. not exposed), the Mantel-Haenszel stratified estimator is the method of choice. In a typical study, investigators match on a limited number of risk factors (e.g., frequency-matching on age and gender) and measure other potential confounding factors. If the data are matched individually, then the Mantel-Haenszel estimator can be used with the strata defined by the matched subjects. An important disadvantage of this method is that other factors cannot be incorporated into the analysis. For frequency-matched studies, the Mantel-Haenszel estimator can be used for the matching variables and other covariates. As discussed in Chapter 18, powerful regression methods are available, including logistic regression for unmatched data and conditional logistic regression for matched data.

Cross-Sectional Studies

Cross-sectional studies (surveys) are used in health research to measure at one point in time the prevalence of a health outcome or a risk factor and estimate associations between prevalence and other factors. Examples are the percentage of persons who smoke or who have some health condition, such as childhood asthma. Surveys are used in many fields; for example, polling during elections is essentially a cross-sectional study of political issues. For surveys that are used to estimate associations between prevalence of a health outcome and other factors, valid inferences can be obtained only if the sampling of subjects is independent of both exposure status and health status. These studies can be nested within an explicitly defined cohort or can be a sample from the general population. Some cross-sectional studies focus on correlations between the prevalence of a health state and concurrent or antecedent exposures in an attempt to identify etiological factors.

Thus, surveys are used to estimate the distribution of current or past traits in populations, including variables that are considered typically as "exposures" or "health states." Health states and antecedent variables are placed on the same footing in the sense that one can estimate the prevalence of a health state or an exposure from the population, because the sampling of subjects is independent of these (Figure 9). This scenario is rather different from cohort and case-control studies, which follow subjects through time for the occurrence of a health event.

Of course, the target population, the sampling frame, and the selection of subjects in cross-sectional studies depend on the objective. If the objective is to estimate parameters of health and exposure in a specific cohort, then the sample will be defined at a point in time and, usually, all subjects in view will be sampled. An example is a survey to determine unmet needs for chronic health care. This approach assumes that the sub-population studied is representative

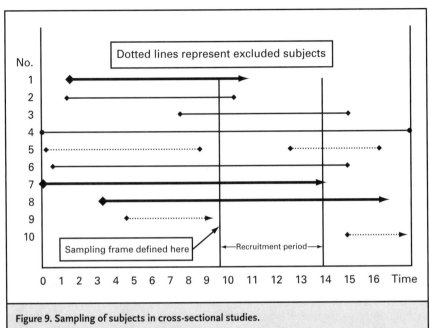

Figure 9. Sampling of subjects in cross-sectional studies.

Subjects are selected randomly from an explicitly defined cohort or from the general population, independent of exposure and outcome. A line ending in an arrow represents a subject who had a health event, and a dotted line represents a subject who was not included in the survey. Health outcomes (prevalence) or exposures can refer to any time prior to the date at which the sampling frame was defined, or the date at which the study was initiated, or the time of interview.

of the total population that would be available if there were no losses to follow-up. Moreover, interpretation of the results is based on the available living population, and this may not be representative of the entire population if they could have been surveyed. Thus, the surviving study population may or may not have the same characteristics as the total cohort (e.g., the prevalence estimated at two points in time may differ).

Similar arguments apply to cross-sectional studies sampled from regional or national populations, except that the dynamics of the population (e.g., mortality, migration) will not be known explicitly as in a cohort. If the population can be considered stationary (that is, although individuals may change, there are no important changes in the characteristics of the population) over a period of time, then external validity is widened.

In general, subjects have a fixed probability of selection that depends on the type of sample taken (e.g., random, stratified, clustered, hierarchical). A census is a special kind of survey in which all potential subjects are selected (sampling fraction of 100%). The survey and the target population for which inferences are to be drawn dictate whether the sampling will be simple or complex. Prevalence surveys within well-defined cohorts usually entail a random sample or a census of the population. For example, a cross-sectional survey in the Norwegian county of Nord-Trondelag[111] used a census approach in an attempt to recruit all residents age 25 years and above in 1984–1986 ($n = 74,599$, 88.1% response rate). This study was used to assess the association between the prevalence of gastric reflux disease, body mass index, and smoking.

In national and regional studies, simple random sampling (with equal and independent probabilities of selection for each member of the population) is generally infeasible, so more-complex sampling methods are usually used. The valid use of such samples requires that the probability of selection of any person is known, that it is not zero, and that any correlations of selection probabilities are known. Often, these methods are based on clustered or hierarchical samples; for example, the Third National Health and Nutrition Examination Survey (NHANES-III) used a nationwide sample of 33,994 (86% response rate) civilian non-institutionalized persons in the U.S., age two months and over. The general objectives were to estimate information on the health and nutritional status (e.g., high blood pressure, *Helicobacter pylori* infection, nutritional blood measures) of this population. (See http://www.cdc.gov/nchs/products/elec_prods/subject/nhanes3.htm.)

Thus, NHANES-III used a four-stage sample design that involved primary sampling units of single counties, area segments within the primary sampling units, households within these area segments, and persons within the households.[112] There were 81 primary sampling units, 89 survey locations, and 2144 area segments. The number of households screened for potential eligible subjects was 93,653, and 19,528 of these were designated for interview. The analysis of these data requires special statistical techniques that account for the sampling strategy, so that the sample population can be built up in such a way as to represent the larger target population. The resulting sample weights reflect the number of persons that each observation represents. Software programs such as SUDAAN (http://www.rti.org/sudaan/index.cfm) are often used for this purpose.

Cross-sectional studies can be exceedingly complex, as exemplified in a prevalence study of advanced colonic neoplasia.[44] The authors had an implicit cohort of patients at 13 U.S. Veterans Affairs medical centers, and during the period 1994–1997 they attempted to enroll all potential subjects visiting the hospitals. Subjects were selected independent of exposure or disease status (colorectal neoplasia). Figure 10 shows the populations for this study, and Figure 11 shows the source and final populations used in the analysis. The findings and interpretation of this study are discussed in Chapter 18.

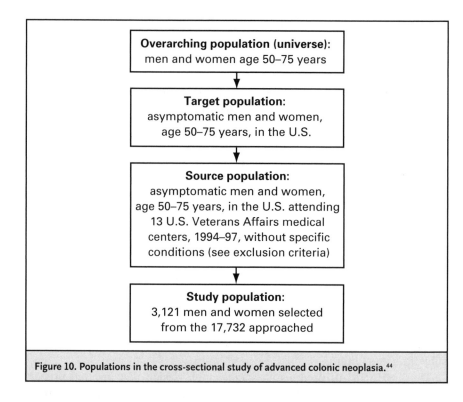

Figure 10. Populations in the cross-sectional study of advanced colonic neoplasia.[44]

In the end, most surveys require regression methods for analysis. However, if the distribution of a continuous variable is to be estimated and compared to subjects with other characteristics, then one simple analysis is a comparison of mean values, using *t*-tests and confidence intervals. In such an analysis of mean values, it is usually assumed that the outcome variable is derived from an independent set of observations, that it is normally distributed, and that its variance can be estimated (taking into account the weights and sample design). For example, among 65% of children and adolescents recruited into a cardio-vascular health program trial (1991–1994) a risk factor survey was conducted in 1997: individual-level variables and homocysteine levels from blood samples taken at that time were measured and compared.[113]

If the parameter of interest is a binary variable (e.g., prevalence of asthma), then proportions are estimated, and inferences on the difference between or ratio of the proportions use chi-squared tests and confidence intervals. For example, in four identical national surveys in the UK conducted over a four-year period, households were selected randomly and an interview was conducted if a smoker lived in the home.[114] In all, 7766 current smokers were recruited, and 1126 (16%) were classified as "hardcore" smokers. The relationships between

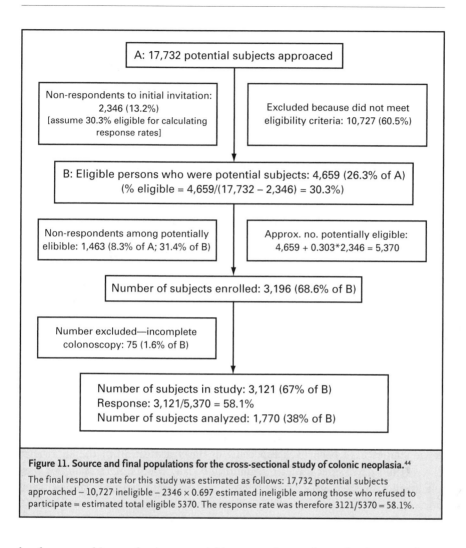

Figure 11. Source and final populations for the cross-sectional study of colonic neoplasia.[44]

The final response rate for this study was estimated as follows: 17,732 potential subjects approached – 10,727 ineligible – 2346 × 0.697 estimated ineligible among those who refused to participate = estimated total eligible 5370. The response rate was therefore 3121/5370 = 58.1%.

hardcore smoking and relevant variables were then estimated using prevalence odds ratios. There are no unexposed "controls" in this study; the associations are based on comparing the prevalence odds of various conditions between hardcore smokers and other smokers.

A word of warning about the interpretation of cross-sectional studies. Surveys are frequently conducted to identify risk factors for a health outcome (i.e., to identify factors that might be used to prevent new cases of disease). Cross-sectional surveys provide estimates only of prevalence. Assuming a one-compartment, steady-state model,[63, 99] the relation between prevalence odds ratios, incidence rates, and the ratio of duration of the outcome between the exposed groups can be derived; but only under the strong assumption that duration of the condition is independent of exposure will the prevalence odds ratio estimate the incidence rate ratio. Thus, etiologic factors cannot always be identified, because the factors may be related to incidence, duration of disease (i.e., prognostic indicators), or both.

Ecological Studies

Ecological studies do not use samples of individual subjects but are used to compare rates of a condition (e.g., disease) among geographic areas with average characteristics of these regions (e.g., average radon levels in each county and lung cancer mortality in that county). Thus, the joint distribution of exposure and outcome does not use individual values. Although these designs may be useful in generating hypotheses and in measuring attributes that refer to whole populations rather than individuals,[115] they cannot be guaranteed to provide unbiased estimates of effects that are interpretable at the individual level (referred to as the ecological fallacy). Morgenstern[116] provides a detailed discussion of ecological studies.

Time-Series Studies

Time-series studies are used most often to investigate short-term effects of exposures on health outcomes. They are usually used when an explicit cohort cannot be assembled and are often analyzed by correlating counts of events on average levels of exposure across the population. Over the past ten years, these studies have been used especially in the investigation of the short-term (i.e., within days) effects of air pollution on daily counts of mortality or hospitalization in fixed geographic areas[117] and in other types of studies (e.g., adverse health events with changes in health care prescription programs[23]). Under certain conditions, these studies can be considered to be equivalent to cohort studies.[118]

Consider the example of investigating the short-term effects of air pollution on health. The unit of analysis is the day, and the outcome data are counts of deaths, hospital discharges, emergency department visits, etc. These data are administrative and are usually obtained from published or private sources. Often, one can subdivide these outcomes by specific disease entities, such as using underlying causes of death or reasons for stay in the hospital. The exposure data usually consist of routinely available measurements of concentrations of particles and gaseous pollutants from fixed-site monitoring stations in a circumscribed geographic area, and these are usually averaged to represent daily values. As daily fluctuations in weather affect mortality, daily averages of mean temperature, relative humidity, and other weather variables routinely measured may also be included in the model.

The essential characteristics of the outcome data dictate the type of analysis that is required. In particular, the outcomes usually display a high degree of seasonality and sub-seasonality that makes the outcomes statistically dependent (e.g., a winter increase in pneumonia). Thus, the statistical analysis of these data is complex and requires special types of regression models (over-dispersed Poisson models) that account for this clustering in time and other features of the data. These studies are not discussed further; a review article gives details.[117]

SUMMARY AND CONCLUSIONS

This chapter has stressed the importance of defining objectives in a clear and operational way so that the epidemiologic study can be used to identify the relevant target population, select the appropriate design that leads to the identification of the source and study populations, and analyze appropriate health outcome variables, exposure variables, and other covariates. It is important that readers have some familiarity with these matters so that they can evaluate the reports that they read. Of special importance is the minimization of potential selection biases into and out of the study population. These biases can impose important limitations on a study, and it is sometimes exceedingly difficult to assess whether the study population is indeed representative of the target population. Confounding, also an important issue in any epidemiologic study, needs to be addressed by measuring the main risk factors and accounting for them either in the design or in the analysis. Another important consideration is that the analysis should conform to the study design.

REFERENCES

1. Last JM. A dictionary of epidemiology. 4th ed. Oxford, UK: Oxford University Press; 2001.

2. Doll R, Gray R, Hafner B, Peto R. Mortality in relation to smoking: 22 years' observations on female British doctors. Br Med J 1980; 280(6219):967–71.

3. Gillman MW, Cupples LA, Gagnon D, et al. Margarine intake and subsequent coronary heart disease in men. Epidemiology 1997; 8(2):144–9.

4. Land CE, Tokunaga M, Koyama K, et al. Incidence of female breast cancer among atomic bomb survivors, Hiroshima and Nagasaki, 1950–1990. Radiat Res 2003; 160(6):707–17.

5. Grabrick DM, Hartmann LC, Cerhan JR, et al. Risk of breast cancer with oral contraceptive use in women with a family history of breast cancer. JAMA 2000; 284(14):1791–98.

6. Verghese J, Lipton RB, Hall CB, et al. Abnormality of gait as a predictor of non-Alzheimer's dementia. N Engl J Med 2002; 347(22):1761–8.

7. Thio CL, Seaberg EC, Skolasky R Jr, et al. HIV-1, hepatitis B virus, and risk of liver-related mortality in the Multicenter Cohort Study (MACS). Lancet 2002; 360(9349):1921–6.

8. George L, Mills JL, Johansson AL, et al. Plasma folate levels and risk of spontaneous abortion. JAMA 2002; 288(15):1867–73.

9. Connor J, Norton R, Ameratunga S, et al. Driver sleepiness and risk of serious injury to car occupants: population based case control study. BMJ 2002; 324(7346):1125.

10. Corne JM, Marshall C, Smith S, et al. Frequency, severity, and duration of rhinovirus infections in asthmatic and non-asthmatic individuals: a longitudinal cohort study. Lancet 2002; 359(9309):831–4.

11. Petersen LA, Normand SL, Daley J, McNeil BJ. Outcome of myocardial infarction in Veterans Health Administration patients as compared with Medicare patients. N Engl J Med 2000; 343(26):1934–41.

12. Verghese J, Lipton RB, Katz MJ, et al. Leisure activities and the risk of dementia in the elderly. N Engl J Med 2003; 348(25):2508–16.

13. Gerstein HC, Mann JF, Yi Q, et al. Albuminuria and risk of cardiovascular events, death, and heart failure in diabetic and nondiabetic individuals. JAMA 2001; 286(4):421–6.

14. Hylek EM, Go AS, Chang Y, et al. Effect of intensity of oral anticoagulation on stroke severity and mortality in atrial fibrillation. N Engl J Med 2003; 349(11):1019–26.

15. Mange KC, Joffe MM, Feldman HI. Effect of the use or nonuse of long-term dialysis on the subsequent survival of renal transplants from living donors. N Engl J Med 2001; 344(10):726–31.

16. Suissa S, Ernst P, Benayoun S, et al. Low-dose inhaled corticosteroids and the prevention of death from asthma. N Engl J Med 2000; 343(5):332–6.

17. Gawande AA, Studdert DM, Orav EJ, et al. Risk factors for retained instruments and sponges after surgery. N Engl J Med 2003; 348(3):229–35.

18. Jackson LA, Neuzil KM, Yu O, et al. Effectiveness of pneumococcal polysaccharide vaccine in older adults. N Engl J Med 2003; 348(18):1747–55.

19. Fleming PJ, Blair PS, Platt MW, et al. The UK accelerated immunisation programme and sudden unexpected death in infancy: case-control study. BMJ 2001; 322(7290):822.

20. Suissa S, Ernst P, Benayoun S, et al. Low-dose inhaled corticosteroids and the prevention of death from asthma. N Engl J Med 2000; 343(5):332–6.

21. Gurwitz JH, Field TS, Harrold LR, et al. Incidence and preventability of adverse drug events among older persons in the ambulatory setting. JAMA 2003; 289(9):1107–16.

22. Juurlink DN, Mamdani M, Kopp A, et al. Drug-drug interactions among elderly patients hospitalized for drug toxicity. JAMA 2003; 289(13):1652–8.

23. Tamblyn R, Laprise R, Hanley JA, et al. Adverse events associated with prescription drug cost-sharing among poor and elderly persons. JAMA 2001; 285(4):421–9.

24. Ray WA, Daugherty JR, Meador KG. Effect of a mental health "carve-out" program on the continuity of antipsychotic therapy. N Engl J Med 2003; 348(19):1885–94.

25. Tseng CW, Brook RH, Keeler E, Mangione CM. Impact of an annual dollar limit or "cap" on prescription drug benefits for Medicare patients. JAMA 2003; 290(2):222–7.

26. Sveinbjornsdottir S, Hicks AA, Jonsson T, et al. Familial aggregation of Parkinson's disease in Iceland. N Engl J Med 2000; 343(24):1765–70.

27. Roy S, Knox K, Segal S, et al. MBL genotype and risk of invasive pneumococcal disease: a case-control study. Lancet 2002; 359(9317):1569–73.

28. Shahbazi M, Pravica V, Nasreen N, et al. Association between functional polymorphism in EGF gene and malignant melanoma. Lancet 2002; 359(9304):397–401.

29. Small KM, Wagoner LE, Levin AM, et al. Synergistic polymorphisms of beta1- and alpha2C-adrenergic receptors and the risk of congestive heart failure. N Engl J Med 2002; 347(15):1135–42.

30. Hwang SW. Mortality among men using homeless shelters in Toronto, Ontario. JAMA 2000; 283(16):2152–7.

31. Kuh D, Hardy R, Langenberg C, et al. Mortality in adults aged 26–54 years related to socio-economic conditions in childhood and adulthood: post war birth cohort study. BMJ 2002; 325(7372):1076–80.

32. Mulvany F, O'Callaghan E, Takei N, et al. Effect of social class at birth on risk and presentation of schizophrenia: case-control study. BMJ 2001; 323(7326):1398–401.

33. Waern M, Rubenowitz E, Runeson B, et al. Burden of illness and suicide in elderly people: case-control study. BMJ 2002; 324(7350):1355.

34. Churchill D, Allen J, Pringle M, et al. Consultation patterns and provision of contraception in general practice before teenage pregnancy: case-control study. BMJ 2000; 321(7259):486–9.

35. Horwitz SM, Kelleher K, Boyce T, et al. Barriers to health care research for children and youth with psychosocial problems. JAMA 2002; 288(12):1508–12.

36. Schlenger WE, Caddell JM, Ebert L, et al. Psychological reactions to terrorist attacks: findings from the National Study of Americans' Reactions to September 11. JAMA 2002; 288(5):581–8.

37. Buchholz U, Mermin J, Rios R, et al. An outbreak of food-borne illness associated with methomyl-contaminated salt. JAMA 2002; 288(5):604–10.

38. Crump JA, Sulka AC, Langer AJ, et al. An outbreak of Escherichia coli O157:H7 infections among visitors to a dairy farm. N Engl J Med 2002; 347(8):555–60.

39. Olsen SJ, DeBess EE, McGivern TE, et al. A nosocomial outbreak of fluoroquinolone-resistant salmonella infection. N Engl J Med 2001; 344(21):1572–9.

40. Jones JM, Lawson ML, Daneman D, et al. Eating disorders in adolescent females with and without type 1 diabetes: cross sectional study. BMJ 2000; 320(7249):1563–6.

41. Amowitz LL, Reis C, Lyons KH, et al. Prevalence of war-related sexual violence and other human rights abuses among internally displaced persons in Sierra Leone. JAMA 2002; 287(4):513–21.

42. Turner CF, Rogers SM, Miller HG, et al. Untreated gonococcal and chlamydial infection in a probability sample of adults. JAMA 2002; 287(6):726–33.

43. Must A, Spadano J, Coakley EH, et al. The disease burden associated with overweight and obesity. JAMA 1999; 282(16):1523–9.

44. Lieberman DA, Prindiville S, Weiss DG, Willett W. Risk factors for advanced colonic neoplasia and hyperplastic polyps in asymptomatic individuals. JAMA 2003; 290(22):2959–67.

45. Lawlor DA, Patel R, Ebrahim S. Association between falls in elderly women and chronic diseases and drug use: cross sectional study. BMJ 2003; 327(7417):712–7.

46. Simon JA, Hudes ES. Relationship of ascorbic acid to blood lead levels. JAMA 1999; 281(24):2289–93.

47. Moss ME, Lanphear BP, Auinger P. Association of dental caries and blood lead levels. JAMA 1999; 281(24):2294–8.

48. Rebbeck TR, Lynch HT, Neuhausen SL, et al. Prophylactic oophorectomy in carriers of BRCA1 or BRCA2 mutations. N Engl J Med 2002; 346(21):1616–22.

49. Davidson MB, Schriger DL, Peters AL, Lorber B. Relationship between fasting plasma glucose and glycosylated hemoglobin: potential for false-positive diagnoses of type 2 diabetes using new diagnostic criteria. JAMA 1999; 281(13):1203–10.

50. Veldink JH, Wokke JH, van der Wal G, et al. Euthanasia and physician-assisted suicide among patients with amyotrophic lateral sclerosis in the Netherlands. N Engl J Med 2002; 346(21):1638–44.

51. Marvel MK, Epstein RM, Flowers K, Beckman HB. Soliciting the patient's agenda: have we improved? JAMA 1999; 281(3):283–7.

52. Landon BE, Epstein AM. Quality management practices in Medicaid managed care: a national survey of Medicaid and commercial health plans participating in the Medicaid program. JAMA 1999; 282(18):1769–75.

53. Redinbaugh EM, Sullivan AM, Block SD, et al. Doctors' emotional reactions to recent death of a patient: cross sectional study of hospital doctors. BMJ 2003; 327(7408):185.

54. Bogardus ST Jr, Concato J, Feinstein AR. Clinical epidemiological quality in molecular genetic research: the need for methodological standards. JAMA 1999; 281(20):1919–26.

55. Ribisl KM, Williams RS, Kim AE. Internet sales of cigarettes to minors. JAMA 2003; 290(10):1356–9.

56. Stewart WF, Ricci JA, Chee E, et al. Lost productive time and cost due to common pain conditions in the US workforce. JAMA 2003; 290(18):2443–54.

57. Aguayo VM, Ross JS, Kanon S, Ouedraogo AN. Monitoring compliance with the International Code of Marketing of Breastmilk Substitutes in west Africa: multisite cross sectional survey in Togo and Burkina Faso. BMJ 2003; 326(7381):127.

58. Birch DW, Eady A, Robertson D, et al. Users' guide to the surgical literature: how to perform a literature search. Can J Surg 2003; 46(2):136–41.

59. Tanis BC, van den Bosch MA, Kemmeren JM, et al. Oral contraceptives and the risk of myocardial infarction. N Engl J Med 2001; 345(25):1787–93.

60. Bailar JC III, Louis TA, Lavori PW, Polansky M. A classification for biomedical research reports. N Engl J Med 1984; 311:1482–7. [Updated in the second edition of this book.]

61. Gordis L. Epidemiology. 3rd ed. Philadelphia, PA: Elsevier Saunders; 2004.

62. Rothman KJ. Epidemiology: an introduction. Oxford, UK: Oxford University Press; 2002.

63. Rothman KJ, Greenland S. Modern epidemiology. 2nd ed. Philadelphia, PA: Lippincott-Raven Publishers; 1998.

64. Koepsell TD, Weiss NS. Epidemiologic methods: studying the occurrence of illness. Oxford, UK: Oxford University Press; 2003.

65. Ascherio A, Zhang SM, Hernan MA, et al. Hepatitis B vaccination and the risk of multiple sclerosis. N Engl J Med 2001; 344(5):327–32.

66. Zammit S, Allebeck P, Andreasson S, et al. Self reported cannabis use as a risk factor for schizophrenia in Swedish conscripts of 1969: historical cohort study. BMJ 2002; 325(7374):1199.

67. Vessey M, Painter R, Yeates D. Mortality in relation to oral contraceptive use and cigarette smoking. Lancet 2003; 362(9379):185–91.

68. Lichtenstein P, Holm NV, Verkasalo PK, et al. Environmental and heritable factors in the causation of cancer—analyses of cohorts of twins from Sweden, Denmark, and Finland. N Engl J Med 2000; 343(2):78–85.

69. Fearon P, Hotopf M. Relation between headache in childhood and physical and psychiatric symptoms in adulthood: national birth cohort study. BMJ 2001; 322(7295):1145.

70. Schatz IJ, Masaki K, Yano K, et al. Cholesterol and all-cause mortality in elderly people from the Honolulu Heart Program: a cohort study. Lancet 2001; 358(9279):351–5.

71. Calle EE, Rodriguez C, Walker-Thurmond K, Thun MJ. Overweight, obesity, and mortality from cancer in a prospectively studied cohort of U.S. adults. N Engl J Med 2003; 348(17):1625–38.

72. Pandey DK, Shekelle R, Selwyn BJ, et al. Dietary vitamin C and beta-carotene and risk of death in middle-aged men: the Western Electric Study. Am J Epidemiol 1995; 142(12):1269–78.

73. Dawber TR, Kannel WB, Lyell LP. An approach to longitudinal studies in a community: the Framingham Study. Ann N Y Acad Sci. 1963; 107:539–56.

74. Evans JM, Wang J, Morris AD. Comparison of cardiovascular risk between patients with type 2 diabetes and those who had had a myocardial infarction: cross sectional and cohort studies. BMJ 2002; 324(7343):939–42.

75. Andersson RE, Olaison G, Tysk C, Ekbom A. Appendectomy and protection against ulcerative colitis. N Engl J Med 2001; 344(11):808–14.

76. Hoek G, Brunekreef B, Goldbohm S, et al. Association between mortality and indicators of traffic-related air pollution in the Netherlands: a cohort study. Lancet 2002; 360(9341):1203–9.

77. Lydon-Rochelle M, Holt VL, Easterling TR, Martin DP. Risk of uterine rupture during labor among women with a prior cesarean delivery. N Engl J Med 2001; 345(1):3–8.

78. Keenan HT, Runyan DK, Marshall SW, et al. A population-based study of inflicted traumatic brain injury in young children. JAMA 2003; 290(5):621–6.

79. Lubin JH. Case-control methods in the presence of multiple failure times and competing risks. Biometrics 1985; 41:49–54.

80. Longnecker MP. The Framingham results on alcohol and breast cancer. Am J Epidemiol 1999; 149(2):102–4.

81. Gottlieb DJ, Wilk JB, Harmon M, et al. Heritability of longitudinal change in lung function: the Framingham study. Am J Respir Crit Care Med 2001; 164(9):1655–9.

82. Goldberg MS, Giannetti N, Burnett RT, et al. A panel study in congestive heart failure to estimate the short-term effects from personal factors and environmental conditions on oxygen saturation and pulse rate. Occup Environ Med 2008; 65:659–66.

83. Breslow NE, Day NE. Statistical methods in cancer research. Volume II—The design and analysis of cohort studies. Lyon, France: International Agency for Cancer; 1987.

84. Pearce N, Checkoway H. A simple computer program for generating person-time data in cohort studies involving time-related factors. Am J Epidemiol 1987; 125(6):1085–91.

85. Greenland S, Morgenstern H. Matching and efficiency in cohort studies. Am J Epidemiol 1990; 131:151–9.

86. Coffey C, Veit F, Wolfe R, et al. Mortality in young offenders: retrospective cohort study. BMJ 2003; 326(7398):1064.

87. Doll R, Peto R. Mortality in relation to smoking: 20 years' observations on male British doctors. BMJ 1976; 2:1525–36.

88. Wacholder S, McLaughlin JK, Silverman DT, Mandel JS. Selection of controls in case-control studies. I. Principles. Am J Epidemiol 1992; 135(9):1019–28.

89. Wacholder S, Silverman DT, McLaughlin JK, Mandel JS. Selection of controls in case-control studies. II. Types of controls. Am J Epidemiol 1992; 135(9):1029–41.

90. Wacholder S, Silverman DT, McLaughlin JK, Mandel JS. Selection of controls in case-control studies. III. Design options. Am J Epidemiol 1992; 135(9):1042–50.

91. Fored CM, Ejerblad E, Lindblad P, et al. Acetaminophen, aspirin, and chronic renal failure. N Engl J Med 2001; 345(25):1801–8.

92. Cox B, Sneyd MJ, Paul C, et al. Vasectomy and risk of prostate cancer. JAMA 2002; 287(23):3110–5.

93. Nuorti JP, Butler JC, Farley MM, et al. Cigarette smoking and invasive pneumococcal disease. N Engl J Med 2000; 342(10):681–9.

94. Innes KE, Byers TE, Marshall JA, et al. Association of a woman's own birth weight with subsequent risk for gestational diabetes. JAMA 2002; 287(19):2534–41.

95. Inskip PD, Tarone RE, Hatch EE, et al. Cellular-telephone use and brain tumors. N Engl J Med 2001; 344(2):79–86.

96. Lanas A, Bajador E, Serrano P, et al. Nitrovasodilators, low-dose aspirin, other nonsteroidal antiinflammatory drugs, and the risk of upper gastrointestinal bleeding. N Engl J Med 2000; 343(12):834–9.

97. Loomis D, Marshall SW, Wolf SH, et al. Effectiveness of safety measures recommended for prevention of workplace homicide. JAMA 2002; 287(8):1011–7.

98. Fraser S, Bunce C, Wormald R, Brunner E. Deprivation and late presentation of glaucoma: case-control study. BMJ 2001; 322(7287):639–43.

99. Pearce N. Effect measures in prevalence studies. Environ Health Perspect 2004; 112(10):1047–50.

100. Siemiatycki J, Day NE, Fabry J, Cooper JA. Discovering carcinogens in the occupational environment: a novel epidemiologic approach. J Natl Cancer Inst 1981; 66(2):217–25.

101. Gerin M, Siemiatycki J, Kemper H, Begin D. Obtaining occupational exposure histories in epidemiologic case-control studies. J Occup Med 1985; 27(6):420–6.

102. Siemiatycki J, Wacholder S, Richardson L, et al. Discovering carcinogens in the occupational environment: methods of data collection and analysis of a large case-referent monitoring system. Scand J Work Environ Health 1987; 13(6):486–92.

103. Siemiatycki J. Discovering occupational carcinogens in population-based case-control studies: review of findings from an exposure-based approach and a methodologic comparison of alternative data collection strategies. Recent Results Cancer Res 1990; 120:25–38.

104. Hernandez-Diaz S, Werler MM, Walker AM, Mitchell AA. Folic acid antagonists during pregnancy and the risk of birth defects. N Engl J Med 2000; 343(22):1608–14.

105. Phillips MR, Yang G, Zhang Y, et al. Risk factors for suicide in China: a national case-control psychological autopsy study. Lancet 2002; 360(9347):1728–36.

106. Pierfitte C, Macouillard G, Thicoipe M, et al. Benzodiazepines and hip fractures in elderly people: case-control study. BMJ 2001; 322(7288):704–8.

107. Lenz SK, Goldberg MS, Labreche F, et al. Association between alcohol consumption and postmenopausal breast cancer: results of a case-control study in Montreal, Quebec, Canada. Cancer Causes Control 2002; 13(8):701–10.

108. Labreche F, Goldberg MS, Valois MF, et al. Occupational exposures to extremely low frequency magnetic fields and postmenopausal breast cancer. Am J Ind Med 2003; 44(6):643–52.

109. Band PR, Le ND, Fang R, Deschamps M. Carcinogenic and endocrine disrupting effects of cigarette smoke and risk of breast cancer. Lancet 2002; 360(9339):1044–9.

110. Scarabin PY, Oger E, Plu-Bureau G. Differential association of oral and transdermal oestrogen-replacement therapy with venous thromboembolism risk. Lancet 2003; 362(9382):428–32.

111. Nilsson M, Johnsen R, Ye W, et al. Obesity and estrogen as risk factors for gastroesophageal reflux symptoms. JAMA 2003; 290(1):66–72.

112. Westat, Inc. National Health and Nutrition Examination Survey III. Weighting and estimation methodology. Executive summary. Rockville, MD: National Center for Health Statistics; 1996.

113. Osganian SK, Stampfer MJ, Spiegelman D, et al. Distribution of and factors associated with serum homocysteine levels in children: Child and Adolescent Trial for Cardiovascular Health. JAMA 1999; 281(13):1189–96.

114. Jarvis MJ, Wardle J, Waller J, Owen L. Prevalence of hardcore smoking in England, and associated attitudes and beliefs: cross sectional study. BMJ 2003; 326(7398):1061.

115. Ross NA, Wolfson MC, Dunn JR, et al. Relation between income inequality and mortality in Canada and in the United States: cross sectional assessment using census data and vital statistics. BMJ 2000; 320(7239):898–902.

116. Morgenstern H. Ecologic studies. In: Rothman KJ Greenland S. Modern epidemiology. 2nd ed. Philadelphia, PA: Lippincott-Raven Publishers; 1998.

117. Goldberg MS, Burnett RT, Stieb D. A review of time series studies used to evaluate the short-term effects of air pollution on human health. Rev Environ Health 2004; 18:269–303.

118. Burnett RT, Dewanji A, Dominici F, et al. On the relationship between time-series studies, dynamic population studies, and estimating loss of life due to short-term exposure to environmental risks. Environ Health Perspect 2003; 111(9):1170–4.

119. Doll R, Peto R, Boreham J, Sutherland I. Smoking and dementia in male British doctors: prospective study. BMJ 2000; 320(7242):1097–102.

120. Gent JF, Triche EW, Holford TR, et al. Association of low-level ozone and fine particles with respiratory symptoms in children with asthma. JAMA 2003; 290(14):1859–67.

121. Stene LC, Magnus P, Lie RT, et al. Birth weight and childhood onset type 1 diabetes: population based cohort study. BMJ 2001; 322(7291):889–92.

122. Ojo AO, Held PJ, Port FK, et al. Chronic renal failure after transplantation of a nonrenal organ. N Engl J Med 2003; 349(10):931–40.

123. Ziegler AG, Schmid S, Huber D, et al. Early infant feeding and risk of developing type 1 diabetes-associated autoantibodies. JAMA 2003; 290(13):1721–8.

124. Israel E, Banerjee TR, Fitzmaurice GM, et al. Effects of inhaled glucocorticoids on bone density in premenopausal women. N Engl J Med 2001; 345(13):941–7.

125. Thompson JR, Gerald PF, Willoughby ML, Armstrong BK. Maternal folate supplementation in pregnancy and protection against acute lymphoblastic leukaemia in childhood: a case-control study. Lancet 2001; 358(9297):1935–40.

126. Koepsell T, McCloskey L, Wolf M, et al. Crosswalk markings and the risk of pedestrian-motor vehicle collisions in older pedestrians. JAMA 2002; 288(17):2136–43.

127. Siddiqui A, Kerb R, Weale ME, et al. Association of multidrug resistance in epilepsy with a polymorphism in the drug-transporter gene ABCB1. N Engl J Med 2003; 348(15):1442–8.

128. Li CI, Malone KE, Porter PL, et al. Relationship between long durations and different regimens of hormone therapy and risk of breast cancer. JAMA 2003; 289(24):3254–63.

129. Fahey T, Montgomery AA, Barnes J, Protheroe J. Quality of care for elderly residents in nursing homes and elderly people living at home: controlled observational study. BMJ 2003; 326(7389):580.

130. Albert CM, Mittleman MA, Chae CU, et al. Triggering of sudden death from cardiac causes by vigorous exertion. N Engl J Med 2000; 343(19):1355–61.

131. Confavreux C, Suissa S, Saddier P, et al. Vaccinations and the risk of relapse in multiple sclerosis. N Engl J Med 2001; 344(5):319–26.

132. Pell JP, Pell AC, Norrie J, et al. Effect of socioeconomic deprivation on waiting time for cardiac surgery: retrospective cohort study. BMJ 2000; 320(7226):15–8.

133. Jefferis BJ, Power C, Hertzman C. Birth weight, childhood socioeconomic environment, and cognitive development in the 1958 British birth cohort study. BMJ 2002; 325(7359):305.

134. Clancy L, Goodman P, Sinclair H, Dockery DW. Effect of air-pollution control on death rates in Dublin, Ireland: an intervention study. Lancet 2002; 360(9341):1210–4.

135. Lu-Yao G, Albertsen PC, Stanford JL, et al. Natural experiment examining impact of aggressive screening and treatment on prostate cancer mortality in two fixed cohorts from Seattle area and Connecticut. BMJ 2002; 325(7367):740.

Analysis

CHAPTER 8

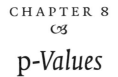

p-Values

JAMES H. WARE, PH.D., FREDERICK MOSTELLER, PH.D.,

FERNANDO DELGADO, M.S., CHRISTL DONNELLY, D.SC.,

AND JOSEPH A. INGELFINGER, M.D.

ABSTRACT   Many scientific studies use p-values to measure the strength of statistical evidence. They indicate the probability that a result at least as extreme as that observed would occur by chance. Although p-values are a way of reporting the results of statistical tests, they do not define the practical importance of the results. They depend upon a test statistic, a null hypothesis, and an alternative hypothesis. Multiple tests and selection of subgroups, outcomes, or variables for analysis can yield misleading p-values. Full reporting and statistical adjustment can help avoid these misleading values. Negative studies with low statistical power can lead to unjustified conclusions about the lack of effectiveness of medical interventions.

We discuss the role and use of p-values in scientific reporting and review the use of p-values in a sample of 25 articles from Volume 316 of the *New England Journal of Medicine.* We recommend that investigators report (1) summary statistics for the data, (2) the actual p-value rather than a range, (3) whether a test is one-sided or two-sided, (4) confidence intervals, (5) the effects of selection or multiplicity, and (6) the power of tests that describe nonsignificant comparisons.

R eaders of the medical literature encounter p-values and associated tests of significance more often than any other statistical technique. In their review of Volumes 350 through 352 of the *New England Journal of Medicine*, Horton and Switzer[1] found that 80 (26%) of the 311 articles classified as Original Articles used the t-test, and 166 (53%) used methods for the analysis of contingency tables. Other articles used p-values in association with nonparametric tests, in life-table analyses, and in the study of regression and correlation coefficients. Only 39 articles (13%) employed no statistical analyses. Of 91 Original Articles published in Volume 350 (excluding Brief Reports), 82 (90%) reported one or more p-values.

Because *p*-values play a central role in medical reporting, medical investigators and clinicians need to understand their origins, the pitfalls they present, and controversies about their use. Calculating *p*-values requires making assumptions about the data, and analyses involving the calculation of many *p*-values can be misleading. Although *p*-values can be useful as an aid to reporting, they are most informative when they are reported with descriptive information about study results.

Investigators compute *p*-values from the measurements provided by the sample of participants included in a scientific study and use these values to draw conclusions about the population from which the observations were drawn. For example, in a study of patients undergoing coronary bypass surgery, Mangano et al.[2] reported that mortality was 1.3% (40 of 2999) among patients who received aspirin within 48 hours after revascularization and 4.0% (81 of 2023) among those who did not receive aspirin during this period ($p < 0.001$). The authors concluded from the small *p*-value that patients who received aspirin during this period were at reduced risk, as compared with patients who did not. This example illustrates a major use of *p*-values: to determine whether an observed effect can be explained by chance, i.e., random variation in patient outcomes. The specific meaning of the statement "$p < 0.001$" is that the observed difference *or a more extreme difference* in mortality rates would occur with probability less than 0.001 if the true mortality rates were identical for patients who did and who did not receive aspirin within 48 hours after revascularization. We return to these concepts below.

The frequent reporting of *p*-values attests to a wide belief in their usefulness in communicating scientific results. Moreover, the *p*-value associated with the primary results of a scientific study can be a factor in an editorial decision about publishing those results.[3] Thus, clear and consistent practices in the calculation and citation of *p*-values are important elements of good scientific reporting. The interpretation of a *p*-value can depend substantially on the design of the study, the method of collecting data, and the analytic practices used. Scientific reports frequently underemphasize or omit information that readers need to assess an author's conclusions. As a result, readers sometimes misunderstand the importance of either a highly significant or a nonsignificant *p*-value.

This chapter describes the basic ideas in a *p*-value calculation. The actual calculation of *p*-values is discussed in many textbooks.[4-7] We also discuss the value of confidence intervals as a complement to *p*-values, review controversies regarding the use of *p*-values in medical reporting, and recommend six specific practices for the reporting of *p*-values.

To sharpen our understanding of the current role of *p*-values in medical reporting, we reviewed the use of *p*-values and related statistical information in 25

Original Articles selected over 20 years ago from the *New England Journal of Medicine* (Volume 316, January–June 1987). In discussions of controversies and recommendations regarding current use of p-values, we discuss how the issue was managed in these 25 articles and in articles chosen from recent literature.

WHAT ARE *p*-VALUES?

p-values are used to assess the degree of dissimilarity between two or more sets of measurements or between one set of measurements and a standard. A p-value is a probability, usually the probability of obtaining a result as extreme as, or more extreme than, the one observed if the dissimilarity is entirely due to random variation in measurements or in subject response—that is, if it is the result of chance alone. For example, Yanovski et al.,[8] in reporting a study of holiday weight gain, state that "the perceived weight gain (1.57 ± 1.47 kg) was significantly greater than the measured weight gain by an average of 1.12 ± 1.79 kg ($p < 0.001$ by paired t-test)." Here, the p-value indicates that an average difference between the measured and perceived weight gains of study participants at least as great as that observed would occur with probability less than 0.001, or in less than 1 in 1000 trials, if there were no true difference between the average measured and perceived weight gain in the population represented by the study participants and if the assumed probability model were correct. The p-value depends implicitly on three elements: the test statistic, the null hypothesis, and the alternative hypothesis.

The Test Statistic

To summarize the dissimilarity between two sets of data, we choose a statistic that reflects the differences likely to be caused by the treatment or condition under study, such as the difference in means, which may use a t-statistic, or a difference in death rates, which may use a chi-squared statistic. Yanovski et al.[8] determined the perceived and measured weight gain for each study participant and calculated the paired t-statistic from these changes to test for a difference between perceived and actual weight gain. In the study of cardiac surgery cited earlier, Mangano and colleagues used a different statistic, the chi-squared test for association between death and receipt of aspirin, which they computed from the numbers of subjects and deaths in each of the two groups.

The p-value properly reflects the relative frequency of getting values of the statistic as extreme as the one observed when the pattern of results is due entirely to random variation. When systematic effects are present, such as treatment increasing length of life or increasing probability of survival in a surgical operation, the statistic should tend to reflect this by being more likely to produce extreme, usually small, *p*-values. When small *p*-values occur, they signal either that a rare random event has occurred or that a systematic effect is present. In a well-designed study, the investigator usually finds the systematic effect more plausible.

The Null Hypothesis

The information needed for the calculation of the *p*-value comes from expressing a scientific hypothesis in probabilistic terms. In the analysis mentioned above from the study by Yanovski et al., the scientific hypothesis to be tested statistically (though not necessarily what the authors expected or hoped to find) was that the true average perceived holiday weight gain was equal to the true average measured weight gain in the study population. Such a hypothesis is called a null hypothesis, the "null" implying that no effect beyond random variation is present. If this null hypothesis were true, the mean difference between the perceived and measured weight gain would vary around zero in repeated sampling.

Although the null hypothesis is central to the calculation of a *p*-value, only 4 of the 25 articles we reviewed from Volume 316 of the *New England Journal of Medicine* stated the null hypothesis explicitly. In most articles, the null hypothesis was defined implicitly by statements such as "calorie-adjusted potassium intake [was] significantly lower in the men and women who subsequently had a stroke-associated death, as compared with all other subjects ($p = 0.06$)."[9] Although such implicit definitions could, in principle, be ambiguous, we found no instances of such ambiguities in the 25 articles we reviewed.

One might ask why small or large *p*-values give us any feeling about the truth of the null hypothesis. After all, if chance alone were at work, a small *p*-value would merely tell us that a rare event has occurred, just as a large *p*-value goes with a likely event. This argument calls attention to another concept needed to understand *p*-values: the alternative hypothesis.

The Alternative Hypothesis

When investigators report *p*-values, they have an underlying, but usually unstated, notion that the null hypothesis may be false and that some other situation may be the true one. For example, Yanovski et al. had an alternative hypothesis in mind—that study participants would not accurately estimate their weight gain. (Because this alternative hypothesis includes all of the amounts by which study participants might underestimate or overestimate their weight gain, statisticians sometimes speak of alternative *hypotheses*.) Statistical tests are designed so that small *p*-values are more likely to occur when the null hypothesis is false.

Thus, we reject the null hypothesis not only because the probability of such an event is low when there is no effect, but also because the probability is greater when there is an effect. These two ideas together encourage us to believe that an alternative hypothesis is true when the test of the null hypothesis yields a small p-value for the observed effect.

Notice the similarity between this way of thinking and proof by contradiction. Logicians state as a premise whatever they intend to disprove. If a valid argument from that point leads to a contradiction, the premise in question must be false. In statistics, we follow this approach, but instead of reaching an absolute contradiction, we may observe an improbable outcome.[10] We must then conclude either that the null hypothesis is correct and the improbable has happened, or that the null hypothesis is false. Deciding between these two possibilities can be difficult. One question that arises is how small the probability should be before we can conclude that the null hypothesis is mistaken.

Authors rarely state the alternative hypothesis explicitly. In our review of 25 articles from Volume 316 of the *New England Journal of Medicine*, we found no instances in which authors did so. There is greater potential for ambiguity with implicit specification of alternative hypotheses than with null hypotheses. Nevertheless, we could infer the alternative hypothesis in each of the 25 articles we reviewed.

THE 0.05 AND 0.01 SIGNIFICANCE LEVELS

The p-value measures surprise. The smaller the p-value, the more surprising the result if the null hypothesis is true. Sometimes a very rough idea of the degree of surprise suffices, and various simplifying conventions have come into use. One popular approach is to indicate only that the p-value is smaller than 0.05 ($p < 0.05$) or smaller than 0.01 ($p < 0.01$). When the p-value is between 0.05 and 0.01, the result is usually called "statistically significant"; when it is less than 0.01, the result is often called "highly statistically significant." This standardization of wording has both advantages and disadvantages. Its main advantage is that it gives investigators a specific, objectively chosen level to keep in mind. In the past it was sometimes easier to determine whether a p-value was smaller than or larger than 0.05 than it was to compute the exact probability, but powerful desktop statistical software has made this circumstance rare. The main disadvantage of this wording is that it suggests a rather mindless cut-off point, which has nothing to do with the importance of the decision to be made or with the costs and losses associated with the outcomes.

The 0.05 level was popularized in part through its use in quality-control work, where the emphasis is on the performance of a decision rule in repeated testing. This viewpoint carries over reasonably well to the relatively small and

frequently repeated studies of process and mechanism that represent the building blocks of scientific understanding. In the large, expensive clinical trials and
descriptive studies that are increasingly common in modern science, however,
the protection provided by repetition is rarely available.

Confidence Intervals

Some methodologists argue that medical reports rely too heavily on *p*-values,
especially when the *p*-value is the only statistical information reported.[11–13]
Because no single study determines scientific opinion on a subject, it is incum-
bent upon the investigator to provide a more-extensive analysis of study results.
In particular, these observers recommend that investigators routinely report
confidence intervals rather than *p*-values.[11]

We create confidence intervals for a given degree of confidence, such as 95%.
The 95% tells how often such intervals include the true value of the estimated
statistic, such as the mean or a correlation coefficient. If we assert that the
true value is in the interval, we will be right in 95% of the assertions, barring
breakdowns in the assumptions. In the study by Yanovski et al.,[8] the two-sided
95% confidence interval for the mean perceived weight gain during the holiday
period (assuming a sample size of 195) is 1.36 to 1.78 kg. The confidence interval gives information not given by the *p*-value; it reports information in terms of
the measurements actually used, and the width of the confidence interval gives
an indication of the informativeness of the data. The width is usually closely
related to the standard error of the statistic being assessed, often about four
times as wide. For example, in large samples the 95% confidence interval for
population means extends 1.96 standard errors above the observed mean and
1.96 standard errors below, and therefore is about 4 standard errors wide. Confidence intervals can also be calculated for confidence levels other than 95%,
but this is uncommon.

We agree that sole reliance on the *p*-value is incomplete reporting, especially
when the *p*-value is reported only as a range. The *p*-value does, however, provide
information not provided by the confidence interval. The statement "$p = 0.002$"
gives an indication of degree of extremity that may not be readily apparent from
noting that a null value is outside the 95% confidence interval. Citing both the
actual *p*-value and the confidence interval provides more information than either
report can provide alone. Reporting basic summary statistics, such as the mean
and the standard error, will usually aid readers in understanding the study and
its conclusions. This practice is well established in the *New England Journal of
Medicine*. All but 3 of the 25 articles we reviewed used either confidence intervals
or standard errors to describe the precision of an estimate.

Other Criticisms of *p*-Values

Some statisticians criticize the *p*-value as a measure of strength of evidence. Diamond and Forrester[14] pointed out that, in the language of diagnostic testing, the *p*-value corresponds to the false-positive rate, the probability of the observed result or one more extreme if the null hypothesis is true. It is *not* the probability that the alternative hypothesis is true given the data. They argued that the popularity of the *p*-value as a measure of the strength of evidence results in part from the mistaken belief among many physicians and other scientists that it does have this interpretation.

Diamond and Forrester noted that the probability that an alternative hypothesis is true depends not only on the *p*-value but also on the prior probability that the hypothesis is true, which may not be known. This issue is identical to that encountered in the interpretation of diagnostic test results. For example, if practically no one in the population has the disease, most diagnoses based on fallible tests will be false positives, whereas if the disease is common, fewer diagnoses will be false positives. Similarly, if effects in the real world almost never or almost always happen, then positive findings are usually mistaken in the first case and almost certainly correct in the second. Many statisticians believe that this is not a limitation of the *p*-value, preferring that data should be described using statistics that depend only on the data, not on subjective information such as prior probabilities. In this latter view, readers of scientific reports should provide their own prior probabilities of various hypotheses.

p-VALUES AND SIGNIFICANCE TESTS

p-values are an integral part of the statistical technique known as hypothesis testing or significance testing. Hypothesis testing is a method for choosing between the null hypothesis and alternative hypotheses. To explain the connection between *p*-values and hypothesis testing, we can describe formal hypothesis testing as consisting of the following steps: (1) choose a test statistic; (2) choose the significance level, α, of the test; (3) compute the *p*-value; and (4) if the *p*-value is smaller than α, reject the null hypothesis in favor of the alternative hypothesis or hypotheses; otherwise, do not reject the null hypothesis. For example, when the significance level, α, is 0.05, hypothesis testing leads to rejection of the null hypothesis if the *p*-value is less than 0.05.

Given the test used to compute the *p*-value, the significance level, and the number of observations made, one can determine in advance the set of values of the statistic that would result in rejection of the null hypothesis. This set of values is called the *critical region*. Thus, another description of the fourth step in hypothesis testing is this: (4) if the statistic falls into the critical region, reject the null hypothesis; otherwise, do not reject the null hypothesis. (Statisticians say that we "fail to reject" the null hypothesis to emphasize that the data cannot prove the null hypothesis to be true. Future studies may show that it is highly improbable.)

Mangano et al.[2] used the chi-squared test for association to compare the mortality rates for patients who did and who did not receive aspirin within 48 hours of surgery. In this instance, the critical region consisted of all mortality outcomes that led to a value for chi-squared of more than 3.84, the upper 0.05 critical value of the chi-squared distribution with 1 degree of freedom.

Note that the words "accept" and "reject" are merely formal labels like "success" and "failure"; they do not correspond to any particular action. The implication of the word "reject" is simply that substantial evidence against the null hypothesis has been supplied. The use of the words "accept" and "reject" is an unfortunate convention, possibly a holdover from sampling methods for quality control, in which the sampling was used to determine what to do about a batch of manufactured materials, where options might have included selling the batch at usual prices, selling it at reduced prices, scrapping it altogether, and so on.

ISSUES IN REPORTING AND INTERPRETING p-VALUES

When one considers the frequent use of p-values in the medical literature and the emphasis sometimes placed on the statistical significance of a study's results, it is not surprising that controversies have arisen about the methods used to compute and interpret p-values. The next sections of this chapter discuss some of these controversies.

One- and Two-Sided Tests

In many calculations of p-values the investigator must choose between the one-sided and the two-sided approach. The one-sided p-value, used mainly in comparisons between two treatment groups, is the probability of observing a difference *favorable to the innovation* as extreme as or more extreme than the one observed, if the null hypothesis is true. The two-sided p-value is the probability of observing a difference *in either direction* as extreme as or more extreme than the one observed. The two-sided p-value is often approximately and sometimes exactly twice as large as the one-sided p-value.

In some situations a good argument can be made for reporting the one-sided p-value. In studies comparing an innovation with a standard regimen, for example, the alternative hypothesis of greatest interest may be that the innovation is superior. The distinction between an ineffective and a detrimental innovation may be unimportant for medical practice. When data on patient outcomes are accumulated gradually, it may even be unethical to continue a trial for the purpose of making this distinction. In another circumstance the purpose of the trial may be to show that an innovation is at least as effective as the standard. Such trials, known as non-inferiority trials, are employed when the new agent offers ease of administration, fewer side effects, or other advantages. In that case, the distinction between superiority and therapeutic equivalence may be of limited importance.

Despite these arguments, some statisticians, journal editors, and regulatory officials believe that one-sided *p*-values should never be used in reporting comparisons between treatment groups. First, they argue that readers will benefit from uniform practices in reporting of *p*-values, so that a *p*-value of a given size has the same meaning across all articles. Second, they believe that the situations justifying a one-sided test are rare, and that most uses of one-sided *p*-values are more properly viewed as attempts to exaggerate the strength of a finding. Thus, investigators planning to cite one-sided *p*-values must be prepared to defend them. This is one of the issues that investigators should address while planning a study, and they should defend their decision from the outset. The early decision to use a one-sided test for the specific comparison presented should be documented. Even when this is done, investigators may encounter editorial resistance if they report one-sided *p*-values in scientific articles.

A third concern with one-sided *p*-values arises when a study is important to a scientific or regulatory decision about the efficacy of a drug. To approve the introduction of a new drug, a regulatory group should be convinced that the expected benefits of the drug outweigh its costs and risks. The *p*-value from a scientific study is only one factor in this decision, and the criterion that the *p*-value be less than 0.05 may sometimes appear to be insufficiently stringent for establishing efficacy. Insisting on two-sided tests is one way to be more conservative. When issues like this are behind a debate about "sidedness," the ideal resolution would be for investigators to discuss more directly the criteria for sufficient evidence. Usually, the actual average value of the treatment effect and a measure of its variability will be more helpful than the *p*-value to those who must weigh costs and benefits.

We believe that the distinction between one- and two-sided *p*-values is not of fundamental importance in interpreting the results of a study, provided that the investigator clearly states which type of statistic was used. If readers are told what the test was about, what measure was used, and whether one-sided or two-sided results are being reported, they can usually recalculate the *p*-value, at least approximately, in the form they believe most appropriate. Investigators should be aware, however, that this position is not uniformly held, and that any use of one-sided p-values may be regarded skeptically by some editors and referees.

In our review of 25 articles from Volume 316 of the *New England Journal of Medicine*, we found one use of one-sided p-values[15] to test a null hypothesis. In 11 other articles the information provided was not sufficient to determine whether p-values were one- or two-sided. The remaining 13 articles used two-sided p-values.

One-Sided, Two-Sided, or Three-Sided?

In fact, the usual two-sided formulation of a test for assessing the difference in performance of two treatments offers only two decisions; either the treatments are alike (there is no evidence of a difference) or they differ. From a statistical point of view, the report based on a two-sided p-value should be "alike" (not significantly different) or "different," but not that "the innovation is more effective than standard therapy." Both investigators and readers might be surprised to learn that a study has shown only that two treatments are different, without commenting on directionality, but this is the proper interpretation of the two-sided test.

If we want to know which treatment is preferable, we are in at least a three-decision problem, with one tail representing "innovation preferred," one representing "standard preferred," and the center for "insufficient evidence to declare a difference." It may be useful to keep track of the total probability of declaring a difference, the usual two-sided total, but what matters in the decision is the probability associated with a particular extreme outcome.

Multiplicity

Often investigators report many p-values in the same study, and still other p-value calculations are unreported. Because p-values smaller than 0.05 occur by chance in 5% of tests of true null hypotheses, the probability that at least one p-value will be smaller than 0.05 increases with the number of comparisons, even when the null hypothesis is correct for each comparison. This increase is known as the *multiple-comparisons* problem. When several comparisons are performed simultaneously, both the calculation and the interpretation of p-values must be reexamined.

The rate at which statistically significant results occur in tests of null hypotheses is sometimes called the *false-positive rate*. For tests at the 0.05 level, the false-positive rate is 1 in 20 tests. Consider the investigator who studies several treatments in a single clinical trial. If all pairs of treatments are compared with respect to a single outcome (such as recovery), and if a standard significance test for two groups is used for each comparison, then the probability of finding at least one significant difference increases rapidly with the number of treatments, even when the null hypothesis—that all of the treatments are of equal efficacy—is true. To ensure that the probability of one or more false-positive results is no greater than a specified value, say 0.05, the investigator must use special statistical methods that take into account the number and type of comparisons made. These methods are called multiple-comparisons procedures. Glantz[16] recommends that these procedures be used routinely in the analysis of studies comparing three or more groups, and Godfrey[17] reviews some of the multiple-comparisons procedures for comparing several group means.

When an investigation is complex and involves many different kinds of comparisons and tests of interrelated hypotheses, an attempt to adjust for multiplicity may be inconsistent with the objectives of the study. Indeed, in attempting to decide when to adjust for multiplicity, one encounters a conceptual difficulty with the idea of multiple-comparisons tests. If a scientific paper includes multiple tests of different hypotheses, that set of tests may not be the natural unit for controlling the overall probability of a false-positive result. One might argue, for example, that one should control the probability of one or more false-positive results for all of the tests performed with data collected in a single study or even, to take the argument to an extreme, for all of the related tests performed in many studies by a single scientific investigator. Because of these conceptual difficulties, no consensus has been reached about the appropriate use of multiple-comparisons procedures in the typical multifaceted scientific study. This difficulty has led some statisticians to reject multiple-comparisons procedures entirely in favor of simply recognizing the effects of multiple testing. In that view 1 of every 20 tests will produce a p-value smaller than 0.05 merely by chance, and this likelihood must simply be kept in mind in the interpretation of any collection of hypothesis tests and their p-values.

Although many of the articles reviewed from Volume 316 of the *New England Journal of Medicine* reported numerous p-values, only one[18] made an adjustment for multiplicity. This paper used Bonferroni's method to adjust for multiple comparisons in repeated analyses of a group evaluated on several occasions.

The problem of multiplicity can arise in a variety of ways. Three common practices—repeated analyses of accumulating data, the evaluation of several endpoints, and the selection of subgroups of interest by the results of the analysis—can substantially increase the probability of finding incorrectly at least one comparison that is statistically significant. In a notable example, the Food and Drug Administration refused to approve a claim based on the Anturane Reinfarction Trial[19] that sulfinpyrazone (Anturane) was effective in the prevention of sudden death in the six months after myocardial infarction. One of the reasons given by the FDA officials for this decision was that a reported *p*-value of 0.003 for comparing the frequency of sudden death in the first six months after infarction exaggerated the strength of the evidence against the null hypothesis because the endpoint, the time interval after infarction, and the subset of enrolled patients included in the final analysis had all been identified through repeated analysis of accumulating data rather than by criteria specified before the study began.[20]

Selection of subgroups, endpoints, or analytic methods leads to multiple-comparisons problems because each selection creates opportunities for choice and thus for significance. Selection effects may be difficult to recognize unless the investigators report fully on their methods. For example, if 10 endpoints are studied and only the 1 that changed significantly is reported, the reader cannot recognize the selection problem. The reader may therefore be wise to take a jaundiced view of unusual endpoints offered without justification. A more subtle form of the multiple-comparisons problem, in which investigators inspect the data and actually perform the test only where they think it might yield "positive" results, is discussed below under post-hoc hypotheses.

Accepted methods for managing the multiple-comparisons problem differ among various types of investigations. When investigators design randomized clinical trials intended to be clinically directive or to win regulatory approval of a new drug, they typically develop a testing procedure that maintains an overall Type I error rate of 0.05 for the study as a whole. This is known as the "experiment-wise" error rate. The simplest way to achieve this goal is to declare a single primary hypothesis and indicate that the outcome of the trial will be judged on the results for this single test performed once at the end of the study. A variant of this approach is to declare two or more primary hypotheses and distribute the Type I error rate among the hypotheses, for example, by testing each hypothesis at the α/k level if k is the number of tests. This technique, mentioned earlier, is known as the Bonferroni method. In this approach, the investigators may identify secondary and tertiary hypotheses, but it is understood that the study can not provide a definitive test of these hypotheses. In recent years investigators involved in drug development have made increasing use of so-called "gatekeeping" procedures[21] in which hypotheses are ordered hierarchically and hypotheses lower in the hierarchy can be tested only if hypotheses above them in the hierarchy have been rejected. These procedures also maintain a specified experiment-wise error rate.

In one important example of the multiple-comparisons problem, concerns about patient safety or other issues may require periodic analysis of accumulating data during the course of a clinical trial. Analyses conducted during the course of a trial are called *interim* analyses. These interim analyses induce a multiple-comparisons problem because they provide multiple opportunities to stop the study and draw conclusions from the data about the safety or effi-cacy of study treatments. To manage this problem, statisticians have created a special set of statistical methods known as sequential analysis plans, monitor-ing plans, or stopping rules.[22] These methods stipulate the times or fractions of the data at which analyses will be conducted and the critical values to be employed at each interim analysis so as to achieve the desired error rate over the entire set of repeated analyses. If a study with a sequential analysis plan is continued to the final analysis, a larger critical value is employed at that analysis to ensure that the study design as a whole has the desired Type I error rate, say 0.05. In recent years, these methods have become increasingly flexible to allow additional analyses, analyses at unplanned time points, and the like. Like all multiple-comparisons procedures, however, these methods have their limitations. Most importantly, they are ordinarily designed to monitor only the primary study endpoint. If troubling results emerge for a secondary endpoint or for a safety outcome, the monitoring plan may provide little guidance about the statistical significance of the observed differences.

Observational studies can also raise challenging multiple-comparisons prob-lems. When a large cohort study is conducted over many years, investigators may measure many exposures and many outcomes. As a result, a single study can generate dozens, if not hundreds, of hypotheses. Nevertheless, adjustment for multiple comparisons is uncommon in the reporting of observational stud-ies. In part, this reflects recognition of the fact that it would be difficult in these situations to describe the universe of hypotheses that have been or could have been tested. Given that uncertainty, investigators may choose to accept a test-wise error rate of 0.05 and keep that in mind when interpreting the data. In fact, many epidemiologists believe that the notion of multiple comparisons is of limited utility in the interpretation of observational studies. Instead, they believe that investigators must evaluate each analysis in its epidemiologic and biological context, recognizing that tests for association between different pairs of exposures and outcomes represent different scientific questions.

The development of sophisticated methods for analysis of the human genome has brought new attention to the problem of multiple comparisons. As one exam-ple of this issue, gene chips are now available that can characterize single nucle-otide polymorphisms (SNPs) at up to 500,000 loci for each individual studied. If a study is designed to identify differences between the distributions of SNPs in individuals with and without a disease, up to 500,000 comparisons are possible. Thus, one might expect as many as 25,000 statistically significant associations at the 0.05 level merely by chance. One early strategy for managing this problem focused on the use of a more stringent criterion for statistical significance. If one requires a *p*-value of 0.0001, for example, only 50 false-positive results in 500,000 independent tests of true null hypotheses are expected. Experience has shown, however, that even this level of seeming conservatism has not been sufficient to prevent the proliferation of "discoveries" of genes associated with disease that could not be replicated. Thus, studies designed to identify new genes associated with individual diseases now typically investigate one study population to identify candidate genes and then conduct a confirmatory study in a different population. This effectively builds the well-recognized principle of replication into the design of a single study.

Primary, Secondary, and Post-Hoc Hypotheses

In some studies investigators specify a small set of primary hypotheses to be tested by the study. The methods for testing these hypotheses may be described in detail in the protocol, and statistical procedures are specified that ensure that the probability of any false-positive result does not exceed a specified level, say 0.05, for the set of tests of the primary hypotheses. Additional hypotheses of interest to investigators may also be identified in advance and described as secondary hypotheses. Typically, each test of a secondary hypothesis or of post-hoc hypotheses (those that emerge in the data analysis) is reported with the nominal *p*-value arising when that test is considered alone.

This strategy parallels Tukey's distinction between *exploratory* and *confirmatory* data analysis.[23] The confirmatory analysis tests the primary hypotheses, to justify the use of the results in decision making—for example, regarding the acceptance of a new drug. A thorough exploration of study data often produces additional hypotheses; they may be more or less anticipated when the study is designed, but are interpreted as "post-hoc"; that is, they arise from the data analysis. Post hoc findings must be interpreted cautiously, in light of the regular occurrence of false-positive findings in multiple comparisons. This distinction is useful in both study design and data analysis. It offers a practical strategy for resolving some aspects of the multiple-comparisons problem.

Bias

Although small *p*-values may make chance an unlikely explanation for differences between two groups, they do not necessarily imply that the differences are due to the therapy or exposure. Instead, the differences may result from other characteristics of the study such as differences in participant characteristics, methods of management, or methods of measurement between the groups to be compared. The tendency of groups within a study to respond differently because of such non-comparability is called a nonrandom error or a nonsampling error or bias. It is assumed to be absent in the usual interpretation of both *p*-values and confidence intervals. Methods for reducing bias are discussed elsewhere.[24, 25]

Precise p-Values

In any situation later investigators will find the exact p-value more helpful than a range, such as $p < 0.05$, when they combine the results of one study with those of other investigations. As a practical matter, however, the investigator who determines p-values by reference to statistical tables will find that for many problems, tables are conveniently available for only a few significance levels.

Although practice varied somewhat in the *Journal* articles we reviewed, many authors quoted p-values less than 0.05 as a range, for example, $p < 0.05$, $p < 0.02$, or $p < 0.01$, and values above 0.05 as NS (nonsignificant). Each of these practices, but especially reporting a p-value simply as NS, is a form of incomplete reporting. This is easily repaired by giving the actual p-value. Modern statistical software makes it easy to compute p-values to the desired level of precision. For many simple tests, including the two-sample t-test and Fisher's exact test for 2×2 tables, p-value calculators can be found online.

STATISTICAL POWER AND SAMPLE SIZE

Investigators often ask statisticians to calculate an appropriate sample size for a particular study. Sample size calculations of this kind depend on the endpoint to be analyzed, the statistical method to be used, and the magnitude of the difference that the investigators want to detect. Once a significance level has been chosen, one can calculate the probability that the null hypothesis will be rejected when there is an effect of a given size. This probability is the *power* of the test for that size of effect. Sample size and the power of the statistical test have a close connection.

Statistical power affects both the design and the interpretation of scientific studies. Studies with low power are likely to be negative, and published results may discourage further research in that direction if the limitations of the study are not appreciated. Reviews of papers reporting the results of therapeutic trials have shown that studies frequently have low power for important alternative hypotheses. For example, Freiman et al.[26] found that of 71 randomized trials for which the authors reported "no effect," 67 (94%) had power smaller than 0.9 for an alternative hypothesis of a 25% therapeutic improvement, and 50 (70%) of the trials had power smaller than 0.9 for a 50% improvement. This means that, in 94% of the studies, there was a greater than 10% chance of missing a 25% therapeutic improvement, and in 70% of the studies there was a similar chance of missing a 50% improvement. (Freiman et al. used a one-tailed test with a significance level of 0.05.)

The reluctance of authors and editors to publish the results of studies that describe nonsignificant comparisons can produce the opposite problem. A proliferation of small trials can lead to overrepresentation of the 1 in 20 trials that achieve a *p*-value of less than 0.05 by chance. Zelen[3] estimated that 6000 to 10,000 therapeutic investigations of patients with cancer were in progress during 1982 and that these trials could generate as many as 300 to 500 false-positive reports.

The problem of false-positive findings can be addressed in part by reporting confidence intervals as well as significance levels. The confidence interval identifies the range of values, such as differences in treatment effects, that are compatible with the study results; wide confidence intervals help to identify studies with low reliability. Discussions of power also have a place in reports of study results. For example, the statement that the study had a power of 15% to detect a 50% reduction in mortality conveys information different from the corresponding confidence interval because it says, "We scarcely had a chance," and it facilitates proper weighing of negative studies. Only 1 of the 25 articles from Volume 316 of the *New England Journal of Medicine* provided quantitative information about the power of a negative result,[27] in part because only 4 articles reported negative results for hypotheses of primary interest. In recent years, however, the editors of the *New England Journal of Medicine* have routinely required a discussion of sample size and power in the Methods section of reports of randomized clinical trials. For example, 19 of 21 reports of randomized trials in the first 13 issues of Volume 355 (2006) included an explicit discussion of sample size and power.

STATISTICAL AND MEDICAL SIGNIFICANCE

Statisticians have adopted the word "significance" to describe the results of statistical tests of hypotheses, but confusion between the everyday meaning of the word and its technical meaning muddies the waters. Although *statistical significance* is a technical term, *medical significance* is more difficult to define because it usually means "importance." Four possibilities exist in describing the implications of study results. Some findings are both statistically significant and medically significant; other findings are neither. The more troublesome results are significant in only one of these senses. When samples are very large, small differences may be statistically significant even though they have no importance in clinical practice or possibly even in public health. At the other extreme, small samples may produce large differences so imprecisely determined that they are not statistically significant.

To illustrate this point, we consider a study by Davis et al. of the effect of captopril on cardiac index in patients with congestive heart failure.[28] The investigators found that, at single daily doses of captopril of 25 to 150 mg, "the cardiac index rose from 1.75 ± 0.18 to 2.27 ± 0.39 liters per minute per

Table 1. Two-Sided p-Values for Increases in Mean Cardiac Index Observed in Studies with Several Sample Sizes.

Mean Increase*	Sample Size		
	10	25	100
0.10	$p = 0.29$	$p = 0.09$	$p < 0.001$
0.25	$p = 0.01$	$p < 0.001$	$p < 0.001$
0.50	$p < 0.001$	$p < 0.001$	$p < 0.001$

*Liters per minute per square meter. SD = 0.3 in each instance.

square meter ($p < 0.001$)." Suppose that the standard deviation of change in cardiac index is 0.3 liter per minute per square meter, a value close to the estimated standard deviation of 0.27 reported by Davis et al. Whereas the medical significance of a treatment effect depends on the size of the average increase in cardiac index, the p-value depends on both the observed mean increase and the sample size. Although a mean increase of 0.50 liter per minute per square meter would be statistically significant for any sample size between 10 and 100 patients, an increase of 0.10 liter per minute per square meter would generate a p-value between 0.29 (defined as nonsignificant) and less than 0.001 (highly significant), depending on the size of the sample (Table 1). The point is that p-values are useful for assessing the role of chance in producing an observed effect of treatment, but the medical importance of that effect depends on its magnitude. This example shows once again the value of citing confidence intervals in scientific reports. For instance, a mean increase of 0.10 liter per minute per square meter in a study with sample size of 100 yields the 95% confidence interval (0.04–0.16), whereas a mean increase of 0.50 in a study with 10 patients yields the 95% confidence interval (0.29–0.71).

Although we have recommended that p-values be reported as actual values rather than as a range, we report only $p < 0.001$ in Table 1. We see little value in reporting the exact p-value when it is smaller than 0.001 because the precise p-value associated with very extreme results is sensitive to small biases or departures from the assumed probability model.

RECOMMENDATIONS

One should not equate p-values or the results of hypothesis testing with decisions. p-values are a way of reporting the results of statistical analyses. Similarly, the result of a hypothesis test might be best described as a conclusion, rather than a decision, to emphasize that the results of hypothesis tests are another way of reporting data. Decisions depend on conclusions but also on such factors as costs, risks, size of effect, consequences, and policy considerations. Issues of institutional decision making and many other factors can also affect the decision. Hypothesis tests and p-values give us a form of reporting that has value because it can be standardized. The practical decision is a separate matter that is based on p-values and related information but not on the p-values alone.

Our review of the issues that arise in reporting and interpreting p-values suggests several practices that we think should routinely be followed in scientific reporting (see also the Uniform Requirements for Manuscripts Submitted to Biomedical Journals[29] and Chapter 14 of this book):

(1)   Report basic summary statistics, such as the mean and the standard deviation, not just the results of a statistical test.

(2)   When it is computationally feasible, report the actual p-value (such as $p = 0.03$) rather than an inequality (such as $p < 0.05$). This practice provides additional information, usually at the cost of little added effort.

(3)   State clearly, whenever the distinction is relevant, whether a p-value is for a one-sided or a two-sided test.

(4)   Report confidence intervals or standard errors to communicate the range of values consistent with the study data. Although confidence intervals may not always be necessary, they should be included more frequently in reports of major findings.

(5)   Discuss the effect of multiplicity on the reported p-values. Although formal multiple-comparisons procedures may not be available for a particular kind of analysis, the interpretation of p-values often depends on the extent to which the final results arose from comparisons of several groups or measurements made on several occasions, as well as on multiplicities in data analysis, such as the use of several statistical tests, the exclusion of "atypical" patients, and data exploration.

(6)   Discuss the statistical power of negative studies. Small studies are likely to be interpreted as unduly discouraging about the value of further investigation if the limited power of the study is not reported.

These proposals have implications for the design and conduct of scientific studies. They imply that investigators should consider power in designing studies. They also indicate the importance of specifying the hypotheses to be studied and the associated analyses before the study begins, in order to avoid ambiguities that may arise from analyses that were suggested only by the data. The steps necessary to ensure the validity of p-values are not technically difficult, yet they can substantially improve the prospects of achieving the goals of a scientific study.

REFERENCES

1. Horton NJ, Switzer SS. Statistical methods in the *Journal*. N Engl J Med 2005; 353:1977–9.

2. Mangano DT for the Multicenter Study of Perioperative Ischemia Research Group. Aspirin and mortality from coronary bypass surgery. N Engl J Med 2002; 347:1309–17.

3. Zelen M. Strategy and alternate randomized designs in cancer clinical trials. Cancer Treat Rep 1982; 66:1095–100.

4. Ingelfinger JA, Mosteller F, Thibodeau LA, Ware JH. Biostatistics in clinical medicine. 2nd ed. New York: Macmillan, 1987.

5. Snedecor GW, Cochran WG. Statistical methods. 8th ed. Ames, Iowa: Iowa State University Press, 1989.

6. Colton T. Statistics in medicine. Boston: Little, Brown, 1974.

7. Armitage P, Berry G, Matthews JNS. Statistical methods in medical research. 4th ed. New York: John Wiley, 2001.

8. Yanovski JA, Yanovski SZ, Sovik KN, et al. A prospective study of holiday weight gain. N Engl J Med 2000; 342:861–7.

9. Khaw K-T, Barrett-Connor E. Dietary potassium and stroke-associated mortality: a 12-year prospective population study. N Engl J Med 1987; 316:235–40.

10. Gore SM. Assessing methods—art of significance testing. Br Med J 1981; 283:600–2.

11. Rothman KJ. A show of confidence. N Engl J Med 1978; 299:1362–3.

12. Rothman KJ. The role of significance testing in epidemiologic research. Chapter 9 in Modern epidemiology. New York: Little, Brown, 1985.

13. Walker AM. Reporting the results of epidemiologic studies. Am J Pub Hlth 1986; 76:556–8.

14. Diamond GA, Forrester JS. Clinical trials and statistical verdicts: probable grounds for appeal. Ann Intern Med 1983; 98:385–94.

15. McPherson DD, Hiratzka LF, Lamberth DC, et al. Delineation of the extent of coronary atherosclerosis by high-frequency epicardial echocardiography. N Engl J Med 1987; 316:304–9.

16. Glantz SA. Biostatistics: how to detect, correct and prevent errors in the medical literature. Circulation 1980; 61:1–7.

17. Godfrey K. Comparing the means of several groups. N Engl J Med 1985; 313:1450–6. [Expanded in Chapter 12 of the second edition of this book.]

18. Totterman TH, Karlsson FA, Bengtsson M, Mendel-Hartvig I. Induction of circulating activated suppressor-like T cells by methimazole therapy for Graves disease. N Engl J Med 1987; 316:15–22.

19. Anturane Reinfarction Trial Research Group. Sulfinpyrazone in the prevention of sudden death after myocardial infarction. N Engl J Med 1980; 302:250–6.

20. Temple R, Pledger GW. The FDA's critique of the Anturane Reinfarction Trial. N Engl J Med 1980; 303:1488–92.

21. Dmitrienko A, Offen WW, Westfall PH. Gatekeeping strategies for clinical trials that do not require all primary effects to be significant. Stat Med 2003; 22:2387–400.

22. DeMets DL, Friedman L, Fuberg CD. Data monitoring in clinical trials: a case studies approach. New York: Springer Science + Business Media, 2005.

23. Tukey JW. Exploratory data analysis. Reading, Massachusetts: Addison-Wesley, 1977.

24. Cochran WG. Planning and analysis of observational studies. New York: John Wiley, 1983.

25. Anderson S, Auquier A, Hauck WW, et al. Statistical methods for comparative studies. New York: John Wiley, 1980.

26. Freiman JA, Chalmers TC, Smith H Jr, Kuebler RR. The importance of beta, the type II error, and sample size in the design and interpretation of the randomized controlled trial: survey of 71 "negative" trials. N Engl J Med 1978; 299:690–4. [Updated in Chapter 19 of the second edition of this book.]

27. Riis BJ, Thomsen K, Christiansen C. Does calcium supplementation prevent postmenopausal bone loss? A double-blind, controlled study. N Engl J Med 1987; 316:173–7.

28. Davis R, Ribner HS, Keung E, et al. Treatment of congestive heart failure with captopril, an oral inhibitor of angiotensin-converting enzyme. N Engl J Med 1979; 301:117–21.

29. Uniform Requirements for Manuscripts Submitted to Biomedical Journals. www.icmje.org, updated periodically.

Understanding Analyses of Randomized Trials

NANCY E. MAYO, PH.D.

ABSTRACT   Clinical trials can be deceptively complex to analyze because of dropouts over time, multiple endpoints, multiple time points, covariates, and other features. This chapter presents aspects of analyses that are likely to be familiar to readers, such as the concept of intention-to-treat, as well as other considerations that may be newer, such as response shift, estimation of change over time, biases created by missing data, stopping rules, and sample size considerations. It also tries to demystify the array of statistical tests that permeate research articles on RCTs and presents a framework for matching the measurement scale of the outcome to statistical tests. The rich array of RCTs from the *New England Journal of Medicine* provides examples to illustrate analytical challenges.

C hapter 4 examines aspects of the design of randomized clinical trials that influence whether the information gathered from the trial provides evidence to guide clinical practice. From that chapter, the reader should be able to understand five critical elements of study design and performance: whether (1) the question posed was appropriate for the study's goals, (2) the subjects were allocated to groups in an unbiased way, (3) the outcomes chosen were the relevant ones, (4) the study had sufficient statistical power to support the authors' conclusions, and (5) the study continued to an appropriate end.

In this chapter we provide insights into understanding the results of analyses commonly used in studies of treatment effects. It focuses on five issues, in the order that they are addressed during the conceptualization of a study: (1) dealing with multiple endpoints or multiple time points, (2) dealing with missing data, (3) adjusting for covariates, (4) matching the analysis to the measurement scale of the key variables, and (5) interpreting the results. As in Chapter 4, some illustrations draw on studies summarized in the boxes.

1. Was the question posed appropriate for the study's goals?

2. Were subjects allocated to groups in an unbiased way?

3. Were the outcomes chosen the relevant ones?

4. Did the study have sufficient statistical power to support the authors' conclusions?

5. Was the study continued to an appropriate end?

6. How did the study deal with multiple endpoints or multiple time points?

7. How did the study deal with missing data?

8. Did the study adjust for covariates?

9. Was the analysis matched to the measurement scale of the key variables?

10. Were the results interpreted correctly?

Some Critical Points in Understanding Clinical Trials

Endpoints in randomized clinical trials (RCTs) are of three types: confirmatory, which are meant to confirm or refute a specific hypothesis about a treatment effect; explanatory, which are useful in understanding how and why a treatment has some specific effect; and exploratory, which aid in the development of new understanding and new hypotheses for future study. All are important, but they require different approaches in both study design and statistical interpretation.[1]

INTENTION-TO-TREAT PARADIGM

One basic step underlying all of these analyses specifies the subjects whose data are used and their responses to the treatments. Analyses of RCTs customarily follow the principle of intention-to-treat, stated by Peduzzi et al.[2] as ". . . all randomized subjects are analyzed according to original treatment assignment, and all events are counted against the assigned treatment." Despite good adherence to this principle, the literature contains many examples of subject "slippage"; that is, those who did not complete the treatment regimen prescribed in the protocol.[3] That some of these losses seem quite reasonable and intuitively appealing does not make them any less of a concern. For example, what should the analyst do with subjects who, once randomized, (1) are found to be ineligible; (2) do not receive any of the treatment; (3) reach an endpoint too early, before having "enough" of the intervention to plausibly produce the endpoint; (4) disappear; or (5) otherwise deviate from the specified treatment? To illustrate the problem, imagine an RCT in which every patient assigned to placebo is moved to active treatment if the condition gets worse. Deaths would occur among patients on active treatment, but not among patients continuing on placebo.

The strength of the RCT lies in the "R"—the randomization combined with intention-to-treat analysis. If, during the course of the trial, persons are allowed to select themselves out of the trial or are dropped by the investigator, then randomization is no longer exerting its preventative influence on bias, and the study approaches a cohort study.[3] Tallman et al.[4] evaluated the impact of autologous stem-cell transplantation for women with high-risk breast cancer. They randomized 540 women, but only 511 were analyzed because of exclusions after randomization owing to protocol violations. This number was further reduced to 417 by considering only those with strict protocol adherence; of the original 270 women assigned to the stem-cell-transplant group, 197 (73%) were transplanted, but 18 women in the non-transplant group went on to have a transplant, sometimes elsewhere. For time-to-recurrence, the results in this restricted group favored the transplant group. In contrast, in the whole group analyzed as randomized, and as correctly reported in the journal article, no differences in this or any other endpoint were observed. The most likely reason for the discrepancy in results is that those who remained in the study to get cell transplants were different from those who did not, defeating the purpose of randomization. This example shows why it is critical to adhere to the intention-to-treat paradigm.

STUDIES WITH MULTIPLE ENDPOINTS

RCTs commonly have several relevant outcomes or assess results at multiple times. With our expanding knowledge of the diverse impacts of interventions, the issue of dealing with multiple outcomes frequently arises in trials. For example, Hays et al.[5] (see Box 1) reported 13 health-related quality-of-life outcomes of using hormone replacement therapy (HRT). If these outcomes were perfectly correlated (they are not), the probability of finding a statistically significant difference between groups on all outcomes would be the same as the probability of finding any one of them significant. If the outcomes were statistically independent (they are not), the probability of finding at least one difference with $p < 0.05$ by chance would be $1 - (1 - 0.05)^{13} = 0.487$, or approximately 50%. Thus, some correction for multiplicity should be applied, to control the number of false-positive results. Several methods are available, each with specific strengths. The three approaches in common use are: restrict the focus to only

Hypothesis	Background implied two sided: HRQL could be better or worse in hormone-replacement group in comparison to placebo
Type of study	Effectiveness as women took drugs unsupervised; 74% of women in HRT group and 80% of women in placebo group took at least 80% of prescribed pills; 9.7% and 6.6%, in HRT and placebo respectively, discontinued use; 2-group parallel with a 4-week placebo lead-in to test compliance
Population	16,608 post-menopausal women aged 50 to 79 with an intact uterus
Intervention	HRT with estrogen plus progesterone
Comparison	Look-alike placebo
Outcomes	Impairments: Menopausal symptoms (arbitrarily weighted and summed into a score); depressive symptoms (CES-D); sleep disturbance (WHI Insomnia Rating Scale); cognition (MMSE)
	Primary: generic HRQL using the RAND-36 (SF-36 with different scoring algorithms)
	QOL component: satisfaction with sexual functioning
Effect size	Not stated a priori; a posterori effect sizes were all less than 0.2 (trivial effect) and this magnitude was compared with the smallest increment of change possible on each scale
Sample size / Power	Type I error 0.004 (0.05/13); Bonferroni* correction because 13 outcome variables were assessed for impact of HRT
Randomization	Stratified by site and age, blocked with random block size
Blinding	Subject and treatment team
Timeline	Randomization to 12 months
Missing data	HRQL data missing for approximately 9% per group at 12 months
Analysis	Intention-to-treat with missing data excluded;
	Simple linear regression: Change in each of the 8 RAND-36 subscales and other 5 outcomes modeled as a function of study group; multiple linear regression to explore moderating effects of baseline variables (age, body-mass index, moderate or severe vasomotor symptoms, menopausal symptoms, sleep disturbance, previous use of HRT, and history of cardiovascular disease) and their interactions with study group
Results / Conclusions	**Small but statistically significant effect of HRT on 3 of the 13 outcomes** (physical functioning and bodily pain subscales of RAND-36 and sleep disturbance); no moderating effects of any baseline variables. Subgroup analyses for younger women and those with moderate to severe night sweats and hot flashes showed improvement with HRT but no effect on HRQL. No meaningful effect of HRT on patient-reported outcomes.

Bold type refers to information on the primary outcome.

Box 1. Impact of hormone replacement therapy (HRT) on HRQL from the Women's Health Initiative trial.

Hays et al. 2003[5]

* Bonferroni correction is a conservative way of adjusting for the effect of multiple comparisons; Type I error is made stricter by dividing by the number of comparisons, e.g., 0.05/n.

one or two pre-specified outcomes; adjust the significance level; or create global indices or summary statistics. The first method is a feature of design, discussed in Chapter 4. The latter two have implications for both design and analysis and are illustrated here. Chapter 8 also discusses these issues of multiplicity.

Adjusting the Significance Level

The Bonferroni correction is a conservative way of adjusting for the effect of multiple comparisons. The Type I error rate is allocated among the comparisons by dividing the nominal significance level by the number of comparisons (e.g., $0.05/k$); the result is very close to that for outcomes that are statistically independent, but it requires no assumptions about independence. Not all authorities agree with this adjustment; some feel that if the analysis focuses on estimating parameters (rates, proportions, means) rather than on testing hypotheses, the estimate of the parameter and its corresponding precision (expressed as a confidence interval) have nothing to do with the number of parameters being estimated.[6] Also, if outcomes are positively correlated, the Type I error rate is smaller than 0.05, perhaps much smaller, and useful effects may be missed. Opponents to Bonferroni-type adjustments argue that it is better to identify more associations than fewer, and that the confirmation of false-positive associations is better handled through further study.[6] This discussion more often focuses on studies of associations rather than studies of efficacy and effectiveness; but when an RCT has multiple secondary outcomes, this advice is sound if it is likely that additional studies will be undertaken. On the other hand, in applications for approval of new drugs, for which major studies may not be repeated, regulatory agencies often require an allocation of Type I error rate among primary and secondary hypotheses in which the total does not exceed 0.05. Multiple testing is a common problem in applied statistics, as discussed in Chapter 8.

Global Indices

Another approach combines outcomes into a global index or composite outcome. A key assumption for a meaningful global index is that the outcomes measure much of the same underlying construct. This assumption needs to be based on theory but must also be verified statistically using such methods as factor analysis or principal-components analysis. A well-known example of a global or composite measure is the physical health component score (PCS) from the SF-36.[7] This health-related quality of life (HRQL) measure comprises 36 items in 8 subscales. To avoid the issue of multiplicity, two summary scores were created, one for physical health and one for mental health. Researchers used principal-components analysis to identify the subscales that were most closely related to one another and, hence, are likely to measure a common or similar construct. The score is a weighted sum of the scores on the subscales in which the weights reflect how strongly each subscale is related to that underlying construct. The SF-36 is probably the best-known measure of HRQL in studies of medical interventions, and several of the trials reviewed here used it.[5, 8-13]

In a second example a severity index was created to test the effect of nebulized epinephrine for infants with acute bronchiolitis.[14] Three outcomes with varying numbers of elements contributed to the index: respiratory effort (5 signs); oxygen saturation (1 element); and respiratory rate (1 element). Each element was scored. For example each respiratory sign was rated not present (scored 0), mild to moderate (scored 1), or severe (scored 2). Three signs (intercostal recession, subcostal recession, and substernal recession) each received a weight of 1, and tracheal tug and nasal flaring were each weighted 1.5. The weighted scores for respiratory effort yielded a severity score of 1 (mild: 0 to 4.9), 2 (moderate: 5.0 to 8.9), or 3 (severe: 9.0 to 12.0). Oxygen saturation was also scored 0, 1, or 2 (95% to 100%, 90% to 94%, <90%); respiratory rate scored 0, 1, or 2, according to how many standard deviations the observed rate was above or below the mean for healthy infants of the same age (<2, 2 to 3, >3). The sum of the three severity scores was the overall score, which ranged from 0 to 7 and was categorized as mild (0 or 1), moderate (2 or 3), or severe (4 to 7).

Adding up elements in this way assumes that each (in the presence of the others) contributes equally to the underlying construct "respiratory severity" and that all relevant components have been included. Without verification of the assumptions (content representativeness, common factor, ordering of cutpoints, and weighting), such a global measure may result in a non-systematic misclassification of infants into categories, making it difficult to determine whether intervention is associated with this outcome. Indeed, this study found none. At worst, this type of measure can introduce a bias if the intervention is associated with a change in only a few crucial elements and these are not weighted appropriately.

There are several mathematical ways of summing prognostic variables. Perhaps the best example is the methodology used to develop the Charlson Comorbidity Index.[15] Here the weight for each comorbid condition was determined by the strength of association (measured by the odds ratio, OR) between each comorbid condition and mortality. ORs less than 1.2 were excluded (weighted 0), between 1.2 and 1.49 were weighted 1, between 1.5 and 2.49 were weighted 2, between 2.5 and 3.49 were weighted 3, and greater than 3.5 were weighted 6. This index is very widely used, and its value in predicting other outcomes has been demonstrated.[16] Though comorbidity is often an explanatory variable or covariate rather than an outcome, it is relevant to understand how to weight different elements to arrive at a total score. For example, in the study above[14] on the effect of nebulized epinephrine for infants with acute bronchiolitis, the severity index could have been created by a regression model with mortality or length of hospital stay as the outcome, the latter a proxy for severity, and each of the elements as predictors; the regression parameters would then guide the weighting.

Another way of combining multiple outcomes calculates a z-score for each individual on each measure, essentially how many standard deviations the individual's score differs from the group mean. The z-scores for the measures are unit-free and can be added to produce a combined score for each individual. The assumption that the outcomes measure the same construct would need to be formally tested (again factor-analytic techniques can be useful), and only those outcomes that contribute to the construct should be added. Unlike the SF-36, whose two summary scores are created from subscales that are known to represent the global construct of HRQL, the interpretation of *ad hoc* global indices is sometimes not obvious.

Multivariate methods, such as multivariate analysis of variance, can provide a joint test of hypotheses of the effect of treatment on several measures, but they do not directly indicate which measure was affected. If the joint test is significant, then and only then can each measure be looked at for treatment effect.[17] In a 1999 study of the efficacy of tissue plasminogen activator (t-PA) for improving the outcome of ischemic stroke,[18] the effects at 6 and 12 months were analyzed using a global statistic derived from three measures of outcome. A favorable outcome was defined as minimal or no disability on each of three measures relating to function. As the outcome was binary, favorable or not, a logistic regression model (see Chapter 12) was used, and the parameter estimated was the odds ratio. In the joint test, the OR was 1.7 (95% CI: 1.3–2.3), indicating that it is appropriate to look at effects on specific outcomes. t-PA was found to have a similar beneficial effect on each of the outcomes at 6 months and at 12 months after stroke onset.

Table 1 lists some of the approaches for summarizing data over multiple measures and multiple time points.

These examples have combined outcomes on continuous scales, such as scores on various measures. When the outcomes are events such as development of medical conditions and death, most of which are rare occurrences, there is a substantial benefit to statistical power if the endpoints can be combined into a composite outcome. There is also a benefit to interpretation if any of these endpoints are irreversible and block other endpoints (as death does). If an intervention has a higher risk of death, particularly early death, it may have a paradoxically lower risk on other endpoints. The assumption in using a

Table 1. Common Methods for Reducing Multiple Endpoints.	
Over Measures	Over Time
Factor weights	Change scores
z-scores	Slopes
Multivariate analysis of variance (MANOVA)	Mean of follow-up measures
	Area under the curve
	Minimum value
	Mixed models (hierarchical models, growth-curve models)

composite endpoint is that the intervention has a fairly uniform effect on each component[19]; effects may differ in magnitude among endpoints, but they point in the same direction.

Gaede et al.[20] evaluated the effectiveness of multifactorial team management for people with type 2 diabetes (see Box 2) using a composite outcome summarized in Table 2. The advantage of a composite endpoint is illustrated; although treatments were continued for four years with follow-up to eight years, there were very few events of any one kind. A disadvantage is that, except for death, none of the other components are irreversible and prevent other outcomes, so that the number of events could exceed the number of subjects. In such trials the composite outcome usually counts only the first event on any of the component outcomes. Gaede et al.[20] calculated a hazard ratio that takes into account the timing of the event. The multifactorial intervention had a protective effect on all endpoints, except that, possibly by chance, the intervention group had a higher rate of death, and the two groups had the same rate of surgical intervention.

Wing et al.[21] found that ACE inhibitors for hypertension were associated generally with a lower rate of cardiovascular events or death (HR: 0.89; 95% CI: 0.79–1.00) in comparison to use of diuretics. However, the effect was not consistent across the 10 categories of fatal and nonfatal cardiovascular events: the risk of fatal stroke was higher among persons treated with ACE inhibitors (HR: 1.91; 95% CI: 1.04–3.50). Only 2 of the 11 components had statistically significant effects: (1) fatal stroke, with diuretics superior, and (2) nonfatal myocardial infarction, with ACE inhibitors superior. The advantage of the composite endpoint for statistical power is appealing; but, as happens here, interpretation is not always simple.

MULTIPLE TIMES

Multiple outcomes also arise from assessing patient status at multiple times. Methods for handling such data are well developed and widely applied in

Hypothesis	Background implies one-sided: intensive, targeted intervention would result in lower rates of cardiovascular death, disease, and deterioration
Type of study	Effectiveness; 2-group parallel
Population	Type 2 diabetes and microalbuminuria
Intervention	Intensified, targeted, multifactorial management
Comparison	Conventional care
Outcomes	**Primary: Composite of mortality from cardiovascular causes, nonfatal myocardial infarction, coronary-artery bypass grafting, percutaneous coronary intervention, nonfatal stroke, amputation as a result of ischemia, or vascular surgery for peripheral atherosclerotic artery disease** Secondary: incidence of diabetic nephropathy, development or progression of diabetic retinopathy or neuropathy
Effect size	**35% reduction in expected rate of events** of 6% per year (reduction to 3.9%)
Sample size / Power	160 persons / 70% power; Type I error 0.05 (assumed to be two-sided)
Randomization	Simple
Blinding	Subjects not blinded; adjudicators of secondary endpoints blinded
Timeline for follow-up	Baseline, 4 years, and 8 years in conventional group; biochemical and clinical data every 3 months in intensive group
Missing data	2 withdrew in conventional group, 1 in intervention group
Analysis	intention-to-treat; missing data excluded **Between-group: log-rank test; Cox proportional hazards** (time-to-event) to calculate hazard ratio, adjusted for age, duration of diabetes, sex, smoking status, and endpoint status at baseline Secondary: grouped survival model (binary regression with complementary log-log link), adjusting for age, duration of diabetes, sex, and endpoint status at baseline Other: analysis of covariance for measured variables, Mann-Whitney test, chi-squared test
Results / Conclusions	Intervention resulted in more people reaching established process and outcome targets: better pharmacotherapy, better control of bioclinical parameters leading, by end of study, **to a 50% reduction in risk of cardiovascular death and disease progression in intervention group**

Bold type refers to information on the primary outcome.

Box 2. A pragmatic trial of the impact of intensified, multifactorial team management for persons with type 2 diabetes.

Gaede et al. 2003[20]

Table 2. Summary of the Rates of Occurrence of the Components of a Composite Endpoint Used in the Gaede et al.[20] Trial of the Effectiveness of Intensified, Multifactorial Team Management for Persons with Type 2 Diabetes.

Component	Multifactorial Intensive Team Management ($n = 80$) n (Rate per 100)		Conventional Management ($n = 80$) n (Rate per 100)		Rate ratio	
	Any	1st	Any	1st	Any	1st
Death from cardiovascular causes	7 (8.8)	3 (3.8)	7 (8.8)	1 (1.2)	1.00	3.0
Non-fatal myocardial infarction	5 (6.2)	4 (5.0)	17 (21.2)	8 (10.0)	0.29	0.50
Coronary-artery bypass graft	5 (6.2)	4 (5.0)	10 (12.5)	6 (7.5)	0.50	0.67
Percutaneous coronary intervention	0	0	5 (6.2)	3 (3.8)	0	0
Nonfatal stroke	3 (3.8)	3 (3.8)	20 (25.0)	11 (13.8)	0.15	0.27
Amputation	7 (8.8)	2 (2.5)	14 (17.5)	3 (3.8)	0.50	0.67
Surgical intervention for peripheral vascular disease	6 (7.5)	3 (3.8)	12 (15.0)	3 (3.8)	0.50	1.00
Any CVD death or event	33	19 (24)	85	35 (44)		0.54*

*Hazard Ratio (unadjusted) = 0.47; 95% CI = 0.24 – 0.73; CVD = cardiovascular disease

observational studies. These methods are less widely applied in RCTs, particularly when the outcome is measured on a continuous scale and particularly when the analyst has only two measurements, pre- and post-intervention. When the outcome is binary, the usual way of dealing with multiple time points is to calculate a single cumulative rate of occurrence over a fixed time period.

Studies involving observations at many times bring out the challenges in dealing with change over time. Effective statistical methods permit all of the follow-up measurements to contribute to the estimate of treatment effect. Because the rate of change with time may vary by person, and persons start at different initial values, the estimate of treatment effect should accommodate this variation. To deal with these features, many longitudinal studies use a mixed-model approach in which outcome is a function of treatment (considered fixed), time, and covariates, some with a fixed set of values (at least, in the study) and others with values that represent a random sample of the possibilities (a so-called random effect).

Against this background, when there are only two values, pre- and post-intervention, it would be simplistic to abandon the longitudinal view of the data. Doing so reduces these two meaningful measurements to one, and the analysis reduces to that of change scores. One of the assumptions implicit in a change score is that the average change is a good summary measure for all changes, but perhaps some subjects improve and some get worse, with no change on average. Contrast this with a situation where, without the intervention, no one changed. These two patterns of change are clearly not the same. Yet only the variability associated with the change scores would reveal the disparity.

The other assumption in a change score is that the change is true change in a construct and not a change owing to adaptation or coping, such as a change in the respondent's internal standards of measurement (i.e., scale recalibration), a change in the respondent's values (i.e., the importance of component domains constituting the target construct), or a redefinition of the target.[22] These distinctions do not arise for outcomes that are directly measured (e.g., white blood cell count), but must be considered for outcomes that must be based on subjects' reports (e.g., pain).

In rating pain, a person may adapt to a given level of pain and over time may not rate it as extreme, even in the absence of any actual change. The person appears to have "improved," but in fact they have just recalibrated their internal pain scale. In rating quality of life or HRQL, adaptation or intervention can cause some persons to change the way they value one or more aspects of their life. Thus, after an intervention, family support and freedom from symptoms may be more important than ability to do certain activities or participate in events outside the home. The numerical values of the outcome measure may or may not differ, but what makes up the total score has changed, and hence the mathematical estimate of change does not have its expected meaning. Mayo argues[23, 24] that, for many trials involving interventions to improve the outcome of stroke, the intervention could have altered persons' internal standards for the outcomes, so that no between-group difference was observed.

Response shift in patient-reported outcomes can be induced even by medical or surgical interventions that are not designed to alter coping strategies. Medical interventions that affect symptoms or have unpleasant effects may invoke a response shift as people reconsider these in their outcome rating. Comparisons of surgical and medical outcomes could also involve a response shift owing to the experience produced by surgery itself. For example, in the NETT[13] comparison of lung-volume–reduction surgery to medical care (see Box 3), the proportion of people who evaluated their HRQL as improved was dramatically greater in the surgery group than in the medical care group. Before the investigators concluded that the surgery group experienced true positive change in HRQL, they could have demonstrated that the life-altering experience of very extensive surgery had not altered patients' calibrations of HRQL, its components, or the value placed on these components. Their data (Supplementary Appendix 4) show that the changes in HRQL were consistent with changes in FEV_1, a

Hypothesis	Background implies two sided: lung-volume–reduction surgery could be beneficial or harmful in comparison to medical treatment
Type of study	Efficacy; 2-group parallel
Population	Individuals with severe COPD successfully completing pulmonary rehabilitation run-in phase; $n = 1218$
Intervention	Lung-volume–reduction surgery
Comparison	Medical care
Outcomes	**Primary: mortality** at mean 29 months post surgery
	Impairment: Maximal exercise capacity at 2 years; pulmonary function, dyspnea
	Activity: Distance walked in 6 minutes (6MWT)
	Disease-Specific HRQL: St. George's Respiratory Questionnaire
	Generic HRQL: Quality of Well-Being
Effect size	**Not stated for mortality; for maximal exercise capacity, increase of 10 watts in maximum workload considered clinically meaningful**
Sample size / Power	Projected 2500 people; based on expected **mortality of 8%** in medical group; this sample size would provide sufficient power to distinguish between 8% for medical group and 4.5% mortality in surgical group; Type I error 0.05
Randomization	Stratified by site
Blinding	Neither subjects nor assessor blinded
Timeline	90-days; 6, 12, and 24 months; and up to 5 years (mean 29 months)
Missing data	On functional and HRQL outcomes for deceased; deceased assigned the lowest category; missing assigned the next-to-lowest category.
Analysis	Intention-to-treat; missing data assigned as not improved (1) **Mortality: Risk ratio** (unadjusted), not survival analysis owing to non-proportional hazard assumption because of increased early mortality risk in surgical group (2) Impairment: % of persons making increase of 10 watts or more on test of exercise capacity, tested using Fisher's exact test; between group comparison of distribution of change using Wilcoxon rank-sum test (3) Functional and HRQL outcomes dichotomized as improved or not and analyzed using logistic regression; subgroups identified by logistic regression with interaction between group and pre-identified covariates
Results / Conclusions	**Overall, no mortality benefit from surgery** Exercise capacity improved: at 6, 12, and 24 months proportions with improvements > 10 watts were 28%, 22%, 15% for persons with surgery compared with 4%, 5%, 3% for persons in medical group; persons with upper-lobe emphysema and low exercise capacity benefited; persons with non–upper-lobe and high exercise capacity were at higher risk of mortality.

Bold type refers to information on the primary outcome.

Box 3. A randomized trial comparing lung-volume–reduction surgery with medical therapy for severe emphysema.
National Emphysema Treatment Trial (NETT) Research Group 2003[13]

measured variable that is largely determined by the physics of airflow and not subject to recalibration; but 40% of persons in the surgery group showed very large improvements in HRQL, whereas the changes in FEV_1 were much more modest (approximately 40% had improvements of 10% or less). This strong change in HRQL persisted over time, whereas the gains in FEV_1 diminished with time. In using patient-reported outcomes (PROs) it is important to consider that a response shift could have occurred and rule it out; with measured variables the only concern about change is measurement error.

Several options are available in situations where response shift is likely. The design phase could build in a "then-test." A person, at the time of re-appraisal, looks back to the prior appraisal period and provides a re-rating.[25] This is considered valid as the standards applying at the second point in time are used to re-consider the earlier rating. Some measures of HRQL include the possibility of people changing their values. The Chronic Respiratory Questionnaire[26] is such an example. In the data analysis phase, it is possible to assess the degree to which re-conceptualization has occurred by using analytical procedures that essentially look at the "weight" of the components of a global construct before and after an intervention. If such an analysis demonstrates re-conceptualization, it is not meaningful to calculate change, but at least the authors avoid erroneous conclusions about the effectiveness of an intervention. Statistical methods are also available for evaluating response shift at the group level[27, 28] and at the individual level.[29] The reader wishing more information on response shift should consult these landmark publications.[22, 23, 25, 30–32]

The importance of considering the patient's perspective on outcome has moved to the forefront of clinical research following the U.S. Food and Drug Administration's (FDA) 2006 guidance for industry on use of patient-reported outcomes in medical product development to support labeling claims. Information to support new products must now include not only the evidence from biological and physiological tests but also evidence from patients themselves on the impact of the new product on their symptoms, function, and health. It is important that investigators incorporating PROs into their research understand the conceptual and statistical underpinnings of these measures.

Response shift notwithstanding, most investigators are not satisfied with simply subtracting the baseline from the final value because of concern that the pre-intervention value exerts strong influence on the post-intervention score and, therefore, on the change. For example, people who have a poor score on the pre-treatment test or measure have, theoretically, more room for improvement and hence can have a chance for greater improvement in their scores, whereas those who start with a good score have little range for improvement. The phenomenon known as regression to the mean may also affect persons at the lower or upper end of the measurement scale. If a measure has constant mean and variance, but with some individual changes up and down over time, those initially in the middle will randomly spread out at re-measurement, and those with more-extreme values will tend to move toward the center. Therefore, there is strong motivation to somehow "adjust" the change for baseline values. Table 3 outlines some of the approaches for estimating the impact of an intervention on change when the outcome variable is measured on a continuous scale.

No mathematical reason requires that change be adjusted for baseline. Indeed, including the initial value in a regression equation (such as $Y = \alpha + \beta_1 x_1 + \beta_2 x_n + \varepsilon$) to estimate the effect of a treatment on change violates a basic assumption of regression, that the "x" variables are measured without error or, if there is measurement error, these errors are not correlated with the error on the "Y" variable. The error term ε in the regression equation refers to sampling variation in "Y"; the people contributing these outcomes are a sample from a

Table 3. Estimators of Change from Pre-intervention to Post-intervention.

Outcome	Adjustment	Areas of Potential Concern
Post-intervention score only	Covariates only	Post value may depend on baseline value
	Pre-test score + covariates	Violation of regression assumption that measurement error of "x" variables is independent of error in "y"
Change: post – pre; or rate of change (slope of regression line)	Covariates only	Regression to the mean; change may depend on baseline value
	Pre-test score + covariates	Violation of regression assumption that measurement error of "x" variables is independent of error in "y"; creating a categorical variable for pre-test score may be a potential solution
% Change [(post–pre) / (pre)]	Covariates only	Biased estimator: 2 sources of measurement error in numerator, 1 source in denominator; change may depend on baseline value
	Pre-test score + covariates	Biased estimator, adjustment can produce paradoxical results[102]
Proportional change [(post – pre) / (mean of post + pre)]	Covariates only	Unbiased estimator of change; sources of error cancel
Proportional change [(post – pre) / (gap between pre and ceiling value)][103]	Covariates only	Needs a pre-defined targeted maximum value; needs to be tested

larger population. When the "Y" variable also has measurement error, it is not possible to distinguish how much of the error ε comes from measurement error and how much from sampling variation; including the baseline value of this error-prone outcome as a covariate will add to the mis-specification of the error. As tests of the hypotheses are based on relating the measure of response to error, a mis-specified error term can lead to a biased test of the hypothesis.

Oldham[33] suggested that the difference could be adjusted for the mean, though this has little intuitive appeal for some observers.[34] Others[34-36] have suggested dividing the difference by the mean as an unbiased estimator of proportional change because the sources of error in the numerator and denominator are balanced. This estimator will also reduce extremes of variation if persons can deteriorate as well as improve. Twisk and Proper[37] supported adjusting the change score for baseline values and showed the need for that, particularly if there are imbalances between the groups at baseline. However, the flurry of commentaries both for and against this approach[38-42] indicates that further work is needed in the area of change scores. One solution could be to create an indicator variable for level at baseline (perhaps based on norm-referenced cut-points or, in their absence, on tertiles or quartiles of the distribution) and use this indicator for adjustment. It would satisfy the proponents of adjustment for baseline and reduce the problem of correlated errors. This parallels the inclusion of stratification variables as covariates. If baseline value is such an issue in a particular trial, perhaps stratification by level of baseline impairment would be an optimal design strategy from the outset rather than having to deal with the issue rather clumsily in the analysis.

Of the 29 RCTs published in the *New England Journal of Medicine* in 2003 that used change scores as the outcome, 18 did not adjust for baseline[5, 11, 13, 43-57] and 8 did.[10, 20, 58-63] Three studies treated the data from the trial as longitudinal and used mixed modeling to estimate the impact of the intervention on rate of change in the outcome over multiple time points.[12, 64, 65] Mixed modeling would be the ideal approach as it permits the random variation in the baseline measure to be incorporated into "growth" in the outcome over time.

When there are more than two time points, there is no reason to abandon the longitudinal structure of the RCT and use a cross-sectional analysis, but the statistical methods are less well-known and a little harder to interpret than a regression coefficient. Several approaches are used to reduce data from multiple time points to one value. The slope of the regression line from the data of each person, interpreted as a rate of change per unit time, could serve as the "Y" variable and could be used in other analyses suitable for continuous data.

Another approach calculates the area under the curve (AUC) for each person (connecting consecutive data points by line segments) and then uses this as the outcome variable. Ghosh et al.[46] (Box 4) took this approach in analyzing the

Hypothesis	Worded as one-sided: 2 infusions of natalizumab at 6 mg per kg would result in a higher proportion of patients in clinical remission (Crohn's Disease Activity Index, CDAI < 150) than would 2 infusions of placebo.
Type of study	Efficacy; protocol violations: 4 patients received no infusions (deemed ineligible); 4-group parallel
Population	Persons with Crohn's disease who had CDAI between 220 and 450 (out of 600); 248 subjects at 35 study centers in Europe
Intervention	2 intravenous infusions 4 weeks apart: both at 6 mg of natalizumab per kg; both at 3 mg per kg; 1 at 3 mg per kg and 1 of placebo (3 groups)
Comparison	2 infusions of placebo
Outcomes	**Primary efficacy measure: CDAI; clinical remission;** clinical response: decrease in score of $\geq$ 70 points; *Serum level of C-reactive protein,* disease-specific HRQL, Inflammatory Bowel Disease Questionnaire *(IBDQ)*
Effect size	Clinical response: 40% in all 3 active drug groups vs. 15% in placebo group; response rate ratio (RR) = 2.67
Sample size / Power	60 persons per group ($\times$ 4); 80% power, Type I error 0.05 (two-sided)
Randomization	Site stratified, blocked (block size unspecified), computer-generated
Blinding	Subjects, investigators, clinical team, assessors
Timeline	Infusions 4 weeks apart; assessments at week 2, 4, 6, 8, and 12; primary outcome was remission at 6 weeks
Missing data	Primary endpoint at 12 weeks missing for 27 of 244 subjects (11%; 4 subjects did not receive either dose); last value carried forward used to impute missing data; declared not different among study groups (statistical testing not reported)
Analysis	Intention-to-treat of 248 subjects; missing data imputed as last value carried forward. **Remission** and response **rates: Mantel-Haenszel chi-squared test (comparing each group vs. placebo);** area under the curve for scores on CDAI; linear mixed modeling of repeated measurements for treatment effects on other endpoints (C-reactive protein, IBDQ) (parameters not shown)
Results	**Remission: no difference at 6 weeks between 6+6 mg per kg and placebo groups,** but significant differences at week 4 and week 8; all three active drug groups had significantly higher remission rate than placebo group at week 4, and 3+3 mg per kg group also had significantly higher rate at weeks 6, 8, and 12. Response: all three active drug groups had significantly higher response rate than placebo group at weeks 4, 6, and 8. Of a total of 30 contrasts 19 were significant at 0.05; 5 out of 30 were significant at 0.0017 (= 0.05/30).

	HRQL: at 12 weeks, scores on IBDQ were significantly higher only if 2 infusions of active drug were given.
	C-reactive protein (indicates degree of inflammation): significant decrease at 6 weeks in groups with 2 infusions of active drug and at 8 weeks in 3+3 mg per kg group (15 contrasts, 3 significant at 0.05)
	Adverse events: serious events were rare, and none were considered causally related to treatment; non-serious events were common, and incidence was similar in the four groups.
Conclusions	From abstract: "*[N]atalizumab increased the rates of clinical remission and response, improved quality of life and C-reactive protein levels, and was well tolerated in patients with active Crohn's disease.*" From text: "*The efficacy of natalizumab for reducing signs and symptoms of Crohn's disease appears to be at least similar to that of the tumor necrosis factor α-inhibitor infliximab*" (data not shown). Evidence of efficacy and tolerability in short term; value relative to other therapies remains to be tested.
Bold type refers to information on the primary outcome.	

Box 4. A trial testing the efficacy of natalizumab in reducing the severity and life impact of Crohn's disease.
Ghosh et al. 2003[46]

impact of infusions of natalizumab on the Crohn's Disease Activity Index. The AUC analysis assumes that the average of a patient's experience during successive intervals can be estimated adequately by the average of the measures at the beginning and end of each interval. This does not require that the intervals be of equal length, nor does it require that the patients all be measured at the same times. If total times under observation differ, however, the analysis should account for that difference (e.g., by dividing the total for each patient by the number of weeks that patient was under observation). The AUC generally behaves like a continuous variable, so it is possible to use a *t*-test, analysis of variance, or some other method for continuous data.

Area under the curve is also a very pragmatic way of thinking about quality-adjusted life years (QALYs), discussed in Chapter 4. The fraction of a year of survival (often all of it) multiplied by the quality of life during this time essentially defines a QALY. Imagine a study with long follow-up and multiple measures of quality of life over time. For each person, each unit of follow-up time would have an associated quality of life, and the sum of these units would be the total number of QALYs. For example, in the first two years of follow-up, an individual reports quality of life to be 0.8 or 80%, yielding 1.6 QALYs; in the next two years, the person's quality of life is 0.75, yielding 1.5 QALYs, for a total of 3.1 QALYs during the four calendar years. For more information the reader is referred to Fairclough's[1] discussion of this method, among others, for dealing with multiple outcomes.

Mixed models, including hierarchical linear models or growth-curve models, are becoming more popular as they permit each subject not only to start at a different point on the outcome scale, but also to have differing rates of change over time (slopes). These models require at least three time points, and more if one needs to estimate patterns such as a plateau or a deterioration.[66] Statistical methods and software are available to handle these features of data.

STUDIES WITH MISSING DATA

As RCTs move beyond asking questions about the impact of interventions on endpoints that are easily determined, such as death or disease recurrence, data are more often missing for some study subjects or for some outcomes. The best way to protect against missing data is to design and conduct the study with procedures that maximize the chance of obtaining complete and accurate follow-up information on all subjects.[3]

The issue of missing data is complex, and the reader who wishes detailed information can consult a variety of texts and articles, such as the short monograph by Allison [67] and the text by Fairclough.[17] The most frequently cited work on the subject is the book by Little and Rubin,[68] which includes descriptions of techniques for handling missing data.

For this chapter, the main issue is whether the absence of an observation may be related to the value of variables that the study aimed to collect, particularly the outcome "Y." If the absence of an observation does not depend on its value of "Y" or on the values of other variables that were collected, perhaps because the observation is missing as a result of administrative error or an accident (e.g., a lost laboratory sample), then analyses that omit this point will not be biased, though power will be reduced, particularly if more than 5% of the sample has missing data. This type of missing data is called *missing completely at random*. Missing follow-up data for patients who entered a study too late for long-term analyses are often treated this way. When the absence of an observation is not related to "Y" but is related to observed covariates, which could be used in the analysis, then the missing data are called *missing at random*. When the missing data *do* depend on the value of "Y," such as when the poorest values on the outcome are missing because the subjects are ill or experienced the most negative side effects of the treatment, then ignoring these data will introduce a bias. (In some studies, those doing well are more difficult to entice back for follow-up.) Such missing data are termed *missing not at random*.

In an example of analysis when data are *missing not at random*, Foster et al.[58] compared a popular low-carbohydrate diet to a conventional low-calorie/ high-carbohydrate/low-fat diet (see Box 5). No information was gathered on

Hypothesis	Background implies two sided: low-carbohydrate diet could induce a greater or lesser weight loss than conventional diet
Type of study	Effectiveness as subjects were not provided with support from research team; 2-group parallel
Population	Obese individuals without clinical comorbidity; $n = 63$
Intervention	Instruction to follow low-carbohydrate diet
Comparison	Instruction to follow conventional high-carbohydrate, low-fat, low-calorie, diet
Outcomes	**Primary: change in body weight 3, 6, and 12 months,** % testing positive for urinary ketones at each assessment point; blood pressure, serum lipoproteins, plasma glucose, insulin sensitivity at 3, 6, and 12 months
Effect size	Not stated a priori; study effect size: 3 mos., 4.1/18; 6 mos., 3.8/18; 12 mos., 1.9/18.
Sample size / Power	Not estimated a priori
Randomization	Simple, stratified by site
Blinding	Subjects and assessors *not* blinded but probably little opportunity for measurement bias
Timeline	Follow-up to 12 months, with assessments at 10 intervals
Missing data	41% missing by 12 months, greater in conventional group but not statistically significantly so; baseline value carried forward for intention-to-treat analysis; missing excluded from secondary analysis
Analysis	(1) intention-to-treat with baseline value carried forward (assumes no change from last measurement) using **repeated-measures analysis of variance for weight change;** (2) 12-month completers only (on-protocol) using analysis of covariance adjusting for baseline weight.
Results / Conclusions	Both analyses yielded the same results; persons on low-carbohydrate diet lost significantly more weight than persons on conventional diet at 3 and 6 months, but two groups the same at 12 months; persons on low-carbohydrate diet had greater increases in high-density lipoprotein and greater decreases in triglycerides than persons on conventional diet.

Bold type refers to information on the primary outcome.

Box 5. A trial comparing low-carbohydrate and low-fat diets for people with obesity.
Foster et al. 2003[58]

adherence to the diet, and weight loss was monitored by self-report. A substantial proportion (41%) of persons in each group did not report their weight at 12 months. The authors assumed that people with missing data had regained the weight they lost. In other words, if those missing had the poorest outcomes, the absence of a follow-up data point *did* depend on "Y." As ignoring this information could result in a biased estimate of the effect of diet, the authors assumed no change and carried forward the baseline weight. Results from the analysis using "baseline carried forward" were very similar to those obtained by including data on persons who completed the study and data obtained at the last follow-up visit for those who did not complete the study—the low-carbohydrate diet induced a greater weight change at 3 and 6 months, but this difference disappeared by 12 months. A customary assumption is that the mechanism responsible for missing data was the same for each group. As both groups were assigned to a diet, and the numbers of subjects with missing weight were similar for the two diets, this assumption may well be valid. This approach to imputing missing data, "last value carried forward," is generally conservative but seems reasonable in this study.

A similar situation arose in the study by Ghosh et al.[46] (Box 4) when some Crohn's disease patients did not complete the study as planned; the investigators filled in the missing data by carrying forward the last value observed. This approach assumes that, had the persons been assessed, their value would have been the same as the one before. Under this assumption, if someone was a responder (i.e., had a reduction of at least 70 points on the Crohn's Disease Activity Index) earlier, they would remain a responder even though there is no information to support this. The investigators also assumed that the mechanism for absence of data was the same in the groups. The data presented suggest that most withdrawals occurred because of no response or adverse events; thus, the "no response" status would be carried forward. In general, however, because of the potential for bias, it is risky to use these types of imputations unless the assumptions can be verified.

Other options are available for dealing with missing data. By default most statistical packages delete all subjects with one or more missing values. This approach can sacrifice considerable efficiency, even when the missing data are missing completely at random. It is conceivable that, in a large and complicated trial, each subject would have at least one important observation missing; the investigator could hardly exclude all of them. Casewise or listwise deletion (analysis restricted to people with complete data on all variables), as this is called, can also give a biased result if the mechanisms by which the data are missing differ among groups, among variables, or over time. As data are usually missing for many reasons, analyses of "completers only" are not optimal. It is important that an article report the number of people who started the treatments and the number who contributed data at each point in each of the analyses.

When data are missing completely at random, it is possible to use simple methods to impute values for the missing data and salvage power. Unfortunately, some of these simple solutions (give everyone the mean or a value derived from similar people) can seriously underestimate the variability and lead to lower (more significant) p-values. Some statistical packages have options that permit multiple imputation for each missing value, with the aim of introducing appropriate variability, but these methods are computationally complex and require statistical expertise.

Multiple imputation may appear to be "making up the data," but results are generally closer to being correct than with simple-imputation techniques. Multiple imputation provides an estimate of the value of a missing variable that would have been recorded if the person had been assessed. The estimated value incorporates the data that are available, cross-sectionally and over time, as well as variation in the multivariate distribution of the existing data. In the analysis both the estimate and the associated error, within and between imputed data sets, are used, and the model error term thus includes the usual sources of error as well as error arising from imputation. Without this process, the p-value tends to be underestimated and more likely to cross the conventional threshold for significance.[67, 68] When prevention of drop-outs fails, the best solution to reduce bias may often be multiple imputation, using covariates and any outcome data that are available.

Wood et al.[69] and Fielding et al.[70] provide an overview of methods and assess the extent to which missing data are adequately handled in RCTs published in major medical journals. The Wood systematic review covered studies published in 2002 and found that missing data were common: 63 of the 71 trials (89%) had some missing data, and 13 of these had data missing on more than 20% of the sample. The majority of trials with missing data (41/63) excluded from the analyses those subjects with missing data. When missing data were imputed, the methods were crude: last value carried forward, worst-case scenario, or simple imputation using regression techniques. Only 5 of the 37 studies with repeated measures used statistical approaches permitting imputation. Clearly, missing data are a weakness of many clinical trials, a flaw that should be reduced sharply or prevented through imaginative data collection and, failing prevention, through statistical approaches that attempt to create a data set as close as possible to that which would have been observed if the assessment had been completed, including estimated variances as well as individual values, means, and other statistical measures.

ADJUSTING FOR COVARIATES

As randomization is expected to balance groups on all variables, known and unknown, measured or not, RCT investigators have had a tendency to use simple tests of effect by comparing group means or other simple measures. Achieving this balance is a feature of large studies. Most smaller studies cannot rely on randomization alone, so investigators often use statistical procedures that take covariates into account.

Adjustment for covariates in practice does not usually have a dramatic effect on the estimate of effect because randomization protects against serious group imbalances and most covariates are not strongly associated with outcome.[71, 72] When the outcome is continuous, variables other than the treatment group can be used in a statistical model to increase the precision of the estimate of treatment effect by removing some of the known sources of variability in the outcome.[71] These variables are not under study; they are included because of their known importance, and no hypotheses are tested on their contributions. Inclusion of these prognostic variables is not based on whether they are unbalanced across groups, as their purpose is to "soak up" and remove known variance from the analysis. In a stratified study the indicator variables for strata should be included if they are correlated with the outcome.[73] For example, if a multi-institution study is stratified by hospital, including hospital as an adjustment variable would not be needed as hospital is not expected *a priori* to correlate with outcome. In instances when stratification is on initial severity of the outcome, including the stratum indicator provides an adjustment for baseline but without introducing additional sources of error that are correlated with the measurement error of the outcome variable.

The situation differs somewhat when the outcome is an event (a dichotomous variable). Including a covariate that is strongly associated with outcome will increase the error associated with treatment effect[71, 74, 75] and can increase the estimate of the treatment effect as well.[71] In Cox models, biased results of treatment effect can occur if covariates are entered in an exploratory manner rather than as a prespecified set. This holds true despite imbalances in the groups.[76] When these models include many prognostic variables, the estimate of treatment effect can approach a subject-specific effect. When no or only a few variables are included, the estimate of treatment effect is for the group, averaged over the *omitted* variables.[72, 74] The simpler model is not "biased" with respect to the more-detailed model; they answer different questions. Most public health or population applications require an estimate of the treatment effect for the "average" person. However, in many clinical applications the focus is on estimating a treatment effect for more-typical persons such as those included or even for individual persons with specific characteristics,[72, 74] and the more-detailed model can provide an estimated probability of the outcome for an individual and improve power to detect effects of treatment.[77] Thus, the choice of method depends on the question and the intended application of the results. The statistical and methodological literature is consistent and convincing that the treatment effects from RCTs should be adjusted for a carefully selected and pre-specified set of covariates.

Subgroup Analysis

Including covariates in the model is not the same as subgroup analysis. A subgroup analysis aims to test hypotheses and provide estimates of effects for the subgroups; in other words, the subgroup variables are under study (see Chapter 15). With covariate adjustment, the aim is to improve the precision of estimates of overall treatment effect; the adjustment variables are not under study, and no hypotheses about their effects are being tested. Subgroups in RCTs are best identified by including a variable for the interaction between the group and the covariate and examining its size and statistical significance.[78, 79] These two situations, covariate adjustment or subgroup analysis, have different sample size considerations, and the optimum choice depends on the measurement scale of the outcome.

No matter what role the covariate plays in the analysis, the sample size needs to be augmented for the variable; additional sample size considerations apply when a covariate is being used for a subgroup analysis.[78, 79]

The sample size needed for a given trial depends on the size of the effect to be detected (a larger effect size, as a ratio of desired difference to expected standard deviation, requires fewer subjects), the power of the study, and the inclusion of covariates for adjustment or for subgroup analyses. Sample size estimates are best carried out using appropriate statistical software, which will require the investigator to specify the model, the number of groups, the effect size to be detected if it is present, power, the distribution of the covariate, and the strength of the covariate's relation to the outcome.

There are often advantages in having preliminary sample size estimates to judge feasibility and the wisdom of pursuing the trial. A number of rules of thumb have been developed for how many additional subjects are needed for covariate adjustment in regression analyses.[80, 81] For purposes of statistical modeling (which is not the purpose of the primary analysis of a trial, although it might be a secondary objective), Green[80] indicates that adequate power (80%) can be achieved for moderate effect sizes with a sample size $n > 50 + 8m$, where m is the number of covariates to be modeled. If covariates are included only for adjustment purposes, no parameters are estimated for them, and no hypotheses tested, to maintain the same degree of power, only one additional subject is required per level or per degree of freedom (df) inherent in the covariate, remembering that a continuous variable has only 1 df, but a categorical variable with k categories has $k-1$ df.[80, 81] The addition of the covariate in this situation is expected to reduce the standard error of the treatment effect, balancing out the effect of enlarging the model.

In an analysis of an event outcome, a ratio of at least 10 events (not subjects) for each covariate has been recommended,[82] but this is based on modeling purposes rather than covariate adjustment. Recently, this rule of thumb has been revisited[83] for the situation where the aim is to control for confounding rather than prediction. Vittinghoff and McCulloch[83] identify several scenarios where this rule can be relaxed and acceptable power is achieved with event-per-variable ratios ranging from 5 to 9. The strength of the association between the outcome and the covariate as well as other design features affects the optimal ratio.[83] For example, in the Gaede et al.[20] study on the effectiveness of multifactorial team management for people with type 2 diabetes (see Box 2), the analysis of the time to the first cardiovascular event involved 54 first events in the 160 subjects randomized (the total number of cardiovascular events was 118 because some subjects had more than one event). This study could have supported adjustment for 5 to 9 covariates in addition to group, and the authors indicated that the estimate of the effect of group was adjusted for 5 covariates: age, sex, duration of diabetes, smoking, and presence or absence of cardiovascular disease at baseline. The effect of adjustment on the estimate of the hazard ratio for group was nil (HR: 0.47 for both), and adjustment increased the width of the 95% CI by 6% (to 0.22 to 0.74). In this example, the average effect and the subject-specific effects were identical, which can be typical in a clinical setting where the average patient can be fully characterized by the measured variables.

In general, the effects of subgroup analysis on sample size are substantial; to attain the same power for comparing two subgroups as for the main effect, the sample size must be increased by a factor of four or more.[78] With more than one subgroup, the study is powered for the one with the lowest hypothesized effect size, which requires the most subjects. The NETT trial of surgery for emphysema[13] used logistic regression to search for subgroups with differential mortality response to surgery. Variables with a significant interaction were then tested in a multivariate model and tested for other pairwise interactions. This analysis showed that the subgroup of persons with upper lobe emphysema and low exercise capacity responded differently to surgery than the group as a whole and had significantly lower mortality with surgery than with medical treatment. Over all subjects the total mortality was 26%, equivalent for both groups; in the subgroup with upper lobe emphysema and low exercise capacity the mortality rate in the surgical group was 19% compared with 34% for the medical group.

It is possible to both adjust for covariates and do subgroup analyses, but the investigator needs to be very careful in setting up these situations *a priori* to avoid the perception of hunting for an association. In addition to including the specifics in the statistical methods section, when presenting the data, the estimates for the adjustment variables should not be featured in the body of the table to avoid confusion as to their role in the analysis, but the variables should be clearly named in an appropriate place in the manuscript. The information presented in the tables of results should include only the estimates of the treatment effect, the effects for the variables defining the pre-specified subgroups, and the interaction terms between treatment and subgroup. The data layout should also show the effect for each subgroup to avoid the perception of "statistical hocus-pocus."

The box provides a memory aid for adjusting sample size for covariates in RCTs.

Adjustment only	Subgroup analysis
Continuous = + 1 per covariate df Dichotomous = 5–9 events per covariate	Sample size for main effect × 4 for interaction with group

MATCHING THE ANALYSIS TO THE MEASUREMENT SCALE OF THE KEY VARIABLES

Many readers of research reports skip over the Methods section, including the statistical material, and rely on the authors' interpretation of the results. In doing so, they miss much material that could enlighten the results. The role of the statistical analyses commonly used in RCTs need not be mysterious. This section shows the link between the type of data collected, the type of analysis, and numerical results. For many combinations of the measurement scale of the outcome (continuous, categorical, or time-to) and the measurement scale of the exposure variable(s), Table 4 lists common statistical tests.

One of the most overwhelming aspects of statistical analysis is the vast array of tests available. The array becomes much easier to deal with, however, when we note that the choice of statistical analysis is driven, first, by the measurement scale of the outcome variable and then by the measurement scale of the exposure variables. Though the measurement scale of the outcome varies among clinical trials, the exposure (group assignment) is always categorical, usually with 2 categories and rarely more than 4.

Apart from the measurement scale of the outcome, the number of repeated measurements is also a factor in the choice of analysis. A study with a baseline and a post-intervention measurement would have two measures. If the analysis uses only the post-intervention measure or the change score, then there is only one measurement. Many studies collect data at multiple time points. For example, Ghosh et al.[46] measured disease activity and disease-specific HRQL at baseline and at 2, 4, 6, 8, and 12 weeks. A repeated-measures statistical procedure would make maximum use of these data, as opposed to picking one time point for analysis or comparing each time point against baseline (which would create a problem of multiple comparisons, as discussed above).

The third column of Table 4 shows the measurement scale(s) for the exposure variable(s). Here "exposure" refers to any variable that is being studied for its

Table 4. Relation of Common Analyses to the Measurement Scales of the Outcome and the Exposure.

Outcome	N_{rm}	Exposure (n categories)	N_e	Possible analysis or test
Continuous	1	Continuous	1	Pearson correlation
Continuous	1	Categorical (2)	1	Two-sample *t*-test, *Wilcoxon** or *Mann-Whitney U*†
Continuous	2	Categorical (2)	1	Paired *t*-test, *Wilcoxon**
Continuous	1	Categorical (>2)	n	*n*-way ANOVA, *Kruskal-Wallis*
Continuous	≥2	Categorical (>2)	1	Repeated-measures ANOVA
Continuous	1	Any	1	Simple linear regression
Continuous	1	Any	Any	Multiple linear regression
Categorical (2)	1	Categorical (2)	1	Chi-squared (Fisher's exact test when any cell size <5)
Categorical (2)	1	Categorical (≥2)	n	Chi-squared, Mantel-Haenszel chi-squared (*n* is small)
Categorical (≥2)	1	Categorical (≥2)	1	Spearman correlation; chi-squared
Categorical (2)	1	Any	Any	Logistic regression
Categorical (≥2)	1	Any	Any	Polytomous (ordinal or nominal) logistic regression
Time-to	1	Categorical (≥2)	1	Kaplan-Meier, log-rank test
Time-to	1	Any	Any	Cox proportional-hazards
Any	>2	Any	Any	Mixed models (hierarchical models, growth-curve models)
Any	Any	Any	Any	Generalized estimating equations

ANOVA = analysis of variance

N_{rm} indicates number of (repeated) measurement points; a measure before and after treatment would be considered two measures; to compare only these two measures (they would be considered paired), a paired *t*-test or Wilcoxon rank sum test would be appropriate.

N_e indicates number of exposure or explanatory variables under consideration; time-to indicates survival time as the outcome.

* Wilcoxon rank-sum test for independent (or matched pairs) and the † Mann-Whitney U test (unpaired) are nonparametric tests for use with variables that are not normally distributed in the current, usually small, sample. Where both apply, either one is simply a mathematical transformation of the other.

effect on outcome. In an RCT the main exposure variable is group assignment. However, sometimes other variables are also considered, either for adjustment or for explanatory or exploratory reasons (as indicated by N_e in Column 4). Some statistical tests are for very specific types of data and restricted to only two variables—one outcome and one exposure. For example, a two-group RCT with mortality within a fixed time period as the outcome (a categorical variable with two levels: deceased or not) and complete follow-up to the end of the observation period could be analyzed using a chi-squared test; for a continuous outcome, such as a measure of disease severity, a t-test could be used.

Several types of statistical analyses are general enough to accept many forms of exposure variable and can handle any type of measurement scale, including both categorical exposures (like gender) and continuous exposures (like age). In addition, these statistical procedures can handle any number of variables simultaneously (up to the number of subjects). In RCTs these other variables are usually added only for adjustment, and only the effect of the treatment group is of interest. In other types of studies (e.g., studies of etiologic factors), and in explanatory or exploratory analyses of data arising from trials, several exposure variables are of interest, and sample size restricts the number of variables that can be examined simultaneously for association.

The final column of Table 4 lists some of the statistical analyses or tests that could be appropriate for the measurement scales of the outcome and exposure. Various statistical reference sources give more details on the use and interpretation of these methods. The table, however, shows most of the approaches one is likely to find in the medical literature and provides a basis for asking whether other reported analyses might be more appropriate.

An Example Involving Several Outcome Measures and Analyses

The study by Ghosh et al.[46] (Box 4) on drug therapy for Crohn's disease illustrates some of these complex statistical decisions. Table 5 summarizes the statistical methods and results. The primary outcome, remission (a score of < 150 on the Crohn's Disease Activity Index), was assessed at one point in time (6 weeks—that is, 2 weeks after the second infusion). The statistical test matched the outcome (dichotomous: remission or no remission), and the analysis made exposure dichotomous by converting the 4-level variable for group into the 3 pairwise comparisons between each active treatment and placebo. Each country in which patients were treated served as a stratum, and the Mantel-Haenszel chi-squared test took the strata into account in comparing remission rates.

One of the three pairwise comparisons corresponded to the authors' primary hypothesis, that patients who received two infusions of 6 mg of natalizumab per kilogram (abbreviated 6+6) would have a higher rate of remission than those

Table 5. An Illustration of Matching Measurement Scale of the Outcome to Analyses and Statistical Results.

Data Structure	Stated Analyses	Analyses Presented
Exposure is categorical with 4 levels (1 placebo and 3 active drug groups with varying doses)		
Primary outcome #1 – remission at 6 weeks Categorical: (2 levels) remission: value below 150 on disease severity index	Mantel-Haenszel chi-squared test with country of treatment as strata (provides one summary statistic across all countries; assumes homogeneity across countries)	One *p*-value for primary efficacy hypothesis, 6+6 mg/kg vs. placebo at week 6; two *p*-values for the other active drug groups vs. placebo at week 6; 12 *p*-values for the active drug groups vs. placebo at weeks 2, 4, 8, and 12
Secondary outcome #1 – clinical response: decrease of $\geq$70 points on disease severity index		15 *p*-values (one for each comparison of an active drug group vs. placebo at each of weeks 2, 4, 6, 8, and 12); no adjustments for multiplicity (as specified)
Secondary outcome #2 – scores on severity index Continuous score with 6 time points	Area under the curve	$p < 0.02$ for each natalizumab group (significant after Bonferroni adjustment)
	Linear mixed modeling of repeated measurements	$p < 0.05$ for all pairwise comparisons of the three active drug groups vs. placebo group at weeks 2, 4, 6, 8
Secondary outcome #3 – HRQL Continuous score with 6 time points	Change from baseline, compared between each active drug group and placebo group by Mann-Whitney-Wilcoxon test	Median scores (and range) at baseline, 6 and 12 weeks; *p*-values refer to change in score for each active treatment group from baseline, vs. placebo group ($k = 3$), for a total of 6 contrasts (5 with $p < 0.05$); no adjustments for multiplicity
Secondary outcome #4 – C-reactive protein Continuous with 6 time points	Change from baseline, compared between each active drug group and placebo group by Mann-Whitney-Wilcoxon test; also compared in subgroup with baseline value above normal range	Mean change from baseline to 2, 4, 6, 8, and 12 weeks, shown as a bar graph; each active treatment group compared with placebo group ($k = 3$), for a total of 15 contrasts (3 with $p < 0.05$); no adjustments for multiplicity

Ghosh et al. 2003[46]: A trial testing the efficacy of natalizumab in reducing the severity and life impact of Crohn's disease.

who received two infusions of placebo. Its p-value, 0.533, however, was far from statistical significance. The other two comparisons at 6 weeks (3+0 vs. placebo and 3+3 vs. placebo) yielded p-values of 0.757 and 0.030. For these and other secondary analyses, the authors chose not to adjust for multiplicity, so the difference between 3+3 and 0+0 could be regarded as statistically significant ($p = 0.030$). A reader who asks why 3+3 might be more effective than 6+6 might prefer to make the Bonferroni adjustment with a threshold of 0.025 ($= 0.05/2$) for each of the two p-values, and would reach the opposite conclusion; no difference in remission rate at 6 weeks for any of the doses of natalizumab in comparison to placebo.

Similar pairwise comparisons, all secondary, were based on the remission rates at 2, 4, 8, and 12 weeks (12 p-values) and on the rates of clinical response at 2, 4, 6, 8, and 12 weeks (15 p-values). Of the 12 p-values for remission rates, six were < 0.05. Interpreting these informally, as indications, three involved the 3+3 group, three were at week 4, and two were at week 8. The Bonferroni adjustment would apply a threshold of $0.05/12 = 0.0042$ and find statistical significance (at a simultaneous 0.05 level) only at week 8, where the p-values reported for 3+3 and 6+6 were < 0.001. Of the 15 p-values for the pairwise comparisons of rates of clinical response, 12 were < 0.05. Now the adjustment would use a threshold of $0.05/15 = 0.0033$, and only three comparisons would remain significant: 3+3 at weeks 4, 6, and 8.

Other secondary analyses of the disease activity scores (post-hoc) used the area under the curve and (separately) applied linear mixed modeling for repeated measures to the scores, with the aim of bringing together all the data to evaluate treatment effects. On the area under the curve the differences for the 3+3 and 6+6 groups were significant at 0.05/3. From the repeated-measures analysis all pairwise comparisons of the three natalizumab groups with the placebo group had $p < 0.05$ at weeks 2, 4, 6, and 8 (the article does not report the actual p-values, nor does it mention any adjustment for multiplicity involving them).

For the last two secondary outcome measures (the scores on the Inflammatory Bowel Disease Questionnaire and the levels of C-reactive protein), the analyses used the Wilcoxon-Mann-Whitney test to assess change from baseline. A further analysis of C-reactive protein focused on the subset of patients whose baseline value was above the normal range. Of the six comparisons of changes in IBDQ scores (the three active drug groups vs. the placebo group at weeks 6 and 12), only 3+0 vs. placebo at week 12 did not have $p < 0.05$ (individual); taking multiplicity into account, only the three comparisons at week 6 were significant at 0.05/6. On serum levels of C-reactive protein the authors reported a significant decline ($p < 0.05$) at week 6 for the 3+3 and 6+6 groups (vs. the placebo group, which did not show a decline), both in all patients and in the elevated subset. Patients in the elevated subset of the 3+3 group also showed a decline ($p < 0.05$) at week 8. The authors do not report the actual p-values, so we cannot consider adjusting for multiplicity. Apart from issues of multiplicity, the analyses of IBDQ scores and C-reactive protein levels have a potential shortcoming: each comparison uses only the data from two treatment groups at a single time (e.g., the placebo group and the 3+3 group at week 6). Such comparisons can often be more precise when they are part of an analysis that includes all the data (as in the repeated-measures analysis of the disease activity scores) and, if necessary, considers transformation of the outcome variable. Overall, the conclusions of the authors seem correct; the somewhat irregular pattern of non-significant results seems more likely to be a result of limited statistical power than real variations in effectiveness. This complex set of analyses might have been simplified if the research question had been posed differently.[84] Does dose matter? If this is indeed what the authors wanted to know, a simple test for linear trend across dose groups using a regression model would have answered the question. However, in this article,[46] no research question was spelled out in the text; rather the reader is left to infer the exact nature of the question posed. Chapter 4 on design of clinical trials emphasizes the importance of getting the question right from the outset.

When the outcome is ordinal, such as counts of events or graded responses, the analysis seldom properly matches the measurement scale. For example, in two colorectal cancer prevention trials comparing aspirin with placebo,[85, 86] the primary outcome was colorectal adenomas, and subjects could have more than one. The most common (but not preferred) way of dealing with such data creates a dichotomous outcome, none vs. any, and compares rates between the two groups.[85] In the trial reported by Sandler et al.,[86] the distribution of 0, 1, 2, and 3 or more polyps was 216, 26, 9, and 8 subjects in the aspirin group and 188, 37, 19, and 14 subjects in the placebo group. The authors also calculated mean and SD (aspirin, 0.30 ± 0.87; placebo, 0.49 ± 0.99) and range (0–6) for this discrete numerical variable. The simple chi-squared test produced a non-significant p-value. The authors chose to conduct a nonparametric test, a Wilcoxon test, based on the ranks of the data (discussed in Chapter 13). The p-value from this test was significant. The authors present various dichotomizations of the data (0 vs. 1 or more, 0 or 1 vs. 2 or more) and find statistically significant differences. A more-effective approach for such counted data might analyze the outcome variable (here the number of polyps, without collapsing to "3 or more") in a generalized linear model (such as Poisson or negative-binomial regression), which could include subject-level covariates in addition to the treatment effect.

In a study of the effects of memantine for improving cognitive function of persons with moderate-to-severe Alzheimer's disease,[49] the authors treated their primary response variable, a 7-point graded scale of the clinician's impression of change (from 1 for markedly improved to 7 for markedly worse), as a numerical variable. The mean change for the memantine group after 28 weeks, 4.5 (SD: 1.12), was not statistically different ($p = 0.06$) from the mean change for the placebo group, 4.8 (SD: 1.09) when missing data were imputed as the last value carried forward. (With missing data excluded, the difference in means reached statistical significance.) Analyzing this outcome as an ordered categorical variable and using a proportional odds model[87] might have provided a different view of the impact of this drug; at the very least, the parameter from an ordinal logistic regression model is an odds ratio for better improvement, which is easier to interpret than an average improvement. A possible advantage is that missing data can be designated a separate category, and the odds of missing according to group can be estimated as an outcome category. This analysis can be useful if "missingness" is correlated with endpoints.

When a study has more than two groups, the investigators are challenged to decide which comparisons are the most relevant. It may be tempting to examine all $k(k - 1)/2$ pairwise comparisons, but this approach has a number of flaws. First, with k groups, only $k - 1$ statistically independent comparisons ("orthogonal contrasts") can be made, and more will exact a price, usually as more stringent thresholds for finding p-values significant. In addition, when one group is used in more than one comparison, the comparisons are not independent, and problems in that group can jeopardize all the comparisons involved.[88] Ghosh et al.[46] (Box 4) compared each of the three active treatment groups with placebo. If the placebo group had an unexpected response (as may have happened for change in C-reactive protein from baseline to week 6), then results from all contrasts are in danger of arriving at the wrong answer. One way to reduce this risk is to make the common comparison group larger. For $k - 1$ active treatment groups, one comparison group (e.g., a placebo), and a fixed total number of subjects, an optimum split is $\sqrt{k}$ comparison subjects for each one on an active treatment; with three active treatments, this would mean twice as many in the placebo group as in any of the active treatment groups.[89]

A warning is essential. "Shopping" among various methods and reporting the most "favorable" results severely undermines the statistical theory that supports the use of p-values and confidence bounds. It is important that the original protocol specify in detail how the primary analyses will be done, and that the protocol be followed. Statistical procedures that are not specified before the first look at the data may be of great value in exploring unexpected findings, but their evidentiary value is substantially lower.

The analysis of RCTs has evolved over time,[90, 91] and this process is ongoing with heightened interest in using Bayesian approaches to analyzing RCTs.[71, 92-94]

INTERPRETATION OF RESULTS

A review of statistical methods in papers published in the *New England Journal of Medicine* in 1978 and 1979[95] indicated that a reader who knew 11 categories of methods would have access to the statistical methods reported in 90% of those articles. The results in Chapter 3 show that this would not be true in 2007–2008. This change is due in part to developments in statistical methods, but more to growth in the complexity of the data, attributed to the increase in the number of outcomes and the number of time points and to the need to deal more appropriately with missing data. This section discusses simple interpretations of statistical tests and parameters common in reports of RCTs and other parallel comparisons of treatments.

Summaries of results often combine statistical tests of hypotheses and estimates of parameters. The tests yield numbers, such as a *p*-value or a test statistic, that do not translate into the scale of the data. For example, for continuous data, a *t*-statistic for a difference (a ratio of the difference between groups to the standard error of that difference) is less informative than the difference and its confidence interval. In addition, means and variances are generally much easier to combine in meta-analyses than are *p*-values. As a general rule, estimates of parameters, with confidence bounds, are much more informative than *p*-values, and statistical software can now calculate confidence bounds for nearly every statistical test. Their use is strongly recommended.

Table 6 lists interpretations of common parameters. With the exception of regression analyses of linear or mixed models that did not present regression coefficients, all of these parameters were commonly cited in the 73 reports of RCTs published in the *New England Journal of Medicine* in 2003. For categorical data the most prevalent analysis rendered the endpoint binary and carried out some form of survival analysis on the time to reach the endpoint, not just cumulative rates. When cumulative rates were the outcome and the event was rare, logistic regression was appropriately used because the odds ratio approximates the risk ratio, which is more easily interpretable for clinical decision making. (The odds ratio has strong theoretical and computational advantages over the risk ratio, though it is harder to interpret.) When events were common,[85, 86, 96] log-linear models (such as Poisson regression) were appropriately applied, yielding estimates of relative risk rather than relative odds.

The number needed to treat (NNT) was rarely presented,[97] but it is easily calculated from the crude rates[98, 99]; it equals 1 divided by the difference in rates. Table 7 shows calculations of NNT for five studies involving persons with serious medical conditions where treatments were effective in improving outcome in at least one subgroup. McConnell et al.[97] calculated the NNT for three pharmaceutical combinations and placebo from the difference in life-table

Table 6. Interpretation of Common Statistical Parameters.

Parameter	Interpretation
Continuous Data	
95% confidence interval	If this study were to be repeated many times, the true value would fall within this (random) interval 19 times out of 20. For estimates of change, the 95% CI needs to exclude 0 for the result to be considered "statistically significant"
Slope (β from regression line) also called a regression coefficient	People who differ by one unit on the x variable will differ on the Y variable by β units on average.
Area under the curve (AUC)	Outcome-time (e.g., severity-days, pain-days), quality-adjusted life-years (QALY)
Categorical Data	
Rate	Proportion of people who had an event
Risk	An individual's probability of having an event in a specified time; derived from the rate
Relative risk or relative rate (RR)	Average risk or rate in one group relative to average risk or rate in another group; RR of 1.5 indicates that the average risk or rate of one group is 50% higher than the average risk or rate of the other group
Odds	Ratio of the probability of having an event to the probability of not having the event; odds of 2:1 indicate that 2/3 persons will have an event and 1/3 will not
Odds ratio (OR)	Ratio of odds in one group to odds in another group (often a reference group); if the first group has odds of 3:1 and the second group has 1.5:1 odds, ratio of odds is 3.0/1.5, giving OR = 2.0; for the corresponding risks the ratio is 0.75/0.60, yielding RR = 1.25. When the outcome is very rare, the OR approaches the RR.
Hazard rate	Risk of developing an event at a point in time
Hazard ratio	Ratio of hazard rates between two groups
Number needed to treat (NNT)	Number of people who need to be treated with the intervention to prevent one additional negative outcome
Number needed to harm (NNH)	Number of people whose being treated will produce one additional adverse event

estimates of the cumulative incidence probability at four years. To illustrate, the data presented in their Table 2 indicate that the rate of clinical progression of prostate cancer was 17% in the placebo group, but only 5% in the combination doxazosin and finasteride group. The reciprocal of the difference in cumulative incidence is $1/(0.17 - 0.05) = 1/0.12 = 8.3$. Therefore, the number needed to treat with this combination of drugs to prevent one additional clinical

Table 7. Comparison of NNT among Serious Medical Conditions Where Treatments Were Effective in Improving Outcome.

	Colorectal cancer[86]	High risk for pre-term delivery[104]	High risk for prostate cancer[97]	Coronary revascularization[47]	Upper lobe emphysema / low exercise capacity[13]
Intervention shown to be effective	Aspirin 325 mg. per day vs. placebo	Weekly injections of progestational agent vs. placebo	Combination of finasteride/doxazosin vs. placebo	Coated stent vs. uncoated stent	Lung-reduction surgery vs. medical care in subgroup†
Time frame of Rx	3 years	16 weeks	4 years	One-time intervention with follow-up to < 1 year	One-time intervention with follow-up average of 29 months
Outcome	Adenoma	Pre-term delivery	Clinical progression	Vessel failure	Mortality
Rate in control	27%	54.9%	17%	21%	33.8%
Rate in intervention	17%	36.3%	5%	8.6%	18.7%
Risk difference	10ppt	18.6ppt	12ppt	12.4ppt	15.1ppt
Reciprocal of risk difference	1/0.10	1/0.186	1/0.12	1/0.124	1/0.151
NNT (95% CI)	10 (6 to 29)	5 (4 to 11)	8 (7 to 11)	8 (6 to 12)	6 (4 to 20)
$ per unit	$0.02	$25***	$1.94[105]	$3500[106]	$49,011[107]
$ per person	<$30	$400	$2920	$3500	$49,011[107]
$ to prevent one	<$300	$2160	$24,236	$28,350	$294,066
NNH	294 (included 0)	Not estimable	11 (10 to 14) (1858)*	Not estimable	Not estimable

ppt = percentage points

NNT = 1/(risk difference of benefit) (rounded)

NNH = 1/(risk difference of adverse event) (rounded)

†in subgroup with most favorable outcome: upper lobe emphysema and low exercise capacity

*for breast cancer in men: 95% confidence interval included 0

***http://www.fluvaccine.com/Item/HTFINJ.htm

progression in four years was 8.3. For the other two groups with single agents the NNT was 1/(0.17–0.10) = 14.3. (Differences between these values and the ones given by McConnell et al.[97] are due to rounding.) Using this approach, it is possible to calculate the NNT for any study. Like any other parameter, NNT is only an estimate, so presenting it with its corresponding 95% confidence interval yields the most information. Based on the work of Newcombe,[100] Tandberg has developed a very helpful spreadsheet (available at http://www.cebm.net/index.aspx?o=1159).

The NNT is helpful in thinking about relative effectiveness, particularly with respect to costs of intervention. In Table 7 aspirin clearly has the lowest cost per negative outcome prevented. For the other interventions the cost per negative event prevented ranged enormously. NNT is relevant to comparisons among competing interventions for the same condition or among conditions when decisions need to be made about allocation of scarce resources. However, as noted earlier, estimating the costs of medical care is substantially more complicated than it may appear to be, and skilled professional help will generally be needed, in part because the distribution of costs is often severely asymmetric, and special procedures are needed to calculate confidence bounds.

In situations where a widely used treatment has negative as well as positive effects, one can also estimate the "number needed to harm" (NNH). For example, three of the studies summarized in Table 7 also reported adverse event rates. In the study of finasteride and doxazosin for prostate cancer,[97] the absolute adverse event rate difference was not presented overall but rather for 10 side effects. If these are summed, the adverse event rate for placebo was 14.25 per 100 person-years compared with 23.11 for the two groups with finasteride alone or in combination. The risk difference, 0.0886 (= 0.2311 – 0.1425), yields a NNH of 1/0.0886 or 11 (95% CI: 10 to 14). Not included in their table but mentioned in the text was that four men in the two groups where finasteride was an active ingredient developed breast cancer. This translates to a rate of 5.3 per 10,000 (4/7432) or a NNH of 1858 (with a 95% CI that included 0). Most people would consider breast cancer to be more serious than erectile dysfunction, dizziness, or peripheral edema. Zermansky[101] suggests separating adverse events and calculating number needed to kill, number needed to disable, number needed to make the patient ill, and number needed to annoy. Thus, with finasteride,[97] the number needed to annoy was between 10 and 14, and the number needed to make the patient ill was 1858 but with a confidence interval that included 0.

Generally, expected benefits drive power calculations and sample sizes, and potential adverse outcomes are substantially less common. Thus, studies rarely have power to detect differences between groups in adverse events, so it is difficult to appreciate the magnitude of these effects. NNH offers a way to balance the negative against the benefits of the interventions under study.

SUMMARY OF PRINCIPAL ANALYTICAL
CHALLENGES IN RCTS

This chapter has built on Chapter 4 by presenting several considerations important in the analysis of RCTs. Some of these considerations, like intention-to-
treat, will be familiar to the majority of readers, but others may be new, like
response shift; and readers may have overlooked still others such as estimation
of change and the biases created by missing data.

Dealing with multiple endpoints is a frequent challenge owing to the expanding
number of outcomes and multiple time points. Choosing only one of multiple
outcomes may be statistically sound (as long as it is done prior to the study)
but often limits clinical relevance. Sorting outcomes into confirmatory, explanatory, and exploratory will provide a richer view of the effects. Global indices are
mathematically possible but require evidence that the components measure a
single construct or are combinable.

Several appealing methods exist for summarizing outcome over time, including a simple change score, slope of the line, or area under the curve. These techniques reduce the data and allow use of cross-sectional statistical procedures
such as analysis of variance and linear regression. With these cross-sectional
indices, it is not necessary (or advisable) to adjust for the baseline variable.
However, powerful modeling techniques permit longitudinal variability unrelated to the treatment to contribute to the estimate.

Dealing with missing data is probably the most challenging aspect of data
analysis, particularly as RCTs move beyond asking questions about the impact
of interventions on mortality or disease occurrence and include measures of
impairment, activity limitation, and HRQL. The fundamental principle is that
endpoints should be available for each study subject; if that cannot be attained,
the missing data must be missing completely at random or missing at random,
and not depend on the value of the outcome. Missing data on measured variables because of mortality would tend to overestimate the mean in the group
with the greatest number of deaths, as most commonly persons in the poorest
health die. Methods of imputing missing data are numerous but need to be
chosen after considering the implications for both the estimate of effect and its
variance. Simple imputation procedures such as last-value-carried-forward can
be biased. Multiple imputation requires advanced statistical help and program-
ming. Excluding subjects with missing data at the very best reduces power, and
it generally introduces a likelihood of bias.

Adjusting for covariates is desirable because known sources of variation in outcome are removed, which reduces the estimated variability and hence increases
the precision of findings. As the covariates are unrelated to the group assignment, their inclusion should not affect the estimate of size of the treatment

effect[72]; the reduction in variance is advantageous in identifying the true effect, if any, of the intervention. The choice of covariates should be based on *a priori* knowledge of their prognostic value, not on imbalances among groups. Adjustment for important covariates will also reduce any residual bias after randomization that occurs from persons dropping out of the trials, as the covariates are likely to explain some of the attrition. With binary data, adjustment depends on the question being addressed, as the estimate of effect in an unadjusted analysis is for the average person; with adjustment the estimated effect is for people with specific characteristics. The only valid way to use adjustment to look for subgroups that may respond differently is to fit interaction terms between all known prognostic variables and treatment group. This requires a substantial increase in sample size (by a factor of 4 or more) to reduce the risk of wrongly concluding that there is no interaction. Commonly, however, one looks for subgroups for purposes of hypothesis generation, and subgroups selected *post-hoc* entail risks of over-interpreting even striking findings. Ordinary statistical tests, however, are not applicable in situations where interactions are being considered.

Matching the analysis to the measurement scale of the key variables comes naturally to persons trained in statistics, but statistical methods sections of research articles are sometimes difficult for the non-expert to read and understand. In practice, the choice of analysis is largely determined by the nature of the data, and the actual range of analyses is narrow and well within the grasp of most readers of the medical literature. A careful analyst will ensure that tables and figures refer specifically to the tests indicated in the methods section, but this is not true of much of today's scientific literature.

Interpreting commonly used statistical tests and parameters would be facilitated if journal articles published estimates of parameters, with confidence bounds, rather than just p-values. If survival time is the outcome of interest, the most common parameters presented are the odds ratio and the hazard ratio. For continuous data, regression parameters are rarely presented but would be equivalent to the difference between groups. When confidence intervals are presented, the null value depends on the parameter; for a rate, odds, or hazard ratio, "no effect" corresponds to a null value of 1.0. For change scores or slopes, the null value is 0. NNT and NNH are not commonly reported in trials but are often calculable and provide a way of appreciating the balance of good and harm.

REFERENCES

1. Fairclough DL. Summary measures and statistics for comparison of quality of life in a clinical trial of cancer therapy. Stat Med 1997; 16(11):1197–209.

2. Peduzzi P, Henderson W, Hartigan P, Lavori P. Analysis of randomized controlled trials. Epidemiol Rev 2002; 24(1):26–38.

3. Schulz KF, Grimes DA. Sample size slippages in randomised trials: exclusions and the lost and wayward. Lancet 2002; 359(9308):781–5.

4. Tallman MS, Gray R, Robert NJ, et al. Conventional adjuvant chemotherapy with or without high-dose chemotherapy and autologous stem-cell transplantation in high-risk breast cancer. N Engl J Med 2003; 349(1):17–26.

5. Hays J, Ockene JK, Brunner RL, et al. Effects of estrogen plus progestin on health-related quality of life. N Engl J Med 2003; 348(19):1839–54.

6. Rothman KJ. No adjustments are needed for multiple comparisons. Epidemiology 1990; 1(1):43–6.

7. Ware JE Jr, Kosinski M, Keller SD. SF-36 Physical & mental scales: A user's manual. Boston, Massachusetts: The Health Institute, New England Medical Center; 1994.

8. Geddes D, Davies M, Koyama H, et al. Effect of lung-volume–reduction surgery in patients with severe emphysema. N Engl J Med 2000; 343(4):239–45.

9. Goss PE, Ingle JN, Martino S, et al. A randomized trial of letrozole in postmenopausal women after five years of tamoxifen therapy for early-stage breast cancer. N Engl J Med 2003; 349(19):1793–802.

10. Heydendael VM, Spuls PI, Opmeer BC, et al. Methotrexate versus cyclosporine in moderate-to-severe chronic plaque psoriasis. N Engl J Med 2003; 349(7):658–65.

11. Kremer JM, Westhovens R, Leon M, et al. Treatment of rheumatoid arthritis by selective inhibition of T-cell activation with fusion protein CTLA4Ig. N Engl J Med 2003; 349(20):1907–15.

12. Lawrence J, Mayers DL, Hullsiek KH, et al. Structured treatment interruption in patients with multidrug-resistant human immunodeficiency virus. N Engl J Med 2003; 349(9):837–46.

13. National Emphysema Treatment Trial Research Group. A randomized trial comparing lung-volume–reduction surgery with medical therapy for severe emphysema. N Engl J Med 2003; 348(21):2059–73.

14. Wainwright C, Altamirano L, Cheney M, et al. A multicenter, randomized, double-blind, controlled trial of nebulized epinephrine in infants with acute bronchiolitis. N Engl J Med 2003; 349(1):27–35.

15. Charlson ME, Pompei P, Ales KL, MacKenzie CR. A new method of classifying prognostic comorbidity in longitudinal studies: development and validation. J Chronic Dis 1987; 40:373–83.

16. Tessier A, Finch L, Daskalopoulou SS, Mayo NE. Validation of the Charlson Comorbidity Index for predicting functional outcome of stroke. Arch Phys Med Rehabil 2008; 89(7):1276–83.

17. Fairclough DL. Design and analysis of quality of life studies in clinical trials. Boca Raton, FL: Chapman & Hall/CRC; 2002.

18. Kwiatkowski TG, Libman RB, Frankel M, et al. Effects of tissue plasminogen activator for acute ischemic stroke at one year. N Engl J Med 1999; 340(23):1781–7.

19. Glynn RJ, Rosner B. Methods to evaluate risks for composite end points and their individual components. J Clin Epidemiol 2004; 57(2):113–22.

20. Gaede P, Vedel P, Larsen N, et al. Multifactorial intervention and cardiovascular disease in patients with type 2 diabetes. N Engl J Med 2003; 348(5):383–93.

21. Wing LM, Reid CM, Ryan P, et al. A comparison of outcomes with angiotensin-converting–enzyme inhibitors and diuretics for hypertension in the elderly. N Engl J Med 2003; 348(7):583–92.

22. Schwartz CE, Sprangers MAG, eds. Adaptation to changing health: response shift in quality-of-life research. 1st ed. Washington, DC: American Psychological Association; 2000.

23. Ahmed S, Mayo NE, Wood-Dauphinee S, et al. The structural equation modeling technique did not show a response shift, contrary to the results of the then test and the individualized approaches. J Clin Epidemiol 2005; 58(11):1125–33.

24. Mayo NE, Nadeau L, Ahmed S, et al. Bridging the gap: the effectiveness of teaming a stroke coordinator with patient's personal physician on the outcome of stroke. Age Ageing 2007; 37(1):32–8.

25. Ahmed S, Mayo NE, Wood-Dauphinee S, et al. Response shift influenced estimates of change in health-related quality of life poststroke. J Clin Epidemiol 2004; 57(6):561–70.

26. Guyatt GH, Berman LB, Townsend M, et al. A measure of quality of life for clinical trials in chronic lung disease. Thorax 1987; 42(10):773–8.

27. Oort FJ, Visser MR, Sprangers MA. An application of structural equation modeling to detect response shifts and true change in quality of life data from cancer patients undergoing invasive surgery. Qual Life Res 2005; 14(3):599–609.

28. Oort FJ. Using structural equation modeling to detect response shifts and true change. Qual Life Res 2005; 14(3):587–98.

29. Mayo NE, Scott SC, Dendukuri N, et al. Identifying response shift statistically at the individual level. Qual Life Res 2008; 17(4):627–39.

30. Allison PJ, Locker D, Feine JS. Quality of life: a dynamic construct. Social Sci Med 1997; 45(2):221–30.

31. O'Boyle CA, McGee HM, Brown JP. Measuring response shift using the schedule for evaluation of individual quality of life. In: Schwartz CE, Sprangers MA, eds. Adaptation to changing health: response shift in quality-of-life research. 1st ed. Washington, DC: American Psychological Association; 2000: 123–36.

32. Osborne RH, Hawkins M, Sprangers MA. Change of perspective: A measurable and desired outcome of chronic disease self-management intervention programs that violates the premise of preintervention/postintervention assessment. Arthritis Rheum 2006; 55(3):458–65.

33. Oldham PD. A note on analysis of repeated measurements of same subjects. J Chronic Dis 1962; 15:969–77.

34. Hayes RJ. Methods for assessing whether change depends on initial value. Stat Med 1988; 7(9):915–27.

35. Mayo NE. The effect of physical therapy for children with motor delay and cerebral palsy. A randomized clinical trial. Am J Phys Med Rehabil. 1991; 70(5):258–67.

36. Salbach NM, Mayo NE, Robichaud-Ekstrand S, et al. The effect of a task-oriented walking intervention on improving balance self-efficacy poststroke: a randomized, controlled trial. J Am Geriatr Soc 2005; 53(4):576–82.

37. Twisk J, Proper K. Evaluation of the results of a randomized controlled trial: how to define changes between baseline and follow-up. J Clin Epidemiol 2004; 57(3):223–8.

38. Twisk J, Proper K. Is analysis of covariance the most appropriate way to analyse changes in randomized controlled trials? J Clin Epidemiol 2005; 58(2):211–2.

39. Twisk J, Proper K. "Analysis of covariance" vs. "residual change." J Clin Epidemiol 2005; 58(5):542.

40. Forbes AB, Carlin JB. "Residual change" analysis is not equivalent to analysis of covariance. J Clin Epidemiol 2005; 58(5):540–1.

41. Boshuizen HC. Re: Twisk and Proper: evaluation of the results of a randomized controlled trial: how to define changes between baseline and follow-up. J Clin Epidemiol 2005; 58(2):209–10.

42. Boshuizen HC. Reaction to: "Re: In response to the correspondence arising from Twisk and Proper: evaluation of the results of a randomized controlled trial: how to define changes between baseline and follow-up" by Siew F. Chan and others. J Clin Epidemiol 2006; 59(3):323–4.

43. Jayne D, Rasmussen N, Andrassy K, et al. A randomized trial of maintenance therapy for vasculitis associated with antineutrophil cytoplasmic autoantibodies. N Engl J Med 2003; 349(1):36–44.

44. Miller DH, Khan OA, Sheremata WA, et al. A controlled trial of natalizumab for relapsing multiple sclerosis. N Engl J Med 2003; 348(1):15–23.

45. Manson JE, Hsia J, Johnson KC, et al. Estrogen plus progestin and the risk of coronary heart disease. N Engl J Med 2003; 349(6):523–34.

46. Ghosh S, Goldin E, Gordon FH, et al. Natalizumab for active Crohn's disease. N Engl J Med 2003; 348(1):24–32.

47. Moses JW, Leon MB, Popma JJ, et al. Sirolimus-eluting stents versus standard stents in patients with stenosis in a native coronary artery. N Engl J Med 2003; 349(14):1315–23.

48. Black DM, Greenspan SL, Ensrud KE, et al. The effects of parathyroid hormone and alendronate alone or in combination in postmenopausal osteoporosis. N Engl J Med 2003; 349(13):1207–15.

49. Reisberg B, Doody R, Stöffler A, et al. Memantine in moderate-to-severe Alzheimer's disease. N Engl J Med 2003; 348(14):1333–41.

50. Samaha FF, Iqbal N, Seshadri P, et al. A low-carbohydrate as compared with a low-fat diet in severe obesity. N Engl J Med 2003; 348(21):2074–81.

51. Terreehorst I, Hak E, Oosting AJ, et al. Evaluation of impermeable covers for bedding in patients with allergic rhinitis. N Engl J Med 2003; 349(3):237–46.

52. Aaron SD, Vandemheen KL, Hebert P, et al. Outpatient oral prednisone after emergency treatment of chronic obstructive pulmonary disease. N Engl J Med 2003; 348(26):2618–25.

53. Park SJ, Shim WH, Ho DS, et al. A paclitaxel-eluting stent for the prevention of coronary restenosis. N Engl J Med 2003; 348(16):1537–45.

54. Lin JL, Lin-Tan DT, Hsu KH, Yu CC. Environmental lead exposure and progression of chronic renal diseases in patients without diabetes. N Engl J Med 2003; 348(4):277–86.

55. Marcellin P, Chang TT, Lim SG, et al. Adefovir dipivoxil for the treatment of hepatitis B e antigen–positive chronic hepatitis B. N Engl J Med 2003; 348(9):808–16.

56. Hadziyannis SJ, Tassopoulos NC, Heathcote EJ, et al. Adefovir dipivoxil for the treatment of hepatitis B e antigen–negative chronic hepatitis B. N Engl J Med 2003; 348(9):800–7.

57. Leonardi CL, Powers JL, Matheson RT, et al. Etanercept as monotherapy in patients with psoriasis. N Engl J Med 2003; 349(21):2014–22.

58. Foster GD, Wyatt HR, Hill JO, et al. A randomized trial of a low-carbohydrate diet for obesity. N Engl J Med 2003; 348(21):2082–90.

59. Hodis HN, Mack WJ, Azen SP, et al. Hormone therapy and the progression of coronary-artery atherosclerosis in postmenopausal women. N Engl J Med 2003; 349(6):535–45.

60. Woodcock A, Forster L, Matthews E, et al. Control of exposure to mite allergen and allergen-impermeable bed covers for adults with asthma. N Engl J Med 2003; 349(3):225–36.

61. Aspelin P, Aubry P, Fransson SG, et al. Nephrotoxic effects in high-risk patients undergoing angiography. N Engl J Med 2003; 348(6):491–9.

62. Lalezari JP, Henry K, O'Hearn M, et al. Enfuvirtide, an HIV-1 fusion inhibitor, for drug-resistant HIV infection in North and South America. N Engl J Med 2003; 348(22):2175–85.

63. Yanovski JA, Rose SR, Municchi G, et al. Treatment with a luteinizing hormone-releasing hormone agonist in adolescents with short stature. N Engl J Med 2003; 348(10):908–17.

64. Finkelstein JS, Hayes A, Hunzelman JL, et al. The effects of parathyroid hormone, alen-dronate, or both in men with osteoporosis. N Engl J Med 2003; 349(13):1216–26.

65. Rowbotham MC, Twilling L, Davies PS, et al. Oral opioid therapy for chronic peripheral and central neuropathic pain. N Engl J Med 2003; 348(13):1223–32.

66. Raudenbush SW, Chan WS. Application of a hierarchical linear model to the study of adoles-cent deviance in an overlapping cohort design. J Consult Clin Psychol 1993; 61(6):941–51.

67. Allison PD. Missing data. Thousand Oaks, CA: Sage Publications, Inc.; 2002.

68. Little RJ, Rubin DB. Statistical analysis with missing data. 2nd ed. Hoboken, NJ: John Wiley; 2002.

69. Wood AM, White IR, Thompson SG. Are missing outcome data adequately handled? A review of published randomized controlled trials in major medical journals. Clin Trials 2004; 1(4):368–76.

70. Fielding S, Maclennan G, Cook JA, Ramsay CR. A review of RCTs in four medical journals to assess the use of imputation to overcome missing data in quality of life outcomes. Trials 2008; 9(1):51.

71. Pocock SJ, Assmann SE, Enos LE, Kasten LE. Subgroup analysis, covariate adjustment and baseline comparisons in clinical trial reporting: current practice and problems. Stat Med 2002; 21(19):2917–30.

72. Hauck WW, Anderson S, Marcus SM. Should we adjust for covariates in nonlinear regression analyses of randomized trials? Control Clin Trials 1998; 19(3):249–56.

73. Maxwell SE. Covariate imbalance and conditional size: dependence on model-based adjust-ments. Stat Med 1993; 12(2):101–9.

74. Kleinbaum DG, Klein M. Logistic regression: a self-learning text. 2nd ed. New York: Springer; 2002.

75. Hauck WW, Anderson S, Marcus SM. Should we adjust for covariates in nonlinear regression analyses of randomized trials? Control Clin Trials 1998; 19(3):249–56.

76. Lesaffre E, Bogaerts K, Li X, Bluhmki E. On the variability of covariate adjustment: experi-ence with Koch's method for evaluating the absolute difference in proportions in random-ized clinical trials. Control Clin Trials 2002; 23(2):127–42.

77. Hernandez AV, Steyerberg EW, Habbema JD. Covariate adjustment in randomized controlled trials with dichotomous outcomes increases statistical power and reduces sample size requirements. J Clin Epidemiol 2004; 57(5):454–60.

78. Brookes ST, Whitely E, Egger M, et al. Subgroup analyses in randomized trials: risks of subgroup-specific analyses; power and sample size for the interaction test. J Clin Epidemiol 2004; 57(3):229–36.

79. Brookes ST, Whitley E, Peters TJ, et al. Subgroup analyses in randomised controlled trials: quantifying the risks of false-positives and false-negatives. Health Technol Assess 2001; 5(33).

80. Green SB. How many subjects does it take to do a regression analysis? Multivariate Behav Res 1991; 26:499–510.

81. Kraemer HC, Thiemann S. How many subjects?: statistical power analysis in research. Newbury Park, CA: Sage Publications, Inc.; 1987.

82. Peduzzi P, Concato J, Kemper E, et al. A simulation study of the number of events per variable in logistic regression analysis. J Clin Epidemiol 1996; 49(12):1373–9.

83. Vittinghoff E, McCulloch CE. Relaxing the rule of ten events per variable in logistic and Cox regression. Am J Epidemiol 2007; 165(6):710–8.

84. Wittes J. Sample size calculations for randomized controlled trials. Epidemiol Rev 2002; 24(1):39–53.

85. Baron JA, Cole BF, Sandler RS, et al. A randomized trial of aspirin to prevent colorectal adenomas. N Engl J Med 2003; 348(10):891–9.

86. Sandler RS, Halabi S, Baron JA, et al. A randomized trial of aspirin to prevent colorectal adenomas in patients with previous colorectal cancer. N Engl J Med 2003; 348(10):883–90.

87. Scott S, Goldberg M, Mayo N. Statistical assessment of ordinal outcomes in comparative studies. J Clin Epidemiol 1997; 50:45–55.

88. Armitage P, Berry G, Matthews JNS. Statistical methods in medical research. 4th ed. New York: John Wiley; 2001.

89. Dunnett CW. New tables for multiple comparisons with a control. Biometrics 1964; 20:482–91.

90. Machin D. On the evolution of statistical methods as applied to clinical trials. J Intern Med 2004; 255(5):521–8.

91. Fisher LD. Advances in clinical trials in the twentieth century. Ann Rev Public Health 1999; 20(1):109–24.

92. Berry DA. Introduction to Bayesian methods III: use and interpretation of Bayesian tools in design and analysis. Clinical Trials 2005; 2(4):295–300.

93. Brophy JM, Joseph L. Placing trials in context using Bayesian analysis. GUSTO revisited by Reverend Bayes. JAMA 1995; 273(11):871–5.

94. Spiegelhalter DJ, Abrams KR, Myles JP. Bayesian approaches to clinical trials and healthcare evaluation. Chichester, England: John Wiley & Sons, Ltd; 2004.

95. Emerson JD, Colditz GA. Use of statistical analysis in the New England Journal of Medicine. N Engl J Med 1983; 309(12):709–13.

96. Thompson IM, Goodman PJ, Tangen CM, et al. The influence of finasteride on the development of prostate cancer. N Engl J Med 2003; 349(3):215–24.

97. McConnell JD, Roehrborn CG, Bautista OM, et al. The long-term effect of doxazosin, finasteride, and combination therapy on the clinical progression of benign prostatic hyperplasia. N Engl J Med 2003; 349(25):2387–98.

98. Laupacis A, Sackett DL, Roberts RS. An assessment of clinically useful measures of the consequences of treatment. N Engl J Med 1988; 318(26):1728–33.

99. Mancini GB, Schulzer M. Reporting risks and benefits of therapy by use of the concepts of unqualified success and unmitigated failure: applications to highly cited trials in cardiovascular medicine. Circulation 1999; 99(3):377–83.

100. Newcombe RG. Interval estimation for the difference between independent proportions: comparison of eleven methods. Stat Med 1998; 17(8):873–90.

101. Zermansky A. Number needed to harm should be measured for treatments. BMJ 1998; 317(7164):1014.

102. Suissa S, Levinton C, Esdaile JM. Modeling percentage change: a potential linear mirage. J Clin Epidemiol 1989; 42(9):843–8.

103. Blair EM, Love SC, Valentine JP. Proportional change: an additional method of reporting technical and functional outcomes following clinical interventions. Eur J Neurol 2001; 8 (Suppl 5):178–82.

104. Meis PJ, Klebanoff M, Thom E, et al. Prevention of recurrent preterm delivery by 17 alpha-hydroxyprogesterone caproate. N Engl J Med 2003; 348(24):2379–85.

105. Bloom BS, Iannacone RC. Internet availability of prescription pharmaceuticals to the public. Ann Intern Med 1999; 131(11):830–3.

106. O'Neill WW, Leon MB. Drug-eluting stents: costs versus clinical benefit. Circulation 2003; 107(24):3008–11.

107. Ramsey SD, Berry K, Etzioni R, et al. Cost effectiveness of lung-volume–reduction surgery for patients with severe emphysema. N Engl J Med 2003; 348(21):2092–102.

Linear Regression in Medical Research

PAUL J. RATHOUZ, PH.D., AND AMITA RASTOGI, M.D., M.H.A.

ABSTRACT   Regression techniques are important statistical tools for assessing the relationships among variables in medical research. Linear regression summarizes the way in which a continuous outcome variable varies in relation to one or more explanatory or predictor variables. This chapter covers the application and interpretation of simple (a single predictor) and multiple (more than one predictor) linear regression. We discuss in detail the estimation and interpretation of regression slopes and intercepts, hypothesis tests, and confidence intervals in simple linear regression models. Then we contrast regression with correlation and discuss how these methods both summarize statistical association, but do not necessarily imply causation among the variables of interest. We then summarize some main points about the careful use of linear regression so that the reader has an appreciation of the data analytic issues involved in carrying out regression analyses. Building on our presentation of simple linear regression, we provide an overview of multiple linear regression, with a strong emphasis on interpretation of the regression slopes. We discuss the differential use of regression for statistical summarization of relationships between the outcome and predictors, for statistical adjustment of the observed relationship of the outcome to one or more key predictors, and for statistical prediction of the outcome from a set of candidate predictors. An example involving the prediction of HbA_{1c} from characteristics of sleep in diabetes patients is carried throughout the chapter for illustrating the key ideas, and other illustrative examples are drawn from the recent medical literature.

The vast majority of statistical analyses in medical research involve relationships among variables. Common examples include coronary artery disease and cholesterol, lung cancer risk and smoking, cognitive function and aging, and so on. Linear regression summarizes the way in which one variable (Y) varies in relation to one or more other variables (X). *Simple linear regression* involves a single X variable, and *multiple linear regression* covers more than one X variable. The Y variable is commonly referred to as the *outcome* or *response*, and the X variables are called *explanatory* or *predictor* variables or, sometimes, *covariates*. (The explanatory variables are often called "independent variables," but it is safer to avoid this terminology because the term "independent" has other meanings in statistics.) In linear regression analyses Y is a "continuous" variable, such as a laboratory measurement or a score on a 0–100 scale; techniques for categorical variables are discussed in Chapter 12.

> Example 1: A study of sleep and endocrine function[1] evaluated 122 diabetic patients for sleep quantity and quality, as well as for diabetes control, as measured by hemoglobin A_{1c} (HbA_{1c}). The hypothesis under investigation was that reduced sleep quantity and/or quality leads to poorer diabetes control, and hence increased HbA_{1c} levels. Sleep quality was measured via a modified version of the previously validated Pittsburgh Sleep Quality Index (PSQI).[2, 3] The PSQI varies from 0 to 21 "points"; higher values represent poorer sleep, and any score greater than 5 indicates poor sleep quality. Percent HbA_{1c}, obtained from patients' medical charts, measures average blood glucose level for the preceding three months; in diabetic populations, values over 7.5–8% are generally considered indicators of poor glycemic control.[4, 5]

In an uncomplicated world, the relationship between HbA_{1c} and PSQI would be exact, so that a single value of Y would correspond to each value of X, and in a scatter plot of Y versus X the points would fall on a straight line, as in Figure 1. The key quantity of scientific interest would be the slope of the line describing how HbA_{1c} varies with PSQI (the rate of change in HbA_{1c} per unit increase in PSQI).

This idealized relationship of HbA_{1c} to sleep quality is, of course, purely hypothetical. In practice, many factors other than PSQI, both measured and unmeasured, both understood and unknown, affect HbA_{1c} levels. The actual data (Figure 2) show that the relationship is much less clear, although still quite evident. Mean HbA_{1c} shows a tendency to increase with PSQI, but variation among individuals is substantial. We develop this example through the remainder of the chapter.

Statistical regression is a procedure for objectively fitting a curve through a set of points, such as those in Figure 2. To allow for variation or "noise" in the data (from differences among individuals or from measurement error), regression focuses on average behavior. Specifically, "the regression of Y on X" refers to the average (mean) value of Y corresponding to each value of X. The diamonds in Figure 2 show the mean value of HbA_{1c} (Y) at each value of PSQI (X). On average, HbA_{1c} tends to increase with PSQI, although individual HbA_{1c} values vary considerably at any given level of PSQI. In general, the regression of Y on X does not prescribe any particular pattern for how the mean of Y varies with X.

Linear regression refers to the common situation in which the average values of Y across the range of X fall on or close to a straight line. Standard ways of estimating a linear regression produce the straight line that is, in a particular mathematical sense, the best fit to the data. Even when those average-value points do not follow a straight line, the computational procedure will deliver a line, which may often be a useful summary of much of the relationship. The key

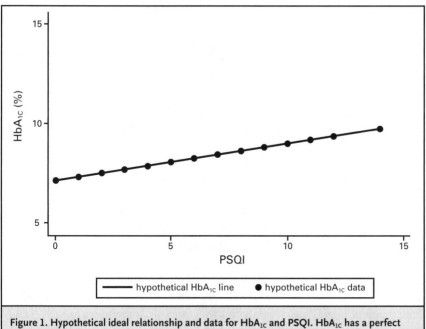

Figure 1. Hypothetical ideal relationship and data for HbA$_{1c}$ and PSQI. HbA$_{1c}$ has a perfect linear relationship with PSQI score, so that all data points fall exactly on a straight line.

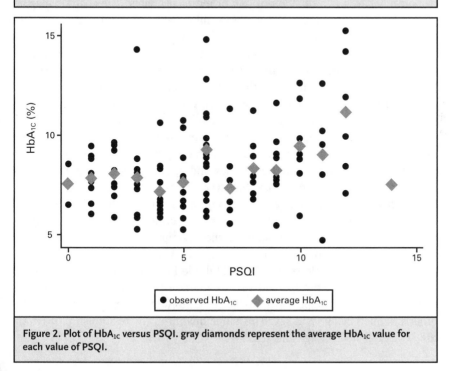

Figure 2. Plot of HbA$_{1c}$ versus PSQI. gray diamonds represent the average HbA$_{1c}$ value for each value of PSQI.

quantity is the *regression slope*, quantifying how many units the average value of Y increases (or decreases) for each unit increase in X.

Examples of simple linear regression are less common in the medical literature than are applications of *multiple linear regression*, involving several predictor variables (X's). The ability to handle multiple X's and predictors that take a variety of forms gives regression methods very broad applicability. Most analyses have one of three aims: summarization and explanation, adjustment, or prediction. These groupings are not hard and fast, but they do provide a sense of the rich diversity of applications.

A *summarization* analysis aims to provide a simple description of how a response Y varies with X or with a set of X's. The obvious appeal of the procedure is that it reduces a potentially complex multidimensional set of relationships to a small set of regression slopes that are easy to understand and straightforward to communicate. For example, it may be of interest to describe how HbA_{1C} varies with a set of sleep characteristics, including a measure of sleep quality such as the PSQI, total sleep obtained, and perceived sleep debt. Placing these three predictors in a single multiple-regression model for HbA_{1C} will yield three regression slopes; adding the effects they summarize provides a parsimonious description of how HbA_{1C} varies with these three sleep measures jointly. A summarization analysis is often motivated by a desire to explain or describe how a response behaves as a function of one or more covariates. The analysis may be guided by hypotheses about these relationships, and it is of interest to evaluate how well these hypotheses are borne out by the data.

Often, explanatory data analysis problems arise in conjunction with a goal of statistical *adjustment*, a compelling need in many medical studies. Suppose, for example, that it is known that both HbA_{1C} and sleep quality vary with age and sex. Ignoring this fact may lead to spurious results, including perhaps an inflation of the relationship of HbA_{1C} to sleep quality. One study design could handle such a problem by sampling only individuals of a single sex and within a narrow age range. More informatively, researchers might perform separate analyses for each of several groups delineated by sex and age, yielding a separate regression slope for each group. It may, however, not be feasible to assemble a useful number of subjects in each such group. Even if the sample sizes are large enough, separate results for each group may be difficult to present and digest. Statistical adjustment aims to simplify the description and clarify the picture when the regression of HbA_{1C} on sleep quality within the various age-by-sex groups yields similar slopes for PSQI. Multiple linear regression that includes explanatory variables for age and sex, in addition to sleep quality, will yield a common regression slope for the relation of HbA_{1C} to sleep quality across the groups defined by age and sex. This slope quantifies the relationship of HbA_{1C} to PSQI, "adjusted for age and sex."

Another purpose of linear regression is *prediction*. Suppose one wants to make reliable clinical predictions of change in HbA_{1c} over a period of a year. Such a prediction model may be critical to setting treatment regimes, targeting individuals for intensified follow-up, etc. Multiple linear regression using predictor variables such as current HbA_{1c}, age, sex, and sleep measures, as well as other cardiovascular risk factors, might figure into such an analysis. The focus is on how well the entire set of predictors together can predict HbA_{1c} one year hence, whereas the interpretation or values of the regression slopes are of somewhat less interest. A later section of this chapter discusses adjustment, summarization, and prediction in more detail.

In addition to the diverse uses for simple and multiple linear regression, related techniques form an important component of modern medical statistics. Special cases of multiple linear regression (sometimes unified under "general linear models") include *analysis of variance* for comparing means among several groups and *analysis of covariance* for comparing such means with adjustment for continuous covariates. Multiple linear regression is primarily applied to data in which the response variable is a continuous quantity. The basic ideas, however, carry over into logistic regression for binary outcome data (Chapter 12), proportional-hazards regression for survival time data (Chapter 11), and random-effects models and generalized-estimating-equations models for longitudinal (repeated-measures) data. Because regression techniques typify the statistical process of separating signal from noise in a set of data, they provide a statistical modeling framework that has proven remarkably useful in focusing attention on the scientific issues under investigation in medical research.

SIMPLE LINEAR REGRESSION

Simple linear regression presents a linear relationship between the response variable Y and the predictor variable X. This relationship is captured by a regression equation, which represents a statistical model. Such models play two important roles in scientific investigation. First, they provide a framework for thinking about the scientific relationships and hypotheses of interest. As such, they aid in narrowing and operationalizing questions of interest. As more variables come into play for purposes of adjustment or prediction in multiple linear regression models, the role of the regression model as a framework for formalizing scientific hypotheses becomes even more important. Secondly, statistical models form the mathematical basis for data analysis. This process includes estimation, as well as inferences such as testing hypotheses and constructing confidence intervals.

In practice, the fitted regression model separates the signal from the noise. It contains estimates of the intercept and slope and thereby traces a line through the cloud of points in a scatter plot of the data. Estimated coefficients are accompanied by standard errors, which express the statistical uncertainty in these estimates. Standard errors in turn are used to conduct hypothesis tests of possible association between Y and X and to construct confidence intervals for the regression slope (and intercept).

The Fitted Line

Figure 1 depicts an idealized linear relationship of HbA_{1c} to sleep quality. If this relationship were to hold, then it would be captured by the well-known algebraic equation for a line

$$Y = a + bX.$$

Statisticians commonly write

$$Y = \beta_0 + \beta_1 X, \tag{1}$$

using β_1 (instead of b) for the slope of Y against X and β_0 (instead of a) for the intercept. The slope quantifies the relationship of Y to X and is usually the key quantity of scientific interest. The intercept is the value of Y when $X = 0$; in most medical research, it is less important than the slope.

In practice, such an ideal relationship never holds, but it may often hold on average:

$$\text{mean}(Y|X) = \beta_0 + \beta_1 X. \tag{2}$$

In this expression $\text{mean}(Y|X)$ refers to the average value of Y among those individuals with a given value of X. Here is the important difference between equations (1) and (2): Equation (1) says that all individuals in the population with a given value of X have the same value of Y, and that this value is exactly equal to $\beta_0 + \beta_1 X$, yielding hypothetical "data" such as those in Figure 1. By contrast, equation (2) says merely that the average (central) value of Y in the population of persons with a given value of X is $\beta_0 + \beta_1 X$. Individuals in that population deviate in both directions from that central value. This deviation is often represented by e, yielding the traditional *simple linear regression equation*,

$$Y = \beta_0 + \beta_1 X + e. \tag{3}$$

This equation is simply another way of writing $Y = \text{mean}(Y|X) + e$ or, in words,

$$\text{response} = \text{signal} + \text{noise}$$

or

$$\text{outcome} = \text{prediction} + \text{deviation}.$$

The reader may adopt the interpretation that is most natural.

We make two important points about equation (3). First, the "noise" or "deviation" component e represents everything that is not included in the "signal," $\beta_0 + \beta_1 X$. It captures the fact that individuals in a population vary around their population mean, and such variation is entirely natural and expected. The e term is sometimes called "error." It is generally not error in the usual sense of the word, although it may include errors of measurement from sources such as imperfect instrumentation, human factors, and diurnal variation. For this reason we discourage the use of the term "error" to refer to individual deviation around the population mean. Second, coefficients β_0 and β_1 in regression equation (3) are unknown in the absence of any data. Data must be used to *estimate* these coefficients, yielding a *fitted regression equation*. Estimated coefficients are denoted by $\hat{\beta}_0$ and $\hat{\beta}_1$.

Example 1 (continued): For the sleep/diabetes study, the HbA_{1C} and PSQI data in Figure 2 are used to estimate the regression coefficients, yielding fitted regression equation $Y = 7.11 + 0.186X + e$, corresponding to the line shown in Figure 3. In terms of the clinical variables, HbA_{1C} and PSQI,

$$HbA_{1C} = 7.11\% + 0.186 \ (\%/\text{point}) \times PSQI + e; \qquad (4)$$

the units of HbA_{1C} are clearly given as percent (%) and of PSQI as PSQI "points." To distinguish between absolute change and relative change, the units of differences between percentages are *percentage points*. In the absence of a standard abbreviation for "percentage points," we use "%" in labels and equations and when referring to regression coefficients; for example, "%/point" in (4) stands for "percentage points of HbA_{1C} per PSQI point." Equation (4) says that a randomly selected subject with PSQI score of, say, 5 points would have, on average, an HbA_{1C} value of

$$7.11\% + 0.186 \ (\%/\text{point}) \times 5 \ \text{points} = 8.04\%.$$

Note that the units of PSQI (points) cancel.

The most important quantity in fitted equation (4) is the estimated regression slope of 0.186 (%/point): It says that, for individuals with PSQI scores separated by 1 point, their difference in HbA_{1C} will on average be equal to 0.186 percentage point. In other words, as PSQI varies by 1 point from person to person, we expect to see corresponding differences in HbA_{1C} between those individuals of 0.186 percentage point.

A necessary part of any regression analysis is the descriptive statistics of the component variables: PSQI in these data ranges from 0 to 14 points, with a mean of 6.0 and a standard deviation (sd) of 3.2 points. HbA_{1C} ranges from 5.7% to 15.2% with a mean of 8.2% and a sd of 2.1 percentage points. Such information allows the reader to assess the clinical significance of the results. For example, the reader can determine that, for subjects whose PSQI scores differ by 2 standard deviations ($2 \times 3.2 = 6.4$ points), the expected difference in HbA_{1C} values is

$$0.186 \ (\%/\text{point}) \times 6.4 \ \text{points} = 1.19 \ \text{percentage points}.$$

Depending on the application, one might then ask whether such a difference in HbA_{1C} values is large enough to be clinically important or even to suggest clinical intervention.

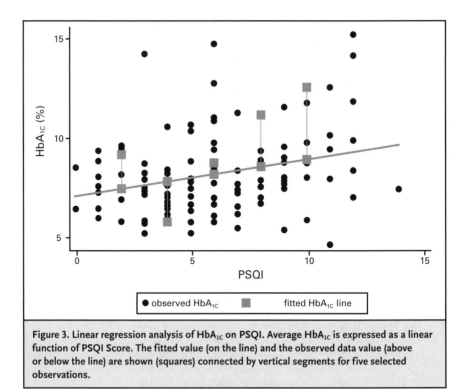

Figure 3. Linear regression analysis of HbA$_{1C}$ on PSQI. Average HbA$_{1C}$ is expressed as a linear function of PSQI Score. The fitted value (on the line) and the observed data value (above or below the line) are shown (squares) connected by vertical segments for five selected observations.

Equation (3) is an example of a statistical model. As such, it states a general form of the relationship of HbA$_{1C}$ to PSQI, but leaves certain details of that relationship unknown; these unknowns are called *parameters*. In this instance the unknown parameters are the coefficients β_0 and β_1. An additional parameter is the population standard deviation σ of the deviations e. Thus, the complete statistical model can be expressed as

$$Y = \beta_0 + \beta_1 X + e \tag{5}$$
$$\text{mean}(e) = 0$$
$$\text{sd}(e) = \sigma$$

The unknown parameters in this model are estimated from the data and have an interpretation that captures the scientific questions of interest in the study. In equation (5), β_0 is the average or mean value of Y for the sub-population for whom $X = 0$ (even if such a person does not, or could not, exist), and β_1 is the difference in average values of Y for two sub-populations separated in their value of X by 1 unit. Finally, individual values of Y vary around the mean $\beta_0 + \beta_1 X$ for each value of X. This deviation or "noise," represented by e, is assumed to be random and to have mean 0, indicating that the individual could be on either side of the fitted line. The amount of variation is measured by the standard deviation σ of e or, equivalently, by its variance σ^2. When the model is fitted, the standard deviation σ is estimated, along with β_0 and β_1.

> Example 1 (continued): In the fitted equation (4) we have estimated values $\hat{\beta}_1$ and $\hat{\beta}_0$. In addition, the estimate of the standard deviation σ is $\hat{\sigma} = 2.03$ percentage points.
>
> First, a line is fitted to the points in the scatter plot, as in Figure 3. Each point in the original scatter plot now has a corresponding "fitted value" on the fitted line. Five such pairs of points are displayed in Figure 3. The arithmetic difference between the actual value and the fitted value—i.e., the segment connecting these two points—is the "residual" for that observation. The residuals are displayed in Figure 4, where their values can be read from the Y-axis and their distribution is displayed in a column at the right. Collecting all of the residuals together, we can present and examine their distribution via a boxplot or a histogram, as in Figure 5. From this distribution we can compute their mean (which is exactly 0 because of the method of fitting the line), their standard deviation, which is 2.03 percentage points, etc.

Plots such as Figure 4 can be very useful. The plot should show random scatter about the zero line if the model is a good fit to the data. Any pattern in the

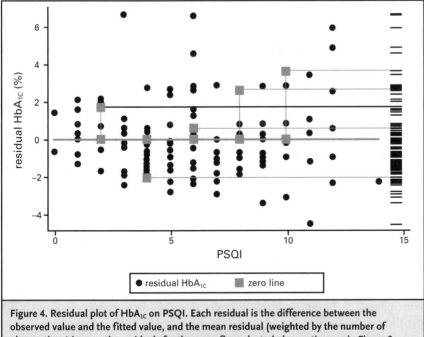

Figure 4. Residual plot of HbA$_{1c}$ on PSQI. Each residual is the difference between the observed value and the fitted value, and the mean residual (weighted by the number of observations) is zero. the residuals for the same five selected observations as in Figure 3 are shown (squares), and the distribution of all residuals is presented with hash marks on a vertical line at the right.

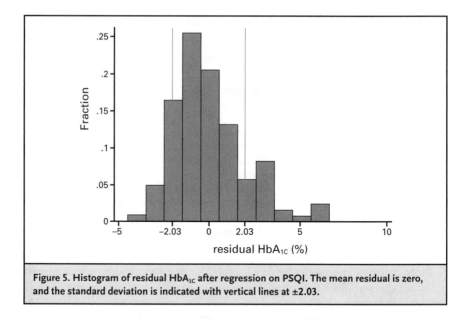

Figure 5. Histogram of residual HbA$_{1C}$ after regression on PSQI. The mean residual is zero, and the standard deviation is indicated with vertical lines at ±2.03.

residuals, for example a U-shaped or inverted-U-shaped cloud, would suggest otherwise. If the degree of scatter increases or decreases with X, this suggests that sd(e) is not constant, as assumed in model (5). Such regression diagnostics are discussed later in the chapter.

Another quantity sometimes reported with fitted regression models is R-squared (R^2), sometimes called the *coefficient of determination*. Briefly, R^2 ranges from 0 to 1 and represents the proportion of total variability in Y (about its mean) that is accounted for or "explained" by X in the linear regression model. The higher the value of R^2, the better is the prediction from the model, although explanatory models with low R^2 are often quite useful as well. In the linear regression of HbA$_{1C}$ on PSQI, $R^2 = 7.9\%$; i.e., PSQI accounts for 7.9% of the total variability in HbA$_{1C}$.

Standard Errors, Tests, and Confidence Intervals

The previous section described the estimation and interpretation of regression coefficients β and of the standard deviation σ of Y around its mean $\beta_0 + \beta_1 X$. In regression analysis, as in other statistical procedures, however, estimation of unknown statistical parameters such as β_0 and β_1 is only one part of the analysis.

Because estimates $\hat{\beta}_1$ and $\hat{\beta}_0$ of β_1 and β_0 are themselves based on data, their values involve statistical uncertainty, called sampling variation, and it is important to quantify this uncertainty. *Sampling variation* is the variability in parameter estimates that arises because we observe a sample from the population, and not the entire population; it is the reason that we cannot make perfectly precise statements about model parameters. Below we discuss the quantification of statistical uncertainty via standard errors, and the role of standard errors in testing hypotheses and constructing confidence intervals.

Standard Errors of Regression Coefficients

Sampling variation of $\hat{\beta}_0$ and $\hat{\beta}_1$ is usually quantified by their *standard errors*. For the study of HbA_{1C} and sleep quality, Table 1 shows the estimates for β_0 and β_1, along with their standard errors. The standard error of the estimate of β_1 is 0.0577 (%/point); this quantity serves as input to hypothesis tests and confidence intervals.

The standard errors of $\hat{\beta}_0$ and $\hat{\beta}_1$ reflect three key features of the data. First, standard errors are proportional to the standard deviation σ of the residuals. This makes intuitive sense because the larger the value of σ, the less precisely we are able to estimate the mean of Y, and the regression model is, after all, a summary of the mean of Y as a function of X.

Second, the standard error of the estimated slope $\hat{\beta}_1$ is inversely proportional to the standard deviation of the X-values. If the values of X vary little about their overall mean, then X cannot tell us much about individual values beyond $\bar{y}$ as a summary of Y. A wide range of slopes will produce regression lines that are reasonably close to the data; that is, the slope of the line is not well determined. For a given value of σ, a larger standard deviation of X yields a more stable estimate of β_1.

Third, the standard errors are inversely proportional to the square root of the sample size n used in fitting the model to the data. That is, the larger the value of n, the more precisely we are able to estimate the regression model.

Table 1. Summary Statistics for Fitted Regression Model of HbA1C (%) on PSQI for $n = 122$ Subjects.

Term	Coef.	Estimate	SE	t	p-value	95% Confidence Limits Lower	Upper
intercept	β_0	7.11	0.391	18.2	0.000	6.34	7.88
PSQI (points)	β_1	0.186	0.0577	3.21	0.002	0.071	0.300

Estimated standard deviation $\hat{\sigma}$ is 2.03 percentage points on 120 degrees of freedom.

Model $R^2 = 7.9\%$.

Hypothesis Tests about Regression Coefficients

The standard error also yields a test statistic t for the null hypothesis that $\beta_1 = 0$. This null hypothesis corresponds to no linear association between Y and X. The hypothesis that $\beta_1 = 0$ is important because, as the scientific hypothesis in many medical studies is one of association between two variables, the corresponding null statistical hypothesis to be tested is that of no association.

The t-statistic is the ratio of $\hat{\beta}_1$ to its standard error. The corresponding p-value comes from a t-distribution whose degrees of freedom (df) equals the sample size minus the number of regression coefficients estimated in the model. Simple linear regression involves two regression coefficients, including the intercept, so that df $= n - 2$. The larger the df, the more precise will be the estimation of σ, and hence the smaller the standard error of $\hat{\beta}_1$.

> Example 1 (continued): Using the estimate and standard error reported in Table 1, the test statistic t for the slope β_1 is computed as
>
> $$t = \frac{\text{estimate}}{\text{standard error}} = \frac{\hat{\beta}_1}{se(\hat{\beta}_1)} = \frac{0.186}{0.0577} = 3.21$$
>
> on 120 df, yielding the two-sided p-value 0.002. This is strong evidence that the measured value of HbA_{1c} is associated with PSQI.

Confidence Intervals on Regression Coefficients

Estimates of regression coefficients are usually accompanied by 95% confidence intervals. Under appropriate (and common) conditions, the confidence interval will include the true but unknown population value with the specified probability. Thus, unless one believes that a rare event has occurred, any parameter value outside the range of values delineated by the confidence interval is considered incompatible with the data.

> Example 1 (continued): Table 1 gives the 95% confidence interval for β_1 as [0.071,0.300] (%/point). This range does not contain 0, again suggesting that $\beta_1 = 0$ is inconsistent with these data and implying that a null relationship of HbA_{1c} to PSQI is also inconsistent with these data. Indeed, for these data, the true slope is likely to lie somewhere between 0.071 and 0.300 (%/point). The bounds of the confidence interval are obtained by computing 0.186 $\pm$ 1.98 $\times$ 0.0577 = [0.071, 0.300]. (The 1.98 is the 97.5th percentile of the t-distribution on 120 df.)

CORRELATION VERSUS REGRESSION

Simple linear regression is a method of describing and quantifying a relationship of one variable Y to another variable X. A related measure, the *correlation coefficient*, summarizes the *direction* and the *strength* of linear relationship between

X and Y on a scale that does not involve the specific units of X and Y (i.e., it is unit-free). Numerous correlation coefficients have been developed as summary measures of association for various types of data. The most common, for continuous data, is the "Pearson" or "product-moment" correlation, denoted by r or r_{YX} to indicate the two variables involved. As with linear regression, Pearson correlation is applicable when the relationship between X and Y is at least approximately linear. The correlation coefficient varies from -1 to $+1$; $r_{YX} = 0$ indicates no linear relationship between Y and X, $r_{YX} = 1$ indicates perfect positive (linear) association, and $r_{YX} = -1$ perfect inverse (linear) association (i.e., the line in Figure 1 would slope downward rather than upward). Neither X nor Y is viewed as the response or the predictor, so the correlation coefficient is a symmetric measure (i.e., $r_{YX} = r_{XY}$). Before using a correlation coefficient to summarize a relationship, the variables should be displayed in a scatter plot. The pattern in the plot can help to determine whether the two variables are linearly associated and, if so, the direction and strength of the association.

By contrast, in regression analysis, the response variable Y is of primary scientific importance, whereas the explanatory variable X is important to the extent that it predicts Y. The regression slope $\hat{\beta}_1$ captures the quantitative relationship of Y to X and helps predict the value of Y for a given value of X. Unlike the correlation coefficient, the regression slope can be any number from $-\infty$ to $+\infty$. Also, the slope is not a symmetric measure: switching the roles of Y and X will generally give a different value for the slope.

The correlation coefficient and regression coefficients capture different aspects of the same relationship. Correlation helps determine whether there is a relationship between X and Y, and how strong the relationship is, whereas the regression coefficient quantifies that relationship. Positive (negative) regression slope corresponds to positive (negative) correlation, and the slope is 0 if and only if the correlation coefficient is also 0. In a scatter plot of Y versus X, the correlation coefficient captures how closely the points (X, Y) follow the regression line, with $r_{YX} = \pm1$ indicating the ideal situation where all the points fall directly on the line. An example of such an ideal relationship is depicted in Figure 1.

Correlation coefficients are most suitable when Y and X are on an equal scientific footing. They might be two measures of the same quantity, neither one necessarily better than the other—for example, two psychiatric assessments using the same structured interview, but made by different clinical raters, or two mammographic breast density readings made by the same rater at different times. Or, they may be two different measures of the same underlying construct, e.g., a urine test and a blood test for a specific hormone, or sleep measured by motion sensors (actigraphy) and by self-report. These are appropriate applications of a symmetric measure of association.

Because the correlation coefficient is symmetric and free of the units of measurement of X and Y, its interpretation is thought to be somewhat portable across settings, permitting comparisons of the strength of association across samples, across studies, or across pairs of variables. Loosely, correlations less than 0.25 indicate fairly weak association, and correlations between 0.25 and 0.50 and above 0.50 reflect moderate and strong associations, respectively. Corresponding interpretations apply to negative values. However, in practice this portability goes only so far, because what is strong association in one context may be weak in another. In the HbA_{1C}–PSQI example, a correlation of 0.30 between HbA_{1C} and PSQI may be considered strong, given the multiple factors that affect each of these variables and the multiple physiological pathways that may link them. On the other hand, 0.30 may be considered weak when it describes the association between two measures of the same construct, such as urine and blood tests of the same hormone. In another example, in a study involving the intelligence quotient (IQ) of children and their mothers,[6] the correlation between children's measured IQ at ages 3 and 5 years was 0.67, which is only moderately strong given that both measures are presumably capturing the same stable characteristic on the same individuals. On the other hand, the correlation between mother's IQ and child's IQ in that same study is 0.52, which seems remarkable in the presence of the many environmental and genetic factors shared across generations.

Despite the benefits of a symmetric measure of association, this feature can be a hindrance in many settings. In most of biomedical science, a symmetric measure ignores the interest in the primary direction of the association. We may associate increasing age with higher blood pressure, but we certainly do not think that higher blood pressure indicates (or even causes) old age. As such, it is natural to model blood pressure as a function of age, but not vice-versa, and to express this relationship using a regression slope instead of a correlation coefficient. In addition, the units of the regression slope carry important clinical information that the correlation coefficient does not. In the HbA_{1C}–PSQI example, the regression slope was 0.186 (%/point); i.e., a one-point difference in PSQI corresponds on average to a 0.186 percentage point difference in HbA_{1C}. The units give a sense of the clinical importance of the relationship of HbA_{1C} to PSQI.

ASSOCIATION AND CAUSATION

The estimated regression slope $\hat{\beta}_1$ and the correlation coefficient r_{YX} quantify the association of the response variable Y to the predictor variable X. Often, however, the underlying scientific issue is whether and to what degree X causes Y. The distinction is evident in two common interpretations of the coefficient β_1. One interpretation says the following:

When comparing two subjects randomly drawn from the population who have X values that differ by one unit, the difference in their Y values, will, on average, be equal to β_1 [association].

The emphasis here is on comparing average pairs of subjects in the population. An alternative and subtly different interpretation is:

If we increase any given subject's X value by one unit, then we will see a corresponding increase in his/her Y value, and that increase will be, on average, equal to β_1 [causation].

The first interpretation, association, simply says that Y and X are associated in the population, but the second, stronger interpretation is one way of formalizing causation (see, e.g., Rubin[7, 8]).

To examine the distinction more concretely, we consider a relationship between intellectual ability and blood lead concentration in young children.

Example 2: Though it is fairly well established that blood lead concentrations above 10 $\mu g/$ dl hinder normal neurobehavioral development in young children, questions remain about the effects of lead at levels below 10 $\mu g/dl$. To address this question, Canfield et al. studied the association of intellectual impairment to lead exposure in children.[6] They collected blood lead concentration data and intelligence quotient (IQ) test results on 172 healthy children, as well as other variables such as maternal IQ, race, maternal education, tobacco use during pregnancy, household income, and the child's sex, birth weight, and iron status. Blood lead concentrations were collected at ages 6, 12, 18, 24, 36, 48, and 60 months and were used to compute a lifetime average blood lead concentration through age 5 years. IQ and other information was complete for 154 of these children. Lifetime average blood lead concentration ($\pm$ sd) for this sub-sample was 7.4 ± 4.3 $\mu g/dl$ (approximate range: 0 to 30 $\mu g/dl$), and IQ was 89.8 ± 11.4 points (approximate range: 64 to 128 points). Linear regression of IQ on lifetime average blood lead concentration yielded an estimated regression slope of $\hat{\beta}_1 = -1.00$ points/ ($\mu g/dl$) with a 95% CI of $[-1.38, -0.63]$ points/($\mu g/dl$) ($p < 0.001$), indicating a statistically and clinically significant inverse association of IQ to blood lead concentration.

In this example, because lead can accumulate in the bloodstream even at very low levels of ingestion, it is possible to imagine an intervention—albeit an unethical one—that increases a child's blood lead concentration while nothing else in that child's environment changes. What will it then take for the regression coefficient to be interpreted as causal?

Fitting the linear regression model allows us to quantify and measure the empirical association between IQ and blood lead concentration. Blood lead concentration is on the right-hand side of the equation because the investigators placed it there and not because the data have anything to say about blood lead concentration preceding IQ in some causal chain of events. From a purely empirical perspective, they could have just as easily regressed blood lead levels on IQ. What they have observed and reported in the data is an association in the population between individuals' blood lead levels and their IQ.

This association may arise because elevated lead in the bloodstream leads physiologically to a decrement in IQ. Or it could be that a variety of other factors contribute to both elevated blood lead and depressed IQ in some persons in the population. For example, children with lower IQ will tend to have parents with lower IQ owing to the documented heritability of IQ. And adults with lower IQ often have fewer economic opportunities to rent or purchase safe and well-maintained housing that is free of decaying, chipping, or flaking lead-based paint. Most likely, the observed association is a combination of such explanations. Because the data themselves hold no evidence about whether the first, second, or some other explanation is most accurate, it is unwise to use these data alone to attach a causal interpretation to any observed association. Other information about the study design and/or the biological processes involved may lend support to an inference of causation. In the absence of such information we would avoid statements such as that in the second, causal interpretation.

Building on this example, one might ask under what conditions will the causal interpretation be valid? The most straightforward one is that of a randomized controlled clinical trial. Suppose that a sample of patients is enrolled in a trial and that each one is randomly assigned a dose X of a drug. The subjects are followed for a response Y, and then the data are analyzed via linear regression of Y on X. In this instance the study protocol has intervened on X. In addition, each subject's value of X is under complete control of the randomization process set out in the study design. Statistically, randomization ensures that, on average, the effects of any factors that may be related to Y will be the same for each randomization group. Thus, it is fair to assign a causal interpretation to an observed association.

CAREFUL USE OF LINEAR REGRESSION

Fitting a linear regression model provides for a simple description of the statistical relationship of Y to X. However, careful analysis examines how well the model captures the patterns in the data and how far we can take it in summarizing the relationship and in making predictions about Y from X. Key questions include: Is the relationship really linear? What is the statistical uncertainty in the model fit and predictions across the range of values of X? Are any data points not well described by the model? Is the story being told by the fitted model dominated or attenuated by a few data points?

Answering these questions is an important part of data analysis; *regression diagnostics* offer a wide array of tools for these tasks.[9, 10] This section illustrates some of the basic ideas in a non-technical manner.

Linearity of Association

Linear regression captures the linear part of the relationship of the mean of Y to X. Such a description is appropriate if the relationship is fairly linear, as in the HbA_{1C}–PSQI example (Figure 3). Can we make the same statement for the IQ–blood lead example? If that relationship is well approximated by a line, then the regression model will provide a parsimonious and accurate description of the data.

Example 2 (continued): Figure 6 reproduces a scatterplot of IQ versus lifetime average blood lead concentration from Canfield et al.[6] A line fitted through these points yielded a regression slope of −1.00 point/(μg/dl). However, the plot reveals that summarizing this relationship as linear is an over-simplification. In fact, the inverse relationship is stronger for blood lead concentrations between 0 and 10 μg/dl, and there is almost no association between IQ and blood lead concentration above 10 μg/dl. The authors of the study recognized this, both from looking at the data and because the research question focused on blood lead concentrations below 10 μg/dl. Thus, they re-fitted the model, restricting the sample to those 86 children (56% of the 154) with lifetime peak blood lead concentration below 10 μg/dl

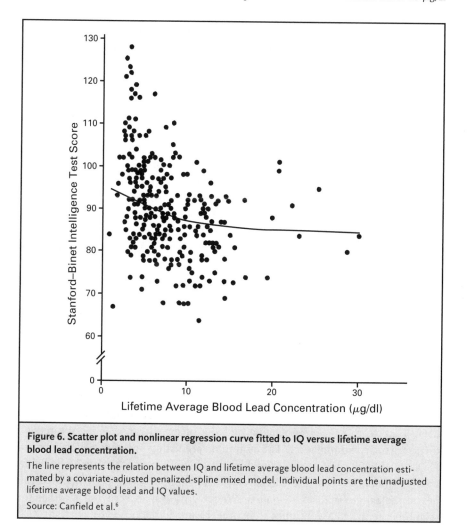

Figure 6. Scatter plot and nonlinear regression curve fitted to IQ versus lifetime average blood lead concentration.

The line represents the relation between IQ and lifetime average blood lead concentration estimated by a covariate-adjusted penalized-spline mixed model. Individual points are the unadjusted lifetime average blood lead and IQ values.

Source: Canfield et al.[6]

at age 5 years. This sub-sample yielded a regression slope of -2.54 points/(μg/dl) (95% CI: $[-4.01, -1.07]$) points/(μg/dl); that is, two children who differ in blood lead concentration by 1 μg/dl will, on average, differ by -2.54 IQ points, so long as both children have blood lead concentrations below 10 μg/dl.

The non-linearity problem highlighted in this example can be handled in several ways. One is the approach that Canfield et al. took. In their study, this was appropriate because the ceiling value of 10 μg/dl was implicit in the study aims. In other settings, using the data themselves to choose a subset on which to focus could introduce additional uncertainty into the analysis. It will be difficult to account for this uncertainty in hypothesis tests and confidence intervals about the regression slope. Another approach is to transform the X variable, perhaps by taking logarithms. This would have the effect of stretching out the points on the left of the plot, and squeezing together the points on the right of the plot, thus rendering the relationship more nearly linear. However, this approach complicates interpretation of the results because blood lead concentrations are now on the logarithmic rather than the natural scale. A third approach is to transform the response Y. But this is not always satisfactory either, because the transformed response might not be as easy to interpret clinically as the untransformed response. The approaches associated with *generalized linear models*[11] offer an alternative (beyond the scope of this chapter) that avoids transforming the response. Yet another approach is to include linear, quadratic (blood lead concentration squared), and even higher-order terms in the regression model. Another family of functions called *splines*, in which line segments or curves join at points to cover the range of X, often yields better results. Use of either higher-order terms or splines expands the regression equation into a multiple linear regression model with its own implications of model fitting, inference, and interpretation. A final note is that, even if the relationship of Y to X is not well approximated by a line, the linear regression procedure will still produce estimates. Though those estimates may be useful, they will oversimplify the relationship in the data.

Extrapolation

Having fitted a regression model relating Y to X, one might wonder whether it should be used to predict Y for values of X outside the range available in the data. That is, can we *extrapolate* beyond the observed range of X? We recommend against extrapolation. For example, predicting mean HbA_{1C} values for PSQI equal to 20 or 25 points would be a problem because the data all lie below 15 PSQI points, so they provide no empirical support whatsoever for fitted values in the range of 20 to 25 points. We have no way of verifying whether the relationship of Y to X continues to be linear outside the observed range of X.

In fact, the relationship of Y to X is almost never exactly linear. Instead, it will often be well approximated by a line *for the observed values* of X. That is, the linear relationship of Y to X is fairly local. Over a large enough range of X, that linearity will almost certainly break down, as we observed in the IQ–blood lead example. The relationship was strong and linear in the range of X from 0 $\mu g/dl$ to 10 $\mu g/dl$, but weakened above 10 $\mu g/dl$. Extrapolation is dangerous because it ventures into uncharted X territory, where statistical uncertainty is high and model form is uncheckable.

An important form of extrapolation can arise when interpreting the regression intercept. In the HbA_{1C}–PSQI example, the estimated intercept of 7.11% in fitted model (4) refers to the mean HbA_{1C} level for individuals with PSQI = 0. This may be a large and important group, or it may represent only a few individuals. In other analyses, the X variable may never be equal to 0; then interpretation of the intercept represents a clear extrapolation outside of the observed range of X. These problems can be avoided by "centering" X at some meaningful value before fitting the model. The value may be the mean of X (or something close to it) or some other scientifically or clinically relevant reference value. For our example, as the mean PSQI is 6 points, and scores greater than 5 points indicate poor sleep quality, it might be reasonable to center X at 5 points. Thus, instead of

$$Y = \beta_0 + \beta_1 X + e,$$

we would fit

$$Y = \beta_0^* + \beta_1(X - 5) + e,$$

which would yield the fitted equation

$$HbA_{1C} = 8.04\% + 0.186 \ (\%/point) \times (PSQI - 5) + e.$$

The estimated regression slope in this new model is the same as that in the original model, and has the same interpretation. But the intercept of 8.04% now refers to the mean HbA_{1C} level among the subpopulation of individuals with PSQI = 5, a scientifically important group on the cusp of poor sleep quality.

Residuals and Outliers

Thorough analysis of a linear regression model seldom appears in the medical literature. Such analysis includes study of the departures of the Y values from the fitted model These are the individual deviations or *residuals*, estimated as

$$(residual) = (observed) - (fitted)$$

and plotted for the HbA_{1C}–PSQI example in Figures 4 and 5. In symbols,

$$\hat{e} = Y - (\hat{\beta}_0 + \hat{\beta}_1 X), \tag{6}$$

where Y is the observed response, $\hat{\beta}_0 + \hat{\beta}_1 X$ is the fitted value for the mean of Y given X, and the regression slope and intercept estimates are denoted by $\hat{\beta}_1$ and $\hat{\beta}_0$.

Ideally, the residuals show no remarkable behavior; they are simply a sample of chance fluctuations. Sometimes, however, a few stand out from the rest. Such *outliers* generally deserve investigation. An effective diagnostic approach, which often reveals outliers more readily, uses a definition of residuals based on the *leave-one-out* principle. The idea is to compare each observation to a regression model estimated from the rest of the data, *leaving out* the target observation. Then the leave-one-out residual is the difference between the Y value and the regression line at the corresponding X, as in equation (6), but obtaining the fitted line from all data *except* the target observation. The resulting residuals are then rescaled so that, at least approximately, each has mean 0 and standard deviation 1. Remarkably, in linear (or multiple) regression it is possible to compute such leave-one-out quantities without actually refitting the model. Discrepant values of Y in the data can then be detected by displaying these rescaled residuals.

Example 1 (continued): For the HbA_{1c}–PSQI example, in a boxplot of rescaled leave-one-out residuals (Figure 7) the largest three values stand out from the rest of the data. These three points are flagged in Figure 8.

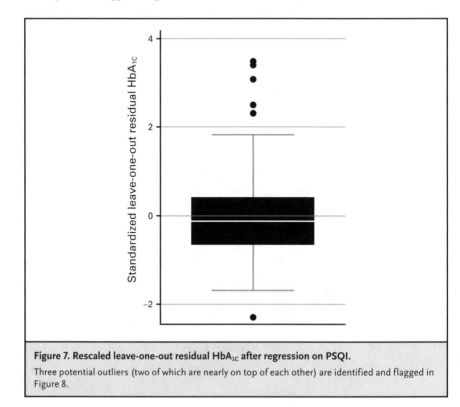

Figure 7. Rescaled leave-one-out residual HbA$_{1c}$ after regression on PSQI.
Three potential outliers (two of which are nearly on top of each other) are identified and flagged in Figure 8.

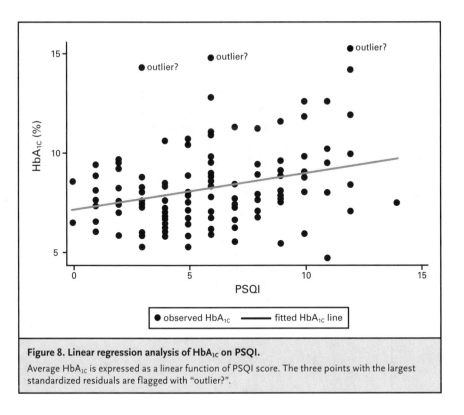

Figure 8. Linear regression analysis of HbA₁c on PSQI.
Average HbA$_{1c}$ is expressed as a linear function of PSQI score. The three points with the largest standardized residuals are flagged with "outlier?".

Outliers raise the question of what should be done about them. First, one should confirm that the data values have been accurately recorded and entered into the data set. Second, it is often worth examining other information on these subjects to gain insight into why their Y values are extreme; perhaps something new can be learned from these subjects. In the HbA$_{1c}$–PSQI example, perhaps the subjects with large HbA$_{1c}$ values have had diabetes for longer periods of time or have other comorbidities that set them apart from the rest of the sample. Usually we do not advise removing these subjects from the analysis, unless a data error is found that cannot be corrected or, upon further inspection, it is discovered that the subject should have been excluded from the study. Rather, it is appropriate to include them in the analysis, perhaps making special note of them. If they are removed (as a form of sensitivity analysis), any report should include both sets of results. Displays of the data go a long way toward letting the reader decide how to interpret any outlying observations.

Influential Observations

Detection of outliers is important because such data points may be interesting in the way in which they depart from the bulk of the data. Data points can also be unusual in their contribution to the estimated regression equation and, in particular, to the regression slope. Such contributions constitute the *influence* of that point. Each point's influence on the slope estimate can be quantified by applying the leave-one-out principle—by taking the difference between the slope estimate computed from the full data set, and the estimate computed with that point removed—and technical criteria exist for flagging points as overly influential. We illustrate the idea with the HbA_{1c}–PSQI example.

> Example 1 (continued): Figure 9 displays the HbA_{1c} versus PSQI regression line with the full data set and a new regression line with two of the strong influence points removed. The new estimate of the regression slope is 0.129 (%/point) with test statistic $t = 2.30$ ($p = 0.023$). This compares with 0.186 (%/point), $t = 3.21$ ($p = 0.002$; Table 1) using the full data set. Although these points are pulling the regression slope upward, even without them we still obtain a statistically significant association of HbA_{1c} to PSQI. The two observations are indicated in Figure 9, providing some insight into why they are influential. In this instance,

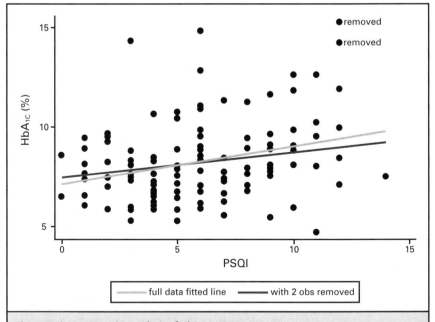

Figure 9. Linear regression analysis of HbA_{1c} on PSQI.

Average HbA_{1c} is expressed as a linear function of PSQI score. The two points with the largest (in absolute value) influence on the regression slope are flagged with the word "removed." The two regression lines are computed with the full data set and with the two points removed.

it is because they have both high values of PSQI (12 points; 99th percentile) and high values of HbA$_{1C}$ (14.2% and 15.3%); the effect is to pull the regression line up for large values of PSQI. Conversely, two of the three outliers flagged in Figure 8 are not points of high influence, because their PSQI values are not extreme.

Points with extreme X values are said to have high *leverage* because their Y values are given more weight in estimating the slope; if their Y values are also large, then that potential to be influential is realized, as shown in Figure 9.

Careful use of regression analysis involves detection and investigation of individual points or small groups of points that may be influential. If any one point has disproportionate influence, it deserves special note. Conversely, if several points have large but relatively equal influence, then none of them by themselves can really be considered influential, relative to the others. On the other hand, if those points form a group for some reason other than their influence—e.g., those points belong to the oldest subjects or to subjects from the same clinic—then the group as a whole may warrant further attention.

MULTIPLE LINEAR REGRESSION

Linear regression extends well beyond examining the relationship of a continuous Y variable to a single continuous X variable, covering situations with predictors that are not continuous and with multiple predictors, each telling part of the story about the response Y. *Multiple linear regression* covers this broader domain. In this section we develop and interpret multiple linear regression models by looking first at a model with one continuous and one categorical predictor, and then at a model with two continuous predictors. We then turn via example to a general formulation and interpretation of multiple linear regression. This general model is the basis for the use of linear regression for summarization, statistical adjustment, and prediction.

One Continuous and One Categorical Predictor

We begin with an analysis of HbA$_{1C}$ and its association with sleep quantity, a continuous variable, and whether a person experiences diabetic complications, a categorical variable. The multiple linear regression model takes the form

$$Y = \beta_0 + \beta_1 X_1 + \beta_2 X_2 + e. \tag{7}$$

Here X_1 is a continuous predictor and X_2 is a binary *indicator* or *dummy* variable, taking value 1 for membership in a given group or sub-population and 0 otherwise. Indicator variables often appear in the clinical and epidemiologic literature because, as we shall see, they capture the difference in the mean response between groups.

Example 3: In the analysis of HbA_{1C} and sleep in persons with diabetes (Example 1), Knutson et al.[1] were interested not only in sleep quality (as measured by PSQI), but also in sleep quantity. To measure sleep quantity, they used the notion of perceived sleep debt, defined as the difference between the preferred and reported sleep duration. Perceived sleep debt ranged from 0 to 6 hours, with a mean (sd) of 1.7 (1.5) hours. The analyses accounted for the history or presence of major clinical diabetic complications (including neuropathy, retinopathy, nephropathy, coronary artery disease, and peripheral vascular disease), which could be associated with elevated HbA_{1C} (from long-term poor diabetes control) and could also lead to decreased sleep quality and quantity. Fifty-two (43%) subjects had at least one diabetic complication. In light of these goals, we fit a multiple linear regression model as in equation (7) where Y is HbA_{1C}, X_1 is perceived sleep debt (DEBT), centered at two hours, and X_2 is an indicator variable (DIAC) taking value 1 for the presence of any diabetic complications and 0 for no diabetic complications. The fitted equation is

$$HbA_{1C} = 8.08\% + 0.39 \ (\%/hour) \times (DEBT - 2) + 0.66\% \times DIAC + e. \qquad (8)$$

Referring to equation (7), we have estimates $\hat{\beta}_1 = 0.39$ (%/hour) and $\hat{\beta}_2 = 0.66\%$ with corresponding standard errors of 0.12 (%/hour) and 0.37% yielding p-values of 0.002 and 0.079. We conclude that greater sleep debt is significantly associated, and the presence of diabetic complications is marginally associated, with higher levels of HbA_{1C}.

The presence of both DEBT and DIAC in fitted model (8) complicates the interpretation of each of their coefficients. Certainly, the slope $\hat{\beta}_1$ is the estimated average difference in Y corresponding to a unit difference in X_1, i.e., the linear effect of X_1 on Y. Similarly, $\hat{\beta}_2$ is the estimated average difference in Y between the two groups defined by indicator variable X_2. (Although $\hat{\beta}_2$ is technically a slope, it turns out to be a difference between groups because X_2 is dichotomous.) Additionally—and importantly—the coefficient corresponding to each predictor must be interpreted as *adjusted* for the other predictor in the model. For example, $\hat{\beta}_1$ expresses the estimated effect of DEBT on mean HbA_{1C}, *adjusting* for differences in HbA_{1C} due to DIAC. This adjustment aims to remove the part of the HbA_{1C}–DEBT association that is due to DIAC. To see how this works, we continue with the example.

Example 3 (continued): To gain a sense of how DIAC (X_2) might be influencing the observed association of HbA_{1C} (Y) to DEBT (X_1), we note that the mean HbA_{1C} level in the presence of (one or more) diabetic complications is 8.69%, but 7.88% in the absence of complications. Additionally, the mean sleep debt is 1.88 hours and 1.49 hours in the presence and absence of complications, respectively. Because HbA_{1C} and DEBT both covary with DIAC, part of the observed association of HbA_{1C} to DEBT could be accounted for by each variable's association with DIAC. Adjustment aims to remove the part of the HbA_{1C}–DEBT association that is due to DIAC.

Examining the data separately in the two diabetic complication groups, Figure 10 plots HbA_{1C} versus sleep debt in each group. Included in that plot are simple linear regression lines for each group. These lines correspond to the fitted equations

$$HbA_{1C} = 8.73\% + 0.42 \ (\%/hour) \times (DEBT - 2) + e$$

for the group with complications, and

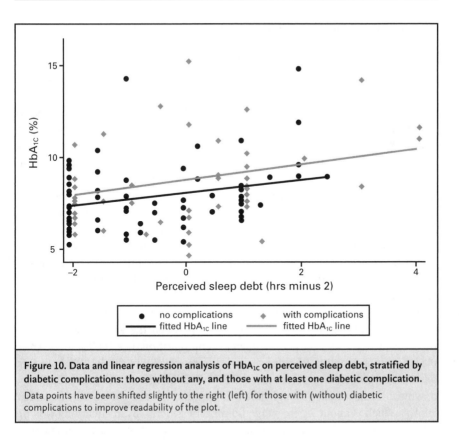

Figure 10. Data and linear regression analysis of HbA$_{1c}$ on perceived sleep debt, stratified by diabetic complications: those without any, and those with at least one diabetic complication.

Data points have been shifted slightly to the right (left) for those with (without) diabetic complications to improve readability of the plot.

$$\text{HbA}_{1C} = 8.06\% + 0.36 \ (\%/\text{hour}) \times (\text{DEBT} - 2) + e$$

for the group without complications.

We make two important observations about this plot and these regression equations. First, the two regression lines are nearly parallel. Second, the intercepts in the two regression equations are 8.73% and 8.06%, representing the mean HbA$_{1c}$ levels in the two groups when sleep debt is exactly two hours. The difference between the two is 0.67 percentage points, indicating higher HbA$_{1c}$ levels in the group with diabetic complications.

Now suppose that the two regression lines were exactly parallel. This fact would have two consequences. First, the regression slope of HbA$_{1c}$ with respect to DEBT would be the same regardless of which group we considered, and only one slope would be needed. Second, the difference in HbA$_{1c}$ between the two groups would be the same at all levels of DEBT.

Model (7) forces these two regression lines to be parallel. Under this restriction, which appears reasonable for these data, β_1 can be interpreted as a within-group regression slope that is common to the two groups, and β_2 is a between-group difference that holds at any given level of X_1. In fitted model (8) the estimated slope of DEBT, 0.39 (%/hour), is *adjusted* for DIAC; it strikes a balance between the two separately estimated slopes, 0.42 and 0.36 (%/hour). Also, the estimated coefficient of DIAC of 0.66% is *adjusted* for DEBT; it is very close to the difference of 0.67% estimated from the separate regressions as the between-group difference when DEBT is fixed at two hours.

The adjustment reflects the presence of both variables in the model, relative to the corresponding slopes in two separate models: the simple linear regression of Y on X_1 and the simple linear regression of Y on X_2. In the first of these models, the slope of HbA_{1C} against DEBT − 2 (i.e., unadjusted for DIAC) is 0.42 (%/hour). From model (8), $\hat{\beta}_1 = 0.39$ (%/hour); the presence of DIAC in the model has only a small impact on this slope. In this example this result is not surprising because the difference in sleep debt in the two complications groups is small (relative to the sd of DEBT), but in some applications the impact is substantial. In general, the regression slope $\hat{\beta}_1$ represents the linear relation of Y to X_1 after accounting for (or "net of") the linear contribution of X_2. In this sense $\hat{\beta}_1 = 0.39$ (%/hour) in fitted model (8) is the estimated slope of Y with respect to X_1, *adjusted* for X_2.

Similarly, in the second of the simple linear regression models, the slope of HbA_{1C} against DIAC (i.e., the difference between the mean HbA_{1C} level in the presence versus absence of diabetic complications) is 8.69% − 7.88% = 0.81 percentage points (the unadjusted difference). From model (8), $\hat{\beta}_2 = 0.66$ percentage points; the presence of DEBT − 2 in the model has produced a downward adjustment (though not a large one, relative to the sd of residual HbA_{1C}, which is about 2 percentage points). In general, $\hat{\beta}_2$ in equation (8) is the estimated slope of Y against X_2, *adjusted* for X_1. This sort of adjustment is typical of observational studies. Because such studies—as distinguished from randomized trials—are not able to control all factors affecting the response, they often focus on the difference between two groups and adjust that difference for the contribution of one or several covariates.

Two Continuous Predictors

A further example analyzes HbA_{1C} as a function of sleep quantity, measured by perceived sleep debt, and subject's age, two continuous predictor variables. The model contains the same symbols as model (7)

$$Y = \beta_0 + \beta_1 X_1 + \beta_2 X_2 + e, \tag{9}$$

but here X_2 is continuous rather than binary.

Example 4: Building on Examples 1 and 3, suppose that the primary focus is on the relation of HbA_{1C} to sleep debt. From preliminary analyses age has quite a wide range, from 24 to 92 years, with a mean (sd) of 58 (13) years. If both sleep debt and HbA_{1C} covary with age, any association of HbA_{1C} and sleep debt could be inflated or attenuated by ignoring the contribution of age to HbA_{1C}. We therefore fit a multiple linear regression model as in (9) with $Y = HbA_{1C}$, $X_1 = DEBT$, and $X_2 = AGE$, centering age at 60 years. The result is

$$HbA_{1C} = 8.26\% + 0.31\ (\%/hour) \times (DEBT - 2) \qquad (10)$$
$$-0.037\ (\%/year) \times (AGE - 60) + e;$$

i.e., estimates $\hat{\beta}_1 = 0.31$ (%/hour) and $\hat{\beta}_2 = -0.037$ (%/year), with standard errors of 0.13 (%/hour) and 0.015 (%/year) and p-values of 0.018 and 0.014. We conclude that greater sleep debt and younger age are both significantly associated with higher levels of HbA_{1C}.

The interpretation of the estimated coefficients $\hat{\beta}_1$ and $\hat{\beta}_2$ of DEBT − 2 and AGE − 60 in the fitted multiple linear regression equation (10) again involves adjusting for the other predictor. Thus, $\hat{\beta}_1$ is the slope of Y with respect to X_1, adjusted for X_2, and $\hat{\beta}_2$ is the slope of Y with respect to X_2, adjusted for X_1. By comparison, in the simple linear regression of HbA_{1C} on DEBT − 2 the slope is 0.42 (%/hour); including AGE − 60 in the model produced an adjusted slope of 0.31 (%/hour). Similarly, the simple linear regression of HbA_{1C} on AGE − 60 yields a slope of −0.050 (%/year); including DEBT − 2 in the model produced an adjusted slope of −0.037 (%/year). In each case, inclusion of the other variable in the model produced a substantial adjustment of the slope toward zero; in particular, age is seen to account for about a quarter of the unadjusted slope in the regression of HbA_{1C} on sleep debt.

Although the models in equations (7) and (9) are generic, in actual applications the meanings of $\hat{\beta}_0$, $\hat{\beta}_1$, and $\hat{\beta}_2$ depend on what other specific variables are in the model. For example, both equation (8) and equation (10) contain DEBT − 2 (along with the constant term); but equation (8) also contains DIAC, whereas equation (10) also contains AGE − 60. Thus, in equation (8) the coefficient of DEBT − 2, 0.39 (%/hour), is the slope of HbA_{1C} against DEBT − 2, adjusted for DIAC, whereas in equation (10) the corresponding coefficient, 0.31 (%/hour), is the slope of HbA_{1C} against DEBT − 2, adjusted for AGE − 60. These are two distinct perspectives on the data, each potentially with its own scientific or clinical implications.

The General Model

Models such as (7) and (9) are instances of a *multiple linear regression* model, so named because it contains multiple predictor variables (X's). The general model may contain any combination of indicator and continuous predictors. The following example, combining the models considered in Examples 3 and 4, serves to illustrate.

Example 5: As in Examples 3 and 4, suppose that the primary focus is on the relationship of HbA_{1C} to sleep debt, but that we also wish to account for subject's age and the presence of diabetic complications in our analysis. We approach this task via a regression model with all three predictors, specifically

$$HbA_{1C} = \beta_0 + \beta_1 (DEBT - 2) + \beta_2 DIAC + \beta_3 (AGE - 60) + e \qquad (11)$$

This model has two continuous predictors and one indicator predictor. The estimated coefficients are presented in Table 2, Model 1. As in separate model fits (8) and (10), perceived sleep debt, the presence of diabetic complications, and younger age are all significantly associated with higher levels of HbA_{1C}, although the slope with respect to DEBT is smaller than in either of the previous models.

Consider interpretation of the estimated version of multiple linear regression equation (11) presented in Table 2, Model 1. First, taken as a whole, this equation can be used to predict the HbA_{1C} levels of an individual with given values of each of the three predictors. For example, suppose we wished to predict the average HbA_{1C} level for a 40-year-old person with three hours of perceived sleep debt and no diabetic complications. This calculation would be

$$\hat{\beta}_0 + \hat{\beta}_1(3-2) + \hat{\beta}_2(0) + \hat{\beta}_3(40-60)$$
$$= 7.94 + 0.271 \times 1 - 0.0397 \times (-20) = 9.00\%$$

If the person had diabetic complications, then this prediction would increase by $\hat{\beta}_2 = 0.726$ percentage point and be equal to 9.73%. These predictions are based on the assumption that the relationship of the response variable HbA_{1C}

Table 2. Summary Statistics for Two Fitted Regression Models of HbA_{1C} (%) on Perceived Sleep Debt, Diabetic Complications, and Age for $n = 122$ Subjects. The Two Models Incorporate Age Differently.

Term	Model 1 Coefficient Estimate	Model 1 95% Confidence Limits Lower	Model 1 95% Confidence Limits Upper	Model 2 Coefficient Estimate	Model 2 95% Confidence Limits Lower	Model 2 95% Confidence Limits Upper
intercept	7.94	7.45	8.42	8.87	8.05	9.69
DEBT* (hrs)	0.271	0.014	0.528	0.321	0.066	0.575
DIAC (any)	0.726	0.011	1.44	0.749	0.025	1.472
AGE* (yrs)	−0.0397	−0.0691	−0.0103			
AGE (yrs)						
24–49				ref.		
50–64				−0.961	−1.892	−0.030
65–92				−1.260	−2.309	−0.211
Standard deviation			1.95	Standard deviation		1.97
Model R^2			16.1%	Model R^2		15.5%

*DEBT is centered at two hours; AGE is centered at 60 years. "ref." denotes the reference category for AGE in Model 2; the estimated intercept predicts the mean of this category, and the coefficients for the other categories, when added to the intercept, predict the means for those categories.

to the predictors DEBT, DIAC, and AGE is *linear* and *additive*. That is, each predictor figures linearly into the regression equation, and the contributions from these predictors are additive.

The estimated intercept $\hat{\beta}_0$ is one such predicted value: it is the estimated mean response Y for persons with a value of 0 for each of the predictors X in the model, accounting for linear and additive effects of each of those predictors. In HbA_{1C} model (11), such persons are 60 years old, with two hours of perceived sleep debt and no diabetic complications, so the indicator variable DIAC is 0. The predicted HbA_{1C} level for such persons based on the model is $\hat{\beta}_0 = 7.94\%$. If we had not "centered" DEBT at two hours and AGE at 60 years, the intercept would refer to persons who are 0 years old and have no sleep debt, a group clearly outside the domain of investigation in this analysis.

The estimated regression coefficients of DEBT, DIAC, and AGE in model (11) reflect adjusted associations. The three coefficients in Table 2, Model 1 quantify the relationship of HbA_{1C} to DEBT, DIAC, and AGE, net of any *linear* and *additive* contributions of the other two predictors.

Before turning to other aspects of multiple linear regression, we consider one final example, which involves a categorical predictor variable with more than two categories. Specifically, we replace continuous age with age groups. Although this approach may not be optimal, and other options are available, it is easy to implement and serves to illustrate the use of multiple linear regression with categorical predictors. It has the further virtue of assuming approximate linearity *within* each age group, but not for the data as a whole; thus it is able to deal with nonlinearity of the age effect.

> Example 6: Suppose, as in Example 5, that our goal was an analysis of the HbA_{1C}–sleep debt association that also accounts for diabetic complications and age, but that we were concerned that age did not act on mean HbA_{1C} in a linear fashion. An alternative approach is to create age groups and treat age as a categorical predictor variable. Examining the distribution of age, we created three groups: 24–49, 50–64, and 65–92 years old. We then choose one group, the youngest, as a reference group and consider a model with an indicator variable for each of the other two age groups:
>
> $$HbA_{1C} = \beta_0 + \beta_1(DEBT - 2) + \beta_2 DIAC + \beta_3 AGE2 + \beta_4 AGE3 + e. \qquad (12)$$
>
> Here AGE2 and AGE3 are indicator variables for membership in the middle and oldest age groups, respectively. AGE2 takes value 1 for persons between 50 and 64 years old and 0 otherwise; AGE3 takes value 1 for persons 65 years and older and 0 otherwise. The estimated coefficients are presented in Table 2, Model 2. As in Model 1, perceived sleep debt and the presence of diabetic complications are significantly associated with higher levels of HbA_{1C}. In addition, the increasingly negative estimated coefficients of the age group indicators reflect a trend of decreasing HbA_{1C} levels with increasing age.

The interpretation of these results is as follows. The estimated intercept $\hat{\beta}_0 = 8.87\%$ is the predicted mean HbA_{1C} level for a person in the youngest age group

(24–49 years) with two hours of sleep debt and no diabetic complications. The estimated coefficients $\hat{\beta}_3 = -0.96$ percentage points for AGE2 and $\hat{\beta}_4 = -1.26$ percentage points for AGE3 are estimated differences between mean HbA_{1C} levels in the middle and oldest age groups, respectively, and the youngest age group, adjusting for sleep debt and diabetic complications. The coefficients of DEBT and DIAC are adjusted for differences in mean HbA_{1C} levels among age groups, as well as for the contributions of DIAC and DEBT, respectively.

The main advantage to model specification (12), with age as a categorical variable, versus model (11), with age as a continuous variable, is that model (12) does not force the slope of mean HbA_{1C} with respect to age to be the same for 30-year-olds as it is for 70-year-olds. On the downside, however, modeling age groups does not account for any differences in mean HbA_{1C} levels that occur by age within a group. Other modeling approaches attempt to gain the advantages of both (11) and (12). These include higher-order functions of age (such as age-squared) or, better, linear or higher-order splines. In some situations, when the number of observations is large enough to support a sizable number of categories, the coefficients of the corresponding indicator variables can guide the choice of the functional form.

When the analysis involves predictor variables for a set of categories, the regression model contains indicator variables for all groups but one. The *reference group* has no indicator variable. Coefficients of each indicator compare the corresponding group against the reference group in terms of the mean value of the response Y. It is up to the analyst to choose the reference group, and this choice affects the interpretation of the coefficients of the indicator variables. In principle, any group can be chosen as the referent, and as long as the model includes indicator variables for each of the other groups, the models are all equivalent. That is, the choice of reference group affects interpretation of the model coefficients, but not the degree to which the model fits the data.

Other Aspects of Multiple Linear Regression Analysis

The interpretation of standard errors, and the computation and interpretation of test statistics, p-values, and confidence intervals in multiple linear regression are analogous to those in simple linear regression. The main difference in multiple linear regression is that the regression slopes represent adjusted associations. In Example 5, interest is on the association of HbA_{1C} to sleep debt, adjusting for age and diabetic complications. The slope estimate and its standard error are $\hat{\beta}_1 = 0.271$ and 0.130 (%/hour). The null hypothesis of no (adjusted) association corresponds to $\beta_1 = 0$. The test statistic for this null hypothesis is $t = 0.271/0.130 = 2.09$. This t-statistic has 118 degrees of freedom (df), which in multiple linear regression equals the sample size ($n = 122$) minus the number of coefficients in the model, including the intercept. The resulting two-sided p-value is 0.039, which indicates a significant HbA_{1C}–sleep debt association, even after accounting for linear effects of age and diabetic complications. The 95% confidence interval for β_1, [0.014, 0.528] (%/hour), indicates the range of values for the adjusted regression slope that are compatible with the data.

The coefficient of determination, or R-squared (R^2) value, also extends directly from simple to multiple linear regression. It represents the proportion of the total variability in the response Y (about its mean) that is accounted for jointly by all the predictor variables X_1, X_2, etc., in the model. In Example 5, $R^2 = 16.1\%$, whereas in Example 6, $R^2 = 15.5\%$, reflecting that the model with linear age had a slightly better fit to the data than did the model with age included as three categories.

Does the Model Fit the Data?

Linear regression involves specifying a model, which includes a response and a set of one or more predictors, and then fitting that model to a set of data. The model fitting, or estimation, step will yield results and parameter estimates whether or not the data conform to the assumptions of that model. What if these assumptions do not hold? What if some observations or other subsets of the data are not well captured by the linear regression model?

Regarding isolated departures of individual data points from the model or from the rest of the data, model diagnostics exist for multiple linear regression. These tools can help to identify data points that are outliers or points of high leverage and/or influence; these are essential steps in studying model adequacy. Of course, the problem is more complicated than with simple linear regression because the joint influence of several predictors must be considered simultaneously.

More-systemic problems arise when the data as a whole appear to violate the assumption that the mean of the response varies as a linear and additive function of the set of predictors. How should we approach this problem? First, statistical tests, graphical procedures and other tools are available to assess the linearity of the relationship of the response to each predictor, accounting for the other predictors in the model, and also to assess whether these variables combine additively or in a more complex way to predict the response.

Second, even if the assumptions of linearity and additivity do not hold exactly, the fitted model is often still a very useful summary of the relationships in the data. It will capture the part of the relationship of the response to the predictors that is linear and additive, and this will often be a main part of the story, even if it is not the whole story. Additionally, such a summary is of use precisely because it glosses over higher-order details in favor of a more parsimonious presentation of the data, yielding an analysis that is easier to interpret and to communicate. Of course, the advantage of including higher-order terms is that the resulting model more faithfully represents the patterns of association in the data.

For instance, in Example 3 (Figure 10), the slopes with respect to sleep debt are slightly different between the two diabetic complications groups. Strictly speaking, this violates the additivity assumption because it suggests that the presence of diabetic complications not only shifts the regression line up or down, but also alters the slope with respect to sleep debt. The two lines are, however, so close to parallel that the difference is unimportant. Indeed, a statistical test could be applied to assess whether this difference is significant. Fitted model (8) simplifies the picture by providing a single slope common to both groups. Good data analysis often requires a compromise between the two competing goals of parsimony and quality of fit to the data.

SUMMARIZATION, ADJUSTMENT, AND PREDICTION REVISITED

The introduction mentioned three broadly construed applications for regression models: summarization, adjustment, and prediction. We now revisit the use of multiple regression for these three purposes.

Summarization

One reason that multiple regression is useful is that it yields a parsimonious description of the nature and strength of the dependence of a response Y on a set of Xs. Consider the following example.

> Example 7: Lauderdale et al.[12] objectively measured various sleep characteristics in a population-based random sample of healthy middle-aged adults. The goal of the study was to provide a description and quantification of sleep in this population, and also to examine whether and how sleep varies by demographic, socioeconomic, and other variables. Sleep parameters included time in bed, sleep latency, sleep duration, and sleep efficiency—all continuous response variables. The analysis used multiple linear regression to examine how each response jointly depends on the predictors. For each response, the authors fitted three regression models. One model included indicator variables for race-by-sex groups and a continuous predictor, age. The next model added income, another continuous variable. The last model added continuous and indicator variables for employment status, body mass index (BMI), alcohol consumption, smoking status, and number of children under 18 years old in the household, among others.

This is an example of using multiple linear regression for data *summarization*. The study is largely descriptive, aiming to provide information on normative sleep patterns in a healthy population. No hypotheses are strongly driving the analyses; interest is more on the joint contributions of the predictors in explaining the variability in sleep, rather than on the coefficient of one specific predictor adjusted for the others. For example, whereas the full model, with all predictors included, provides the regression slope for BMI adjusted for income (and other things), interest on the sleep-BMI association is no more or less important than that on the sleep-income association. The reader also has available the regression slope for income both unadjusted and adjusted for BMI. In a sense, all predictors are on an "equal footing." Taken as a whole, the model is a concise description of the joint impact of race, sex, age, and other factors on sleep in healthy adults. In this sense the regression model is a powerful tool for summarization of this joint effect.

Adjustment

In many applications, not all of the predictor variables will be on an equal footing. Rather, one or more will be of primary importance. The others are included for purposes of statistical *adjustment*. The motivation for adjustment is often that the exposure (predictor variable) of interest is associated with some variables that are also expected to influence the outcome of interest. Such *confounders*, if not properly accounted for, will induce a spurious association between exposure and outcome. We illustrate with the following example.

> Example 2 (continued): In the study of the association of child's IQ to blood lead levels, a major barrier to interpreting the observed inverse association as causal was concern that other variables are associated with both elevated blood lead and depressed IQ in some individuals, and that these variables account for the observed association of IQ to blood lead levels, i.e., that these variables are potential confounders. Such variables may include maternal IQ, level of education, and use of tobacco during pregnancy; family financial status; and the child's gender, birth weight, and iron status. Socioeconomic status is of particular concern because of its link to environments with unstable and uncontained lead-based paint or with lead-contaminated soil, as are perinatal variables such as birth weight and maternal smoking, owing to links with both socioeconomic status and children's development. To handle these problems, the investigators developed a multiple linear regression model that included many of these continuous and categorical covariates as adjustor variables, in addition to lifetime average blood lead concentration. The estimated coefficient of blood lead concentration in this "adjusted" model was -1.52 points/(μg/dl) (95% CI: $[-2.94, -0.09]$) in those with lifetime peak blood lead concentrations less than 10 μg/dl. This compares to an unadjusted blood lead concentration coefficient of -2.54 points/(μg/dl). The adjusted slope was lower in magnitude, but still indicative of a clinically and statistically significant association between blood lead and child's IQ after accounting for potential confounders.

When regression is used primarily for adjustment, the estimated coefficients for all of the adjustor variables are often not even given. Only the coefficients for blood lead are presented in the example. The idea (aside from minimizing journal space!) is to focus the analysis on the blood lead-IQ relationship while accounting for the adjustor variables, rather than to distract from this primary relationship by presenting the regression slopes of all variables.

In this example the adjustor variables such as maternal IQ, education, and household income are potential confounders because they are thought to influence both the exposure (blood lead) and the outcome (child's IQ). Because these variables are included in the regression model, the coefficient of blood lead quantifies the IQ–blood lead association net of any linear and additive relationship of IQ to these variables, thereby eliminating or reducing potential confounding from them. The statistical analyses permit estimation of both unadjusted and adjusted regression coefficients, and these represent two different empirical perspectives on the association of IQ to lead exposure. Conclusions about whether an adjustor variable is truly a confounder and/or whether the adjusted association quantified by the regression model represents a causal link, however, are extra-statistical steps that must be justified by non-statistical considerations including the scientific issues at hand. Confounding and some aspects of causality are discussed in more detail in Chapter 7.

Prediction

Prediction with linear regression has a variety of purposes in medical practice and research. First, it can involve forecasting or prognostication into the future about some responses based on predictors available at present. Second, it may be used to avoid expensive or invasive gold-standard diagnostic measures, instead predicting those measures from easier-to-obtain clinical information. Third, it may involve projection of a given patient into a "what if" situation. Prediction stands in some contrast to summarization and adjustment. In general, models that do a good job of summarization will also be good predictive models and vice versa. However, with prediction, the estimation and testing of regression coefficients are de-emphasized, and predictive accuracy is of primary importance. Therefore, a focus on prediction will sometimes lead to a different regression model than when the focus is on summarization.

Predictive accuracy is the degree to which the fitted value based on a model is close to the actual response. That is, suppose we take a data set and fit a regression model. Now, suppose we have a new observation (e.g., a new patient), with predictors X_1, X_2, etc., and response Y, and that we use the fitted model with these new Xs to predict the unknown Y for this new patient. How close the prediction is to the actual response, on average, is a measure of predictive accuracy. The following example serves to illustrate some of these points.

Example 8: Gulati et al.[13] developed a regression model to predict exercise capacity in healthy women as a function of age. Exercise capacity is measured in metabolic equivalents (MET), defined as the maximal oxygen uptake for a given workload, measured as multiples of the basal rate of oxygen consumption when a person is at rest. The purpose of the study was to establish a nomogram of mean MET-for-age values in a healthy female population. The women were also classified as "active" or "sedentary" on the basis of self-reported participation in a regular exercise or training program. Sample sizes were 866 in the active group and 4643 in the sedentary group. Fitted regression equations were mean(MET) = 17.9 − (0.16/year) × AGE for the active group and mean(MET) = 14.0 − (0.12/year) × AGE for the sedentary group.

Here the modeling objective is to obtain good predictions for input into a nomogram, the driving goal of the project. We make two points about the fitted models. First, the authors were careful to assess whether the relationship of MET to age was linear; it turned out to be. However, if it had not been, their analysis had scope to transform age or to include nonlinear age terms in the regression models. Second, the authors fitted separate models for the sedentary group and the active group; this is equivalent to fitting one model to the entire sample with an indicator variable for being in the active group and an interaction term between active group and age, allowing for different age slopes in the two groups. A simpler approach would have omitted the interaction term. Though the interaction term was most likely significant, its inclusion in the model does not add substantially to the story about the MET-age relationship (MET is higher in the active group and drops with age in both groups), so if the goal had been *summarization*, this term might have been excluded. As the goal was *prediction*, however, both the potential inclusion of nonlinear functions of age and the actual inclusion of the age-by-activity-group interaction rendered the model more faithful to the data and thereby improved its predictive ability. Often good predictive models contain more terms than good explanatory models.

One aspect of predictive modeling is to evaluate and quantify the predictive accuracy. R^2 is a common metric for predictive accuracy in multiple linear regression models, and is more relevant in predictive than in summarization modeling. In the above example, R^2 = 35% in the active model and 24% in the sedentary model, reflecting reasonable but not strong predictive ability.

Additional considerations arise in practice, relating to problems of model selection and of predictive accuracy. Often, there are many candidate predictor variables, and the analyst faces the problem of choosing which ones to include. Prediction is degraded, and the model may be unusable, if any predictor variable is missing for a new patient. Once variables are selected, there is the question of whether to include nonlinear terms. The problem is further complicated by the potential need to include interactions. These choices must be made while recognizing that including too many predictors, including interaction terms (i.e., *over-fitting*), will degrade the generalizability and predictive ability of the model. Taken together, methods for making objective choices about model terms fall in the domain of *model selection*, an area of ongoing statistical research.

REPORTING REGRESSION RESULTS

Reporting on regression modeling is an important step in the analyses. The method used to develop the regression model should be described in sufficient detail that a reader with knowledge of regression and access to the data could reproduce the results (as noted in Chapter 14, point 2).

On the data, sufficient information should be given to enable the reader to digest the analyses and reach conclusions about any fitted model. First, any report should provide sample size(s), univariate descriptions of both the response and all predictors, information on missing data and, importantly, units of measurement for each variable. Second, to the degree that space allows, reports should include plots of the data, so that the reader can see key relationships and the variability in the data. Third, continuous predictor variables should be centered at some relevant value for the analysis at hand, and reasonable reference categories should be chosen for categorical predictors.

The report should present the fitted regression equation either in the text or in a table. The estimated regression coefficients ($\hat{\beta}$s) should be reported with units and be accompanied with standard errors and/or confidence intervals. Reporting only the coefficients and their p-values is rarely adequate. The estimated residual standard deviation should be included as part of the fitted model. When the goal of the model is prediction, it is appropriate to report the R^2 value of the fitted model, but in summarization or adjustment this statistic can often be small and lead the reader to decide that the associations detected via the regression models are not important. We emphasize that a model may very well not be a good prediction model, but may still reveal interesting and important associations. Therefore, R^2 is not always an important statistic to report. Finally, many reports do not include all regression coefficients, especially when those coefficients correspond to adjustor variables. Though this is sometimes unavoidable, it is better to provide this information.

ADDITIONAL READING

For research practitioners who wish to apply regression models and related methods in the analysis of their own data, a now-classic source is Weisberg,[14] whereas a more modern treatment (which includes regression diagnostics) is presented by Chatterjee, Hadi, and Price.[15] Predictive (or "prognostic") modeling is given extensive treatment by Harrell,[16] who also provides guidance on the use of linear and higher-order splines for flexibly modeling continuous variables.

ACKNOWLEDGMENTS

The authors thank Theodore G. Karrison, PhD, for editorial suggestions that improved this material considerably, and Eve Van Cauter, PhD, and Kristen L. Knutson, PhD, for making available the data from their sleep and diabetes outcomes study.

REFERENCES

1. Knutson KL, Ryden AM, Mander BA, Van Cauter E. Role of sleep duration and quality in the risk and severity of type 2 diabetes mellitus. Arch Intern Med 2006; 166:1768–74.

2. Buysse DJ, Reynolds CF III, Monk TH, et al. The Pittsburgh Sleep Quality Index: A new instrument for psychiatric practice and research. Psychiatry Res 1989; 28:193–213.

3. Carpenter JS, Andrykowski MA. Psychometric evaluation of the Pittsburgh Sleep Quality Index. J Psychosom Res 1998; 45:5–13.

4. American Diabetes Association. Standards of Medical Care in Diabetes–2006. Diabetes Care 2006; 29(suppl. 1):S4–S42.

5. Nathan DM, Singer DE, Hurxthal K, Goodson JD. The clinical information value of the glycosylated hemoglobin assay. N Engl J Med 1984; 310:341–6.

6. Canfield RL, Henderson CR, Cory-Slechta DA, et al. Intellectual impairment in children with blood lead concentrations below 10 μg per deciliter. N Engl J Med 2003; 348:1517–26.

7. Rubin DB. Estimating causal effects of treatments in randomized and non-randomized studies. J Educational Psychol 1974; 66:688–701.

8. Rubin DB. Formal modes of statistical inference for causal effects. J Statist Planning and Inference 1990; 25:279–92.

9. Cook RD, Weisberg S. Applied regression including computing and graphics. New York: John Wiley, 1999.

10. Belsley DA, Kuh E, Welsch RE. Regression diagnostics. New York: John Wiley, 1980.

11. McCullagh P, Nelder JA. Generalized linear models. 2nd ed. London: Chapman & Hall, 1989.

12. Lauderdale DS, Knutson KL, Yan LL, et al. Objectively measured sleep characteristics among early-middle-aged adults: The CARDIA Study. Am J Epidemiol 2006; 164:5–16.

13. Gulati M, Black HR, Shaw LJ, et al. The prognostic value of a nomogram for exercise capacity in women. N Engl J Med 2005; 353:468–75.

14. Weisberg S. Applied linear regression. 2nd ed. New York: John Wiley, 1985.

15. Chatterjee S, Hadi AS, Price B. Regression analysis by example. 3rd ed. New York: John Wiley, 2000.

16. Harrell FE. Regression modeling strategies with applications to linear models, logistic regression, and survival analysis. New York: Springer-Verlag, Inc., 2001.

CHAPTER 11

CЗ

Statistical Analysis of Survival Data

STEPHEN W. LAGAKOS, PH.D.

ABSTRACT   A primary endpoint in many medical studies is the time until occurrence of an event, such as disease progression, death, or discharge from a hospital. The statistical analysis of such data, commonly referred to as *survival data* or *failure-time data*, requires specialized statistical methods because the event may not yet have occurred in all subjects by the time the data are analyzed. These techniques can be helpful in identifying factors that influence survival time and in describing the survival experience of a population. This chapter reviews standard statistical methods for analyzing survival data. We describe the Kaplan-Meier method for estimating a survival distribution and the log-rank test for assessing the equality of two or more survival distributions. We also review Cox's proportional-hazards regression model, a popular methodology for assessing the simultaneous effect of multiple baseline factors on survival.

In clinical trials and other medical studies, interest often centers on an assessment of the times until the participants experience some specific event. This may be a clinical outcome such as disease progression, regression of a tumor, or death; or it may be an event related to the patient's clinical course, such as discharge from the hospital, discontinuation of study medication, or development of an adverse reaction to treatment.

Such data are usually referred to as *survival data* or *failure-time data*. Implicit in the definition of survival time is that survival is measured from some well-defined starting point. For example, in a study of survival in patients with AIDS, the starting point might be the time of diagnosis of AIDS. Similarly, in a clinical trial evaluating the use of chemotherapy to prolong remission in women who have received a mastectomy, the starting point might be the time of surgery or the time of randomization into the trial.

A common aspect of nearly all such studies is that some of the subjects will not experience the event defining the end of survival by the time the data are analyzed. For example, if three years have elapsed since an individual was diagnosed with AIDS, his survival time is known only to be something in excess of three years. This is commonly denoted as a survival of 3+ years and referred to as a *censored survival time*.

Medical research often involves survival methods. This chapter introduces the most commonly used statistical methods for analyzing survival data. These are the Kaplan-Meier estimator of the survival distribution, the log-rank test for comparing two or more survival distributions, and Cox's proportional-hazards regression model for assessing the effect of multiple baseline explanatory variables on survival. We also discuss competing-risks data, in which failures belong to one of two or more types (for example, deaths from cancer of the prostate vs. deaths from all other causes).

SURVIVAL AND HAZARD FUNCTIONS

The most common way to describe the survival characteristics of a population is to report the *survival function*, $S(t)$, which is defined as the proportion of individuals who survive beyond time t. For example, if time is measured in years, then $S(5) = 0.35$ means that 35 percent of the population survive beyond 5 years. By specifying the value of $S(t)$ for each t, we can fully describe the survival characteristics of the population. This is often done graphically in a "life table" or "survival plot." To illustrate, Figure 1 gives a hypothetical survival plot describing survival after the diagnosis of AIDS. Like any life table, the curve takes the value 1 at time 0 and then decreases, indicating that the proportion of survivors decreases with time. The median survival is the time at which 50 percent of the subjects have failed. Thus, in Figure 1, the median survival for this population is 1.7 years.

$S(t)$ does not have to decline to zero; for example, cancer-related deaths in a cohort of treated patents would decline only to the estimated proportion of patients cured.

Suppose that someone with AIDS has already survived for one year since being diagnosed. What is this person's prognosis? To answer this question, the hazard function, $h(t)$, extracts information from the survival function. Loosely speaking, the *hazard function* at time t is the proportion of persons who fail shortly after time t from among those who have not failed prior to t; that is

$$h(t) \sim \Pr[t < T < t + dt \,|\, T > t],$$

where Pr denotes probability, T denotes survival time, and dt is a small increment of time. Formally, the hazard function is defined by the expression:

$$h(t) = -\frac{d}{dt}[\ln S(t)].$$

That is, the hazard function is just the negative of the slope of the survival curve when the latter is plotted on a natural logarithmic scale. In epidemiologic

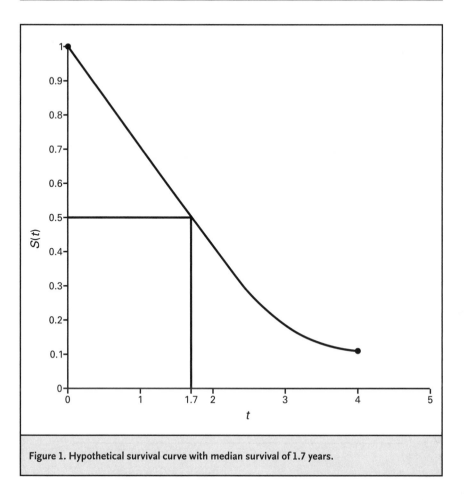

Figure 1. Hypothetical survival curve with median survival of 1.7 years.

studies $h(t)$ is closely related to the concept of age-specific mortality. The main difference is that in epidemiologic studies "t" usually refers to the age of a subject, whereas in clinical trials or other medical investigations it usually refers to time since entry into the study.

To illustrate how hazard functions can be useful in describing the survival characteristics of a population, Figure 2 gives three hypothetical hazard functions. The increasing hazard function reflects a population in which the proportion of persons who fail in a particular year (from among those who have not failed previously) increases with time. This type of distribution appears to describe the time between infection with HIV and the development of AIDS.[1] As an infected person survives each additional year without developing AIDS, his chances of AIDS developing in the subsequent year are greater than in the previous year. In contrast, the decreasing hazard function in Figure 2 reflects

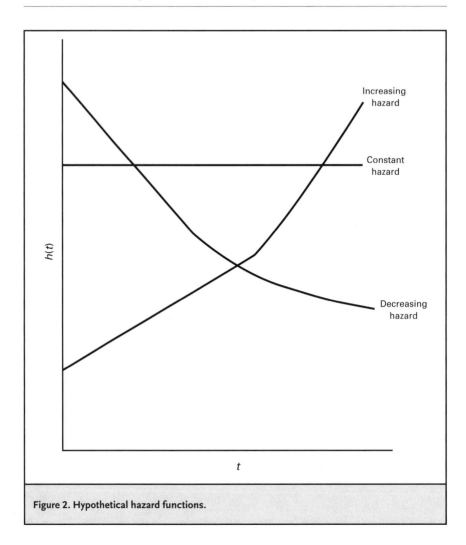

Figure 2. Hypothetical hazard functions.

a population in which the conditional probability of failing becomes less each year; that is, the longer an individual survives, the less his or her chances of failing in the subsequent year. This is the pattern for some forms of cancer—the longer the patient survives the disease, the better the prospects for surviving the next interval. Finally, the constant hazard in Figure 2 describes a population in which the proportion of subjects who are expected to fail in a given year, given that they haven't failed previously, is the same as in any other year. For example, survival from the time of diagnosis of inoperable lung cancer has been shown by several studies to be well approximated by a constant hazard function.[2]

By displaying survival curves on a logarithmic vertical axis, one can also get a qualitative feel for the shape of the hazard function. For example, the survival plots in Figure 3 are approximately linear. Because $S(t)$ is plotted on a logarithmic axis, this means that the hazard functions for these populations are approximately constant, corresponding to the exponential distribution.

CENSORING

A unique feature of survival data is the presence of censored observations. Because of limited periods of follow-up in observational studies, only a portion of the survival time is observed for some participants. Thus, the data available for analysis typically consist of some uncensored observations as well as some that are censored, usually at different time points. To illustrate, Table 1 gives the durations of remission among 42 leukemia patients who were either untreated or treated with the drug 6-mercaptopurine (6-MP).[3] The censored durations of remission, which are denoted with a "+," are smaller than some of the uncensored times and larger than others. Because patients are usually followed for different times, this is typical of censored survival data. Note that the censoring does not occur equally in the two treatment groups; in fact, in Table 1, the control group has no censored data.

Table 1. Durations of Remission (in Weeks) of 42 Leukemia Patients.[3]

6-MP Group ($n = 21$):	6, 6, 6, 6+, 7, 9+, 10, 10+, 11+, 13, 16, 17+, 19+, 20+, 22, 23, 25+, 32+, 32+, 34+, 35+
Control Group ($n = 21$):	1, 1, 2, 2, 3, 4, 4, 5, 5, 8, 8, 8, 8, 11, 11, 12, 12, 15, 17, 22, 23

All the methods described in this chapter, and almost all methods in regular use, assume that censoring is noninformative.[4] Loosely speaking, this means that the mechanism causing censoring at any specific time does not act selectively on subjects who are more (or less) likely to fail at that time. Censoring that arises simply because some subjects have not yet failed by the time the data are analyzed is noninformative because it implies nothing about the subjects' future status. In other situations, however, it is less obvious that censoring is noninformative. For example, suppose censoring occurs because individuals are lost to follow-up. The noninformative assumption means that the lost subjects are representative, with respect to survival after the time of loss, of those who remain under observation. Yet if individuals become lost to follow-up because their disease has progressed, their survival prognosis would be poorer than that of persons not lost to follow-up. Such censoring would be informative and would cause standard statistical methods to be biased.

ESTIMATING $S(t)$: THE KAPLAN-MEIER ESTIMATOR

Many methods have been proposed for estimating the survival function $S(t)$. One approach, called the Kaplan-Meier or Product Limit estimator, can be viewed as an extension of classical life-table methods used in actuarial applications that allows data-dependent time intervals. It enjoys widespread use in medical applications.[5]

Calculation of the Kaplan-Meier estimator of $S(t)$ is relatively simple and now is included as an option in many statistical software packages. At the heart of the method is the fact that the survival function $S(t)$ can be expressed as a product of conditional probabilities, and that each observation, whether it is censored or uncensored, can help to estimate some of these conditional probabilities. To illustrate, suppose that time is measured in whole years, and consider $S(10)$, the probability of surviving at least 10 years. This can be expressed as:

$$S(10) = S(1) \times S(2|1) \times S(3|2) \times \cdots \times S(10|9),$$

where $S(t|t-1)$ denotes the conditional probability of surviving at least t years, given that the individual has survived beyond $t-1$ years. For example, the first two factors on the right-hand side are the probability of surviving one year and the conditional probability of surviving two years, given survival to one year. When multiplied together, they equal the probability of surviving two years. Similarly, the product of the first three factors is the probability of surviving three years. The Kaplan-Meier estimator of $S(t)$ is constructed by estimating the individual factors, say $S(t|t-1)$, by the ratio $(N_t - n_t)/N_t$, where N_t denotes the number of subjects in the sample who are still being followed at time t, and n_t is the number of these who fail between time $t-1$ and time t. That is, the conditional probability of surviving t years, given that the individual has survived at least $t-1$ years, is estimated by the proportion of subjects at risk at t years who in fact survive beyond t years.

An important feature of the Kaplan-Meier estimator is that it makes no assumptions about the shape of $S(t)$ or the corresponding hazard function $h(t)$. The method assumes only that censoring occurs noninformatively.

Figure 3 gives the Kaplan-Meier estimators of $S(t)$ for the two samples described in Table 1. Note the similarities in their shapes. Each consists of a sequence of vertical and horizontal lines—called a step function—that begin at the value $S(t) = 1$ at $t = 0$ and decrease. It is the nature of Kaplan-Meier estimators that the jumps occur at observed times of failure. The greater frequency of jumps at earlier times is typical of survival data. Similarly, the larger jumps at later times are also typical. Because these are estimates, the curves are subject to statistical error. The variability in the Kaplan-Meier estimates tends to be greatest at the largest survival times because usually only a few subjects are still under observation (and few fail) at these times.

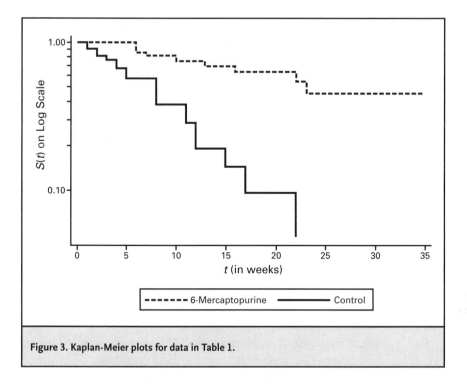

Figure 3. Kaplan-Meier plots for data in Table 1.

Another feature of Kaplan-Meier survival curves is that they do not drop completely to zero if the longest-surviving patient was still alive at the end of the study. This phenomenon occurs whenever follow-up is not sufficient to describe the complete survival experience of the population. Thus, for the 6-MP group in Figure 3, the data provide no information about the distribution of remission times longer than 35 weeks, and hence the Kaplan-Meier curves do not extend beyond this point. In contrast, the Kaplan-Meier estimate for the control group does drop to zero before 23 weeks, though this is not evident from the plot because of the logarithmic vertical scale.

COMPARISON OF TWO GROUPS:
THE LOG-RANK TEST

Suppose that we wish to compare the survival distributions of two groups. For example, we may wish to compare the age-specific mortality rates of males and females, the age-specific rates of stroke for black males and white males, or the results of two experimental treatments being evaluated in a clinical trial. An informal way to carry this out is by plotting the Kaplan-Meier estimators for the groups to be compared. For example, the curves in Figure 3 suggest that 6-MP may prolong the time in remission. To compare these groups more formally, a statistical test is often employed, most commonly the log-rank (or Mantel-Haenszel) test.[5]

The log-rank test is constructed by comparing estimates of the hazard functions of the two groups at each observed time of failure, not just at some fixed time such as five years. Specifically, suppose M_j and N_j denote the numbers of subjects at risk at time t_j in the 6-MP and control groups, respectively. And of these, let m_j and n_j denote the number of failures that occur at time t_j. For example, consider the data in Table 1 and suppose we let $t_j = 22$. It can be verified that $M_j = 7$, $N_j = 2$, $m_j = 1$, and $n_j = 1$. That is, one of the seven subjects at risk in the 6-MP group failed at week 22, compared to one of the two in the control group. If we knew that a total of two failures occurred, and if the two groups had equal hazard functions at this time point, we would expect $E_j = 2(2/9) = 0.44$ of the failures to be in the control group because 2/9 of the persons at risk at this time point are in the control group. In fact, we observed $O_j = 1$ failure in the control group at this time point. In this example, as in practice, the information at each time point may be quite small; but when all points are considered, p-values or confidence bounds may be convincing.

In constructing the log-rank test, O_j and E_j provide a comparison of the hazard functions of the two groups at time t_j. Summing these quantities, for an overall test of the equality of the groups, gives equal emphasis to each time point. As noted below, the log-rank test arises as a likelihood-based test from Cox's proportional-hazards model, and as such it is ideally suited to settings where the hazard functions for the treatment groups are proportional. Alternatively, if we wish to place greater emphasis on earlier time points, a variant of the log-rank test, often called the generalized Wilcoxon test, is used.[5] This is constructed similarly to the log-rank test, but gives greater weight to the observed (O_j) and expected (E_j) numbers of failures at earlier time points when summing.

ASSESSING MULTIPLE EXPLANATORY VARIABLES: COX'S MODEL

When multiple baseline characteristics might be associated with survival time, it is common to analyze each separately using the methods described above. However, it is often of interest to assess the simultaneous effects of several explanatory variables on survival time. For example, we may be interested in the combined effects of age and gender on survival. Or we might want to compare two treatment groups while simultaneously adjusting for other factors that could influence survival. One reason to include explanatory variables in a model when making a treatment comparison is to compensate for bias that might arise when these explanatory variables are not evenly balanced across treatment groups. Another is to increase the precision of the treatment comparison; that is, even if the explanatory variables are balanced across treatment groups, their inclusion in a regression model can lead to more-precise estimates of the treatment's effect on failure time.[6]

The most common approach to this type of analysis is Cox's proportional-hazards regression model.[5] Ordinary regression models usually express the dependent variable as a linear function of several explanatory variables, and the coefficients of these explanatory variables are estimated to assess their joint effect on the dependent variable. Such methods do not easily adapt to censored data. Cox's model overcomes these technical problems by assuming that the explanatory variables are related to survival time by a multiplicative effect on the hazard function. For example, suppose we wanted to analyze the data in Table 1 and allow for the effect of gender. If we let X_1 denote treatment group ($X_1 = 0$ for control and $X_1 = 1$ for 6-MP) and X_2 denote gender ($X_2 = 0$ for females and $X_2 = 1$ for males), then Cox's model would assume that the hazard function for a subject has the form

$$h_0(t)e^{\beta_1 X_1 + \beta_2 X_2}$$

Here $h_0(t)$ is some underlying hazard, and β_1 and β_2 are unknown regression coefficients that are estimated from the data. Expressed another way (remembering that $e^0 = 1$), the hazard functions for the four types of subjects are assumed to be

Female, Control:	$h_0(t)$
Female, 6-MP:	$h_0(t)e^{\beta_1}$
Male, Control:	$h_0(t)e^{\beta_2}$
Male, 6-MP:	$h_0(t)e^{\beta_1 + \beta_2}$

These hazard functions are proportional to one another, and they differ only because of the multiplicative exponential effect. Thus, it is not necessary to know the underlying hazard $h_0(t)$ in order to compare any pair of groups using their hazard ratios. For example, the ratio of the hazard function of a female on 6-MP to a female on control is e^{β_1}. This is also the hazard ratio for a male on 6-MP to a male on control. That is, the relative effect of treatment is assumed to be the same in males as it is in females. The hypothesis that treatment group is not associated with survival is expressed by $\beta_1 = 0$. Similarly, the ratio of the hazard function for a male to that for a female is e^{β_2}, whether both are on control or both are on 6-MP, and the hypothesis that gender is not associated with survival corresponds to $\beta_2 = 0$. The analysis of survival data using Cox's model consists of first estimating the parameters β_1 and β_2 and their standard errors. This allows the estimation of relative risks, the construction of confidence intervals for the parameters or relative risks, and tests of hypotheses about the parameters. The computation of the estimators is somewhat complicated and requires computer programs, but these are readily available in many of the standard statistical packages. An attractive feature of Cox's model is that it allows the coefficients β_1 and β_2 to be estimated from the data without any assumptions concerning $h_0(t)$.

The selection of a multivariate Cox regression model and the interpretation of the results have similarities to ordinary linear regression analyses. For example, step-up or step-down procedures can add or remove explanatory variables, and differential treatment effects across the levels of a baseline prognostic factor can be assessed by adding interaction terms.[5] For example, if we add the explanatory variable $X_3 = X_1 \times X_2$ (with coefficient β_3) to the above model, it would allow the 6-MP:Control hazard ratio in females (e^{β_1}) to differ from that in males ($e^{\beta_1 + \beta_3}$). Thus, the absence of an interaction term ($\beta_3 = 0$) corresponds to a common treatment effect across gender. The issue of heterogeneity of treatment effects, commonly referred to as subgroup analyses, is discussed in detail in Wang et al.[7]

Cox's model readily expands to include more than two treatment groups.[5] Another extension is stratification. To illustrate, consider the modification of the 6-MP/gender Cox model in which $h_0(t)$ and $h_1(t)$ are the underlying hazards for females and males, respectively. $h_0(t)$ and $h_1(t)$ need not be proportional. This stratified Cox model still assumes that the 6-MP:Control hazard ratio is e^{β_1} in either females or males, but it allows the shape of the hazard functions to differ arbitrarily by gender. Thus, when the main focus is on estimating the effect of treatment while adjusting for gender, the greater flexibility of this model makes it preferable to the previous model, in which both treatment and gender are included as exponential factors. Stratification can be extended to more than one explanatory variable, but the need to deal with more than one hazard function has the effect of reducing the amount of information about the variables of interest. Thus, stratification becomes impractical if the number of strata is large.

Two related and important issues in using Cox's model are checking the underlying assumptions and the consequences on making an inference when the underlying assumptions are incorrect. For a thorough discussion of methods for assessing model fit, see Klein and Moeschberger.[8] The robustness of inferences from Cox's model to violations of assumptions has been theoretically studied in detail.[6, 9] When the explanatory variable of interest is independent of the other explanatory variables, such as treatment group in a randomized clinical trial, inferences about this explanatory variable based on fitting a Cox model remain valid, in the sense of preserving Type I error, under a wide range of mis-specifications of the model.[9] However, the power to detect a treatment effect can be greatly reduced when using a Cox model, or log-rank test, if the hazard functions for the comparison groups are not proportional. This is illustrated in the APPROVE trial assessing the safety of rofecoxib.[10]

COMPETING RISKS

In some settings time to failure is naturally accompanied by a qualitative indicator of type (or cause) of failure. For example, (1) a cancer trial may focus on whether a drug affects the time until relapse, yet a patient might die prior to experiencing relapse; (2) the main focus of a study may be the effect of a treatment on the time until death from prostate cancer, but a patient can die from other causes; and (3) there may be interest in whether an anti-infective drug increases the rate of clearance of infection, but patients are also at risk of untoward events, such as death prior to clearance. These examples share the common feature that observation of an outcome of interest (relapse, death from prostate cancer, clearance of infection) may be prevented by another clinical outcome. The latter outcome can be viewed as a "competing risk." It differs qualitatively from our original setting, in which failure is censored simply because the event has not happened by the time the data are to be analyzed. In such competing-risk settings, it is important that the competing type (or cause) of failure be considered in the analysis. For example, a treatment for prostate cancer might reduce the risk of death from prostate cancer, but its overall usefulness will also depend on its effect, if any, on death from other causes. Similarly, an anti-infective drug may enhance clearance of an infection but may not be of practical use if its toxicity adversely affects mortality.

One approach to analyzing such data ignores the type of failure and simply focuses on failure from any cause. For example, cancer trials commonly compare "relapse-free survival"; failure is simply the earlier of relapse or death. Of course, such analyses could fail to distinguish between treatments that have similar effects on the time until the first of relapse or death, but have different effects on the risks of each type (e.g., one treatment may have a higher risk of relapse but lower risk of death than the other treatment).

Often there may be special interest in assessing a treatment's effect on a specific type of failure, such as prostate cancer death. Or, as in the third example, it may be illogical to evaluate time until failure in circumstances where a "positive" outcome is the shortening of one type of failure (e.g., clearance of infection) and the lengthening of the other (e.g., mortality). Here one would want the statistical analysis of the data to take account of the type of failure. Standard statistical methods for analyzing ordinary survival data can also be useful for competing-risk data. However, as noted above, the interpretation of the results must take account of the competing events. To illustrate, suppose that T denotes time until failure and that the indicator variable δ denotes the type of failure, where $\delta = 1$ corresponds to the failure type of interest (e.g., death from prostate cancer) and $\delta = 2$ corresponds to the competing failure type (e.g., death from causes other than prostate cancer). Then, analogous to the hazard function used to describe the distribution of T in ordinary survival data, one can describe the outcome (T, δ) using cause-specific hazard functions, say $h_1(t)$ and $h_2(t)$, that decompose the hazard function $h(t)$ into the two types of failure.

Inferences about cause-specific hazard functions are computationally simple. For example, suppose we wish to compare two treatment groups (say A and B) with respect to the cause-specific hazard corresponding to $\delta = 1$ (e.g., death from prostate cancer). That is, suppose we wish to test the hypothesis $h_1^{(A)}(t) = h_1^{(B)}(t)$. It turns out[5] that this hypothesis can be tested by applying the usual log-rank test after regarding both actual censored observations and failures from the competing event ($\delta = 2$) as censored observations. Cox's model can also be applied here by replacing the underlying hazard function $h_0(t)$ by the cause-specific hazard function $h_1(t)$. To compare treatment groups or conduct a regression analysis focusing on the competing cause of failure, one need only reverse the roles of the two types of failure.

An important distinction, however, between analyses of ordinary survival data and competing-risk data is that the cause-specific hazard function $h_1(t)$ cannot be linked to the survival function $S(t)$ without consideration of failures of both types. Thus, although a computer program for the Kaplan-Meier estimator can be applied to competing-risk data (with failures of one type being regarded as censored observations), the resulting estimated survival distribution cannot be interpreted probabilitistically. Thus, to describe the results, one might instead plot an estimator of the cumulative cause-specific hazard function or the cumulative cause-specific incidence function. The cumulative incidence function[9] corresponding to the first type of failure gives the probability that an individual at risk of failure of either type will experience the first type of failure by time t. For example, Wang and colleagues[11] examine the cumulative incidence of heart failure, in the presence of the competing risk of death, by baseline levels of plasma B-type natriuretic peptide. The cumulative cause-specific hazard function corresponding to the first type of failure is the integral of cause-specific hazard function $h_1(t)$. In another example, Holmberg and colleagues[12] examine the cumulative hazard rates of death from prostate cancer for patients diagnosed with early prostate cancer. Cumulative cause-specific hazard functions can be useful for comparative purposes, but they have the disadvantage of not being interpretable in terms of probabilities of outcomes. Details about estimating cumulative incidence are given in Gray[13] and in Klein and Moeschberger.[8]

ACKNOWLEDGMENT

This work was supported by Grant AI24643 from the National Institute of Allergy and Infectious Diseases.

REFERENCES

1. De Gruttola V, Lagakos S. The value of AIDS incidence data in assessing the spread of HIV infection. Stat Med 1989; 8:35–43.

2. Stanley K. Prognostic factors for survival in patients with inoperable lung cancer. J Natl Cancer Inst 1980; 65:25–32.

3. Freireich EJ, Gehan E, Frei E, et al. The effect of 6-mercaptopurine on the duration of steroid-induced remissions in acute leukemia: a model for evaluation of other potentially useful therapy. Blood 1963; 21:699–716.

4. Lagakos SW. General right censoring and its impact on the analysis of survival data. Biometrics 1979; 35:139–56.

5. Cox DR, Oakes D. Analysis of survival data. London: Chapman and Hall, 1984.

6. Lagakos SW, Schoenfeld DA. On the mis-specification of proportional hazards regression models. Biometrics 1984; 40:1037–48.

7. Wang R, Lagakos SW, Ware JH, et al. Statistics in medicine—Reporting of subgroup analyses in clinical trials. N Engl J Med 2007; 357:2189–94. [Chapter 15 of this book.]

8. Klein JP, Moeschberger ML. Survival analysis. New York: Springer-Verlag, 1997.

9. DiRienzo AG, Lagakos SW. The effects of misspecifying Cox's regression model on randomized treatment group comparisons. Handbook of statistics, 22, 1–15. New York: Elsevier Science, 2004.

10. Lagakos SW. Time-to-event analyses for long-term treatments: The APPROVE trial. N Engl J Med 2006; 355:116–7.

11. Wang TJ, Larson MG, Levy D, et al. Plasma natriuretic peptide levels and the risk of cardiovascular events and death. N Engl J Med 2004; 350:655–63.

12. Holmberg L, Bill-Axelson A, Helgesen F, et al. A randomized trial comparing radical prostatectomy with watchful waiting in early prostate cancer. N Engl J Med 2002; 347:781–9.

13. Gray RJ. A class of K-sample tests for comparing the cumulative incidence of a competing risk. Ann Stat 1988; 16:1141–54.

CHAPTER 12
Cß

Analysis of Categorical Data in Medical Studies

PAUL S. ALBERT, PH.D.

ABSTRACT Many medical studies involve *categorical data*—observations that
are assigned to categories (e.g., gender or hair color). In volume 349 of the *New
England Journal of Medicine,* nearly 70% of papers contained at least one categorical
data analysis. This chapter provides a conceptual view of categorical data analysis in medical studies. We discuss the use of contingency tables to summarize
data. We present various measures for characterizing statistical associations in
contingency tables and discuss which measure is most appropriate for various
types of studies. We further discuss statistical tests for associations between categorical variables. A common problem in medical studies is the examination of
the relationship between the probability of a binary event (such as survival) and
multiple continuous and discrete variables; logistic regression is often used in
this situation. We discuss the use of logistic regression for analyzing data from
prospective and retrospective case-control studies. We illustrate all techniques
with examples from *Journal* articles.

The analysis of categorical data is common in medical studies. Categories
may be dichotomous (e.g., gender or survival), more numerous but unordered (e.g., hair color), or ordered (e.g., educational status categorized
as completing school only through grade 6, completing through grade 12, or
completing higher education). The endpoints of clinical trials are often categorical variables that measure disease activity, such as tumor regression or second
myocardial infarct. The *New England Journal of Medicine* publishes many examples
of categorical variables tabulated by treatment or disease group. The 62 original
articles in volume 349 of the *Journal* (July to December 2003) included 40 (65%)
with at least one such tabulation. Throughout this chapter, we illustrate various
approaches to the summary and analysis of categorical data using examples
from this and other volumes of the *Journal.*

The relationships among categorical variables are often summarized in contingency tables, in which the frequency of one categorical variable is tabulated by categories of another variable. A common example is the frequency of disease status by treatment group or medication status. In a large cohort of patients with nonvalvular atrial fibrillation, Hylek et al.[1] studied incident ischemic strokes. They assessed the effect of the intensity of prior oral anticoagulation on the severity of ischemic stroke, graded in five categories. Medical records provided information on the use of aspirin or warfarin and the international normalized ratio (INR, a laboratory measurement of blood clotting activity, with higher numbers indicating greater anticoagulation) at admission. Hylek et al. classified patients into four groups according to the antithrombotic-medication status and INR at admission: no medication, aspirin, warfarin and INR < 2.0, and warfarin and INR ≥ 2.0. Table 1 reproduces the percentages and column totals from the article and adds cell counts that are consistent with the percentages. The columns correspond to antithrombotic-medication status and INR at admission, and the rows correspond to the categories of severity of stroke. Although not presented in the table, the percentages for the combined warfarin group can easily be calculated. For example, the combined percentage of patients who had a fatal in-hospital stroke is [117(0.09) + 71(0.01)]/188 = 0.06. This calculation illustrates an attractive feature of contingency tables that is not usually possible with data summaries of continuous data. Namely, it is often easy to perform additional analyses, as well as check an author's computations.

The data in Table 1 suggest that outcomes in patients who take warfarin and had INR ≥ 2.0 are better than those in patients taking either aspirin or warfarin with INR < 2.0. Also, patients who take aspirin may have less-severe strokes than those who take no oral anticoagulation. The situation is more complicated when comparing the warfarin groups with the other groups. If the authors had combined the warfarin groups, there would be little difference in the frequency of severe strokes between aspirin and warfarin. For example, in both the aspirin group and the combined warfarin group 6% of patients had fatal in-hospital strokes. Stratified by INR status (INR < 2 or ≥ 2), warfarin is most effective when patients have high INR scores, and for this subset of patients it appears to be more beneficial than aspirin in reducing severe strokes. Thus, important associations can be obscured by collapsing categories in a contingency table.

Not all tables of counts are contingency tables, even though they may seem to be contingency tables at first glance. Table 2 shows data on five different adverse effects reported in a randomized clinical trial evaluating a sublingual-tablet formulation of buprenorphine and naloxone for opiate addiction.[2] The numbers of adverse reactions in each of the three randomized groups (i.e., buprenorphine and naloxone, buprenorphine alone, and placebo) are presented in separate columns, along with the percentage of patients experiencing each adverse event. The

Table 1. Effect of Oral Anticoagulation on Severity of Stroke in Patients with Atrial Fibrillation (Cell Counts with Column Percentages).

Severity of Stroke	Antithrombotic Medication Status			
	None	Aspirin	Warfarin INR < 2.0	Warfarin INR ≥ 2.0
Fatal in-hospital stroke	35 (14%)	10 (6%)	11 (9%)	1 (1%)
Severe stroke, total dependence	20 (8%)	11 (7%)	7 (6%)	3 (4%)
Major stroke, neurologic deficit that prevents independent living	92 (37%)	58 (36%)	51 (44%)	27 (38%)
Minor stroke, neurologic deficit that does not prevent independent living	89 (36%)	78 (49%)	44 (38%)	39 (55%)
No neurologic sequelae	12 (5%)	3 (2%)	4 (3%)	1 (2%)
Total	248 (100%)	160 (100%)	117 (100%)	71 (100%)

Source: Hylek et al.[1]

percentages in Table 2 are actually counted rates: corresponding to each line in the table is another line, not shown, with the number of patients who did not have the adverse event. One could describe Table 2 as a streamlined summary of five contingency tables, each with two rows (e.g., headache and no headache) and three columns (corresponding to the three treatment arms). Thus, Table 1 and Table 2 are inherently different. In Table 1 column percentages add up to 100% for each column, because a patient can be classified in only one category of stroke severity. In Table 2 column percentages do not necessarily add to 100%, because patients could have no adverse events or as many as all five of the adverse events. More generally, in a contingency table each subject is counted exactly once, in one cell. In Table 1, a contingency table, each patient belongs to a single combination of antithrombotic medication status and severity of stroke. In Table 2, on the other hand, each patient belongs to one of the three treatment groups,

Table 2. Toxicity Data for Randomized Trial of Sublingual-Tablet Formulation of Buprenorphine and Naloxone in Treating Opiate Addiction. Number of Events and Percentages by Treatment Arm.

Adverse Event	Buprenorphine and Naloxone (N = 107)	Buprenorphine (N = 103)	Placebo (N = 107)
Headache	39 (36.4)	30 (29.1)	24 (22.4)
Withdrawal syndrome	27 (25.2)	19 (18.4)	40 (37.4)
Insomnia	15 (22.4)	19 (18.4)	20 (18.7)
Diarrhea	4 (3.7)	5 (4.9)	16 (15.0)
Constipation	13 (12.1)	8 (7.8)	3 (2.8)

Source: Fudala et al.[2]

but contributes to each of the five categories of adverse event (either by having an event or not having one).

Informally, the results presented in Table 2 suggest that the rates of headaches and constipation increase from placebo to buprenorphine to buprenorphine and naloxone, and that withdrawal syndrome and diarrhea have higher rates on placebo than on the other two treatment arms.

MEASURES OF ASSOCIATION

Interest often focuses on measuring the association between variables in a contingency table. We begin by considering the association in a 2×2 table with two binary variables such as disease status and treatment group in a two-group clinical trial. The first of these variables is often referred to as a response, which is not subject to the investigators' manipulation, and the second is a "circumstance," subject to the investigators' manipulation. Schreiber et al.[3] present the results of a randomized placebo-controlled clinical trial examining the effect of inhaled nitric oxide during the first week of life on the incidence of chronic lung disease and death in premature infants who were undergoing mechanical ventilation for respiratory distress syndrome. Table 3 presents the 2×2 table showing the distribution of chronic lung disease or death by treatment group.

Table 3. Death or Chronic Lung Disease in Premature Infants with Respiratory Distress Syndrome. Numbers and Percentages within Treatment Group.

Outcome	Inhaled Nitric Oxide	Placebo	Total
Death or chronic lung disease	51 (48.6%)	65 (63.7%)	116
Neither death nor chronic lung disease	54 (51.4%)	37 (36.3%)	91
Total	105	102	207

Source: Schreiber et al.[3]

How do we summarize the association between treatment and outcome in this table? Various measures of association are commonly used for such 2×2 tables. A natural way is to compare the proportion who die or have chronic lung disease in the two treatment groups. This is simply a comparison of 48.6% (51/105) and 63.7% (65/102). A simple measure of association is the ratio of these two percentages, usually called the relative risk. Another measure is the difference between the two percentages, the risk difference. A third measure is the odds ratio. The odds of an outcome in a treatment group is the percentage with that outcome divided by the percentage without; the odds ratio for a treatment group is the odds in that group divided by the odds in the control group.

Table 4. Notation for a Generic 2×2 Table.

Response	Treatment	Control	Total
Positive	a	b	r_1
Negative	c	d	r_2
Total	s_1	s_2	N

As a basis for discussing these measures more systematically, Table 4 shows a generic 2×2 table and related notation. The variables a, b, c, and d represent the counts in the four cells. The variables r_1 and r_2 are the row totals, s_1 and s_2 are the column totals, and N is the total count in the four cells. When each column presents response data by treatment group, r_1 and r_2 are the total numbers of positive and negative responses in the trial. Likewise, s_1 and s_2 are the numbers of patients in the two treatment groups. In this notation, the risk difference is $a/s_1 - b/s_2$, the relative risk is $(a/s_1)/(b/s_2)$, and the odds ratio is $[(a/s_1)/(c/s_1)]/[(b/s_2)/(d/s_2)] = (a/c)/(b/d) = ad/bc$. We discuss these briefly.

The proportions of positive responses (or, more generally, events) in the two treatment arms are a/s_1 and b/s_2. Under a common statistical model the count a follows a binomial distribution with total count s_1 and unknown population proportion P_t. Similarly, the count b follows a binomial distribution with s_2 and P_c. Thus, a/s_1 is an estimate of the unknown P_t, and b/s_2 estimates P_c. Under a binomial distribution the patients' outcomes are statistically independent, and each patient in a treatment group has the same probability of an event. The investigator wants to know whether the underlying probability of an event is the same for the two treatment groups; that is, whether $P_c = P_t$. This is generally the null hypothesis in such work, to be tested using the data a, b, c, and d.

The *relative risk* (RR) is P_t/P_c in the population and is estimated by $(a/s_1)/(b/s_2)$. It can be interpreted as the ratio of the risk of an event in the treatment group to the risk in the control group. Departures from 1 in the relative risk reflect an association between treatment group and response. When the event is a positive outcome, a relative risk greater than 1 reflects positive association, and a relative risk less than 1 reflects negative association. For a negative outcome, such as death, the direction of association is reversed. In the nitric oxide clinical trial (Table 3) the estimate of the relative risk of death or chronic disease in the treatment group compared to the placebo group is $(51/105)/(65/102) = 0.486/0.637 = 0.762$.

Another simple measure, the *risk difference*, is $P_t - P_c$ in the population and is estimated by $(a/s_1) - (b/s_2)$. A risk difference of zero reflects absence of association between the two variables, and a positive difference corresponds to a higher probability of an event in the treatment group than in the control group. In the nitric oxide clinical trial the estimate of the risk difference is $51/105 - 65/102 = 0.486 - 0.637 = -0.152$.

A potential shortcoming of the relative risk and the risk difference as measures of association is that they are not symmetric in the two variables. Specifically, if variable 2 defines the two groups of subjects and variable 1 defines the presence or absence of an event, the relative risk (or the risk difference) is not the same as it is when the roles of the two variables are reversed. Symmetry is not required, or even useful, when variable 1 is an outcome and variable 2 is a "circumstance," as in the nitric oxide trial, where estimating the relative risk of treatment by outcome, $(a/r_1)/(c/r_2)$, does not make sense. However, asymmetry is undesirable when measuring the association between two outcome variables, such as the occurrences of two adverse events in the buprenorphine/naloxone trial. And even when variable 1 is an outcome and variable 2 is a "circumstance," the relative risk of a positive outcome has no simple relation to the relative risk of a negative outcome. The former would be estimated by $(a/s_1)/(b/s_2)$, and the latter, by $(c/s_1)/(d/s_2)$.

In terms of the population proportions, the odds of a positive event in the treatment group is $P_t/(1 - P_t)$ and is estimated by a/c, and the odds in the control group is $P_c/(1 - P_c)$, estimated by b/d. The ratio of these odds, the *odds ratio* (OR), is simply the relative odds of a positive event between the two groups, estimated by $(a/c)/(b/d) = (ad)/(cb)$. Similar to the relative risk, a departure from 1 in the odds ratio reflects an association; an odds ratio greater than 1 reflects positive association, and an odds ratio between 0 and 1 reflects a negative association. Though the odds ratio may be less intuitive than the risk ratio or the risk difference, it has much better mathematical properties, making it more useful in various analyses. In particular, the odds ratio is symmetric in the two variables, making it particularly attractive in measuring associations between outcome variables.

For the nitric oxide trial, the estimated odds ratio measuring the association between treatment and response is $(51/54)/(65/37) = 0.54$. As with the estimated relative risk, an estimated odds ratio of 0.54 suggests that that the odds of having a death or chronic lung disease on inhaled nitric oxide is approximately one-half the odds of this poor outcome on placebo. Thus, the value of the odds ratio suggests a strong association between treatment and outcome. The degree of negative association summarized by an odds ratio of 0.5 is equivalent to the degree of positive association summarized by an odds ratio of 2.0. More generally, the odds ratio for a negative outcome (on one variable) is the reciprocal of the odds ratio for a positive outcome.

Although the odds ratio can be used for summarizing the association between the two variables in a 2×2 table, it cannot generally be interpreted as a relative risk. The exception occurs when the probability of an event is low in both groups (say, less than 10%). In this situation, the odds ratio will be approximately equal to the relative risk. In Table 4 the odds ratio is $(a/c)/(b/d)$, and the relative risk is $(a/s_1)/(b/s_2)$. Thus, for a rare outcome, the estimated odds ratio will be approximately the same as the estimated relative risk, because s_1 will be approximately equal to c and s_2 will be approximately equal to d.

Strom et al.[4] provide an illustration of the odds ratio as a measure of relative risk. The authors conducted a retrospective cohort study to examine the risk of allergic reactions within 30 days after receiving sulfonamide nonantibiotic. Of primary interest was whether the risk was higher among patients who had had prior allergic reactions to sulfonamide antibiotics than among patients who had not had a prior reaction. Table 5 shows the data for this primary objective. The odds ratio for this association can be estimated by $(96/873)/(315/18942) = 6.6$. Similarly, the estimated relative risk can be computed as $(96/969)/(315/19257) = 6.1$. Thus, the odds ratio is a good estimate of relative risk for these rare events.

Table 5. Effect of Prior Hypersensitivity after Sulfonamide Antibiotics on the Risk of Allergic Reaction to Sulfonamide Nonantibiotic within 30 Days.

Outcome	Patients with Prior Hypersensitivity after Sulfonamide Antibiotics	Patients without Prior Hypersensitivity after Sulfonamide Antibiotics
Allergic reaction	96 (9.9%)	315 (1.6%)
Other	873 (90.1%)	18,942 (98.4%)
Totals	969	19,257

Source: Strom et al.[4]

Although either the odds ratio or the relative risk can be used to measure association in a 2×2 table resulting from a prospective or retrospective cohort study, the relative risk cannot be directly estimated from a retrospective case-control study. In such studies the investigator determines the numbers of cases and controls, making direct estimates of risk for cases and controls impossible. However, a great strength of the odds ratio is that it still approximates the relative risk for a retrospective case-control study if the outcome is rare (see Chapter 7 in Fleiss et al.[5] for a mathematical explanation). For example, in a case-control study, Modan et al.[6] estimated the relative risk of ovarian cancer for patients with and patients without either a *BRCA1* or *BRCA2* mutation. Controls were matched to women with ovarian cancer on age, area of birth, and place and length of residence in Israel, where the study was done. Interestingly, even though they started out with two controls for every patient, by the time they removed those who would not give consent or could not answer the questions posed by the investigators or whose DNA samples could not be genotyped, they ended up with slightly fewer controls than cases. The data in Table 6 include all cases of peritoneal or epithelial cancer and controls who had molecular analysis for *BRCA1/BRCA2* mutations. The estimated odds ratio is $(244/596) / (13/738) = 23.2$, suggesting that the risk of ovarian cancer among *BRCA1* or *BRCA2* patients is much higher than that for individuals without these mutations.

Table 6. Effect of a Founder Mutation in *BRCA1* or *BRCA2* on the Risk of Ovarian Cancer.

Mutation	Patients	Controls
Either *BRCA1* or *BRCA2*	244 (29.0%)	13 (1.7%)
None	596 (71.0%)	738 (98.3%)
Totals	840	751

Source: Modan et al.[6]

So far, we have limited ourselves to measuring an association between two dichotomous categorical variables. There are no good single measures for characterizing the association between two categorical variables with more than two categories. However, for variables with more than two categories, one may compare the frequency of an event (the proportion who are in one of the categories) among the categories of the second variable. For example, in the 5×4 table in Table 1, the relative risks of a fatal in-hospital stroke for patients taking aspirin, warfarin with an INR < 2.0, or warfarin with an INR ≥ 2.0 (relative to patients on neither of these medications) are 0.43 (= 6% / 14%), 0.64, and 0.07, respectively. Similarly, the odds ratios of a fatal in-hospital stroke for patients in these groups (again relative to the group of patients on neither of these two medications) are 0.39, 0.61, and 0.06, respectively. For either the relative risks or odds ratios, departures from 1 suggest an association in the contingency table.

Two or More Outcomes for the Same Patient

So far, we have limited our discussion to the association between two binary variables in which one group of patients is observed under one condition (such as a treatment) and another group of patients is observed under another condition (such as a control group). Often, categorical responses are observed under two different conditions on the same individual (e.g., at two times or after two different treatments), and interest is in estimating the association between response and this condition. The generic table displayed as Table 7 looks much like Table 4, but its implications are quite different. We are no longer interested in whether $a/(a+c)$ differs from $b/(b+d)$ or whether a/c differs from b/d, but rather in whether the response rate under condition 2, $(a+c)/N$, differs from the response rate under condition 1, $(a+b)/N$; this is equivalent to asking whether c differs from b. Further, the risk of response in condition 2 relative to that in condition 1 can be estimated as $(a+c)/(a+b)$.

Regamey et al.[7] studied transmission of human herpesvirus 8 (HHV-8) from renal-transplant donors to recipients. They analyzed serum samples from 220 renal-transplant recipients for the presence of antibodies to HHV-8 on the day of transplantation and one year later. In Table 8 the proportion of patients who

Table 7. Schematic for Paired Dichotomous Responses (+/−) under Two Conditions.

Condition 1	Condition 2		
	+	−	Total
+	a	b	$a + b$
−	c	d	$c + d$
Total	$a + c$	$b + d$	$N (= a + b + c + d)$

tested positive for HHV-8 antibodies on the day of transplantation is 14/220 = 0.064, and the proportion who tested positive one year after transplantation is 39/220 = 0.177. The relative risk of HHV-8 reactivity (one year later relative to at day of transplantation) can be estimated as 39/14 = 2.78. It is noteworthy that 25 patients switched from negative to positive, but none switched in the other direction. Unless other critical variables have also changed, this is strong evidence that the conversion is related to transplantation. Another important quantity is the proportion of patients who are positive for HHV-8 antibodies one year after transplantation among patients who are negative on the day of transplantation (i.e., the rate of seroconversion after transplantation), which is 25/206 = 0.121.

Table 8. Presence of Antibodies to HHV-8 in Serum of Renal-Transplant Recipients on Day of Transplantation and after One Year.

Presence or absence of antibodies on day of transplantation	Presence or absence of antibodies one year after transplantation		
	+	−	Total
+	14	0	14
−	25	181	206
Total	39	181	220

Regamey et al.[7]

The example in Table 8 involves paired binary data in which each individual is measured at each of two times; the primary object of study is not the patient (as in Tables 1, 3, 5, and 6) but the *pair* of observations for each patient. Another common application is the matched case-control study, in which each case is matched with a control on important variables such as age and sex (not illustrated here).

Estimates of measures of association for contingency tables are based on samples and hence involve uncertainty. Often, 95% confidence intervals are used to express that uncertainty. Most authors report confidence intervals calculated by software packages, and articles often mention the methods used.

Technical details of most methods are discussed in many textbooks, including Chapter 6 in Fleiss et al.[5] The next section discusses testing for the presence of an association in contingency tables.

TESTING FOR AN ASSOCIATION

The RR and OR are measures of association. When the probabilities of an event are equal in the treated group and the control group, the risk ratio and the odds ratio in the population are both 1, and the risk difference is 0. However, we observe only a sample from the population; the population proportions are unknown. The RR and OR for the sample are subject to some degree of random variability, and we may need to know what population values are compatible with the data. Most often, interest focuses on whether the population RR or OR could reasonably equal 1. In the generic 2×2 table of Table 4, the main question is whether the population proportions are equal (i.e., $P_t = P_c$), which is equivalent to testing whether the odds ratio or the relative risk in the population is equal to 1 (or whether the risk difference is 0).

In a sense, however, this question is artificial. In practice the two population proportions are unlikely to be exactly equal (and hence the corresponding "null hypothesis" is known to be false, without any testing). The assumption of equality provides a basis for estimating the range of values of the RR or OR that are reasonably consistent with the data, as shown by confidence bounds or the statistical significance of the departure.

For 2×2 tables several approaches have been developed for assessing departures and their significance. One common approach works directly with the probabilities of the tables that could have arisen in the sample. Another approach uses a form of distance between the actual table and a hypothetical table corresponding to $P_t = P_c$.

Fisher's Exact Test

If in Table 4 one takes as given the total number of subjects (N), the number in the treatment group (s_1), and the total number of events (r_1), the numbers in the four cells still generally have freedom to vary. Then each of the possible tables corresponds to a particular number of events in the treatment group (because the margins contain enough information to determine the numbers in the other three cells). For example, Table 3 has $N = 207$, $s_1 = 105$, and $r_1 = 116$; if $a = 55$ (instead of the actual 51), then the other three entries must be $b = 61$, $c = 50$, and $d = 41$. When N, s_1, and r_1 have these values, a could take on any value from 14 to 105; each such value of a fixes the values of the other cells in the body of the table. One could in concept calculate the probability of observing each value of a if treatment and outcome are independent. The procedure known as *Fisher's exact test* does just this—it determines the probability of each of those tables (or, equivalently, the probability of each possible number of events in the treatment group) if the two descriptors (treatment and outcome) are statistically independent. The p-value for testing whether $P_t = P_c$ can be calculated as the sum of the probabilities of numbers of events in the treatment group that are at least as extreme as the actual number. In context it is usually clear which values of a are "at least as extreme" as the actual one. In Table 3, for example, the aim of the treatment is to prevent death or chronic lung disease, and so the more-extreme values of a are those less than 51. Such a p-value is one-sided, because "more-extreme" naturally describes departures in only one direction. Several ways have been devised for obtaining a two-sided p-value, and they can give different results. One approach adds up the probabilities of tables that have probability no greater than the observed table.

For the nitric oxide clinical trial data presented in Table 3, the estimated relative risk and odds ratio are 0.76 and 0.54, respectively. Are these estimates compatible with population values of the RR or OR equal to 1 (and therefore also compatible with equality of the two population proportions)? The two-sided p-value from Fisher's exact test is 0.03, suggesting that we would observe cell counts at least as extreme as we actually observed in fewer than 3% of occasions, if the two population proportions were equal. This result provides evidence that the two population proportions are probably not equal.

The nitric oxide clinical trial illustrates the use of Fisher's exact test when one of the two variables is a "circumstance" such as treatment group and the other is a response. In this situation testing equality of the two population proportions P_t and P_c makes sense, because the number of patients in each treatment group is taken as fixed. Fisher's exact test is also appropriate when one is testing for an association between two outcome variables such as in Table 5. For this situation, we are testing whether the two outcome variables are statistically independent (that is, knowing the value of one variable provides no information for predicting the value of the other). Independence corresponds also to the RR or OR being equal to l.

A substantial percentage of the articles in volume 349 of the *New England Journal of Medicine* (25 of 62) use Fisher's exact test for the analysis of either a primary or secondary objective of the study. Originally, Fisher's exact test was applied only to tables whose N was quite small, for which statistical tables were available, because of the effort required to compute p-values. More recently, statisticians have developed ways to streamline the calculations and thus largely remove the restriction on the total count. They have also extended the procedure to tables with more than two rows and columns (Agresti,[8] Section 3.5.8).

Chi-Squared Test

A second, simpler, approach also works with the observed totals in the margins of the 2×2 table (r_1, r_2, s_1, s_2, and N in Table 4), from which one can calculate the counts in the four cells that one would expect if P_t were equal to P_c. Then, for example, the combined event rate is estimated as r_1/N, and the expected number of events in the treated group is $s_1(r_1/N)$ (not necessarily an integer). Table 9 shows the results of this calculation for the data in Table 3. The (Pearson) chi-squared statistic (X^2) uses the difference between the observed count and the expected count in each cell (in this example, 51 observed and 58.8 expected events in the treated group) to determine the probability of observing this value of a or a more extreme value if treatment and outcome are statistically independent.

When $P_t = P_c$ (RR = 1 or OR = 1) and N is large, the distribution of X^2 is well approximated by a member of the chi-squared family (χ^2) of theoretical distributions—specifically the "chi-squared distribution on 1 degree of freedom." (The success of the approximation also requires that the expected count not be too small in any cell.) When all four counts in the table are moderately large, the probabilities from Fisher's exact test (two-tailed) and the chi-squared test are close together. The 1 degree of freedom corresponds to the fact that, when the row and column totals are fixed, a single cell count in the table determines the rest of the 2×2 table. A large value of X^2 relative to the chi-squared distribution provides evidence that the two population proportions are not equal, but does not say anything about the direction of the difference (i.e., this test is two-sided). For Table 9, $X^2 = 4.82$, and the p-value from the chi-squared distribution with one degree of freedom is 0.03.

Table 9. Expected Counts in Table 3 under the Hypothesis of the Two Population Proportions Being Equal (i.e., No Association between Treatment and Response).

Outcome	Inhaled Nitric Oxide	Placebo	Total
Death or chronic lung disease	(116/207) × 105 = 58.8	(116/207) × 102 = 57.2	116
Other	(91/207) × 105 = 46.2	(91/207) × 102 = 44.8	91
Totals	105	102	207

Paired Data (McNemar's Test)

For paired data, as in Table 7, testing for association is equivalent to testing whether the RR is equal to 1, which occurs when the probability of response is the same for the two conditions. The response rates are $(a+b)/N$ under condition 1 and $(a+c)/N$ under condition 2, and the customary statistical test is based on the difference,

$$\frac{a + b}{N} - \frac{a + c}{N} = \frac{b - c}{N}.$$

Because of the pairing, the usual chi-squared test for a 2×2 table and Fisher's exact test are not appropriate. Indeed, the number of subjects in the ++ cell, a, does not contribute to the difference between the rates (except by being part of N). The appropriate test is known as *McNemar's test*, and is available in most statistical software packages. An exact test, based on the binomial distribution, is also possible and is especially useful when $b + c$ is small.

For the data in Table 8 Regamey et al.[7] used McNemar's test to assess whether the relative risk differs from 1. With 25 patients going from negative to positive and none going the other way, the p-value was very small ($p < 0.001$), and the authors concluded that the probability of testing positive for HHV-8 antibodies was substantially higher one year after transplantation than on the day of transplantation.

Larger Contingency Tables

An attractive feature of the chi-squared test is that it easily generalizes to variables with more than two categories and to tables with more than two variables. For example, one can test for an association between two variables with R and C categories (i.e., a contingency table with R rows and C columns). Under the assumption of no association between the two categorical variables, X^2 will have a chi-squared distribution with $(R - 1)(C - 1)$ degrees of freedom. Appropriate computing programs are in many statistical computer packages.

For the 5×4 table of severity of stroke by anticoagulation medication status in Table 1, the test statistic X^2 was 25.4. Compared against the chi-squared distribution with $4 \times 3 = 12$ degrees of freedom, it has a p-value of 0.01, which suggests an association between the two variables.

In contingency tables larger than 2×2 the categories of the row variable or the column variable or both may have an ordering, as severity of stroke does in Table 1. The chi-squared test ignores information by not taking the ordering(s) into account. The choice of method depends on whether the number of rows and the number of columns are both greater than 2 and on whether both variables are ordered. Chapter 13 discusses methods that are appropriate when one variable is ordered and the other has two categories.

SAMPLE SIZE AND POWER FOR
TESTING ASSOCIATION

Ten of the 62 original articles in volume 349 of the *New England Journal of Medicine* had sample size calculations for a 2×2 table. Computing formulas are available in many statistical books and software packages. All of these studies were clinical trials in which the primary analysis was a comparison of proportions between two treatment groups. Sample size calculations always recognize a trade-off between power and significance level. Thus, if an investigator wants to increase power (with fixed sample size), the significance level must be higher (i.e., less stringent). More broadly, required sample size increases as the power increases, the significance level decreases, or the minimal detectable risk difference decreases. The optimal trade-off requires expert judgment and, often, professional help from a statistician.

Schreiber et al.[3] present sample size calculations for the nitric oxide clinical trial (Table 3). The authors assumed an incidence of chronic lung disease or death of 60% for the placebo group and chose to look for a reduction to 40% or lower for the inhaled nitric oxide group. For a chi-squared test of the treatment effect at the 5% level of significance, the sample size per group required for at least 80% power is 94. Thus, approximately 95 patients were required in each group, or 190 patients in all. This was close to the targeted sample size of 207 accrued to this study.

COLLAPSING TABLES: SIMPSON'S PARADOX

Most contingency tables in *New England Journal of Medicine* and other medical journals present the frequency of one categorical variable by another. However, a study may involve three or more relevant variables (e.g., treatment group, outcome, and treatment center, if the outcome may depend on, say, the average severity of disease at each center). Data for the centers could be added together to create a two-dimensional table (treatment and outcome), but this may result in misleading inferences. Table 10 presents a hypothetical example of the relationship between treatment and response in two centers. Each center shows some evidence of a treatment effect. The odds ratio measuring the association between treatment and response is $(1600 \times 600)/(1000 \times 800) = 1.2$ for Center 1 and $(2400 \times 600)/(3000 \times 400) = 1.2$ for Center 2. Further, the risk difference is 0.05 in Center 1 and 0.04 in Center 2. Table 11 shows the 2×2 table resulting from combining the two centers (i.e., collapsing across treatment center). Interestingly, the odds ratio for the collapsed 2×2 table is $(4000 \times 1200)/(4000 \times 1200) = 1$, indicating no association between treatment and response. This behavior illustrates a statistical phenomenon known as Simpson's Paradox, whereby associations between two categorical variables can be eliminated, created, or even reversed by collapsing over a third variable.

For this hypothetical trial, the associations between center and treatment and between center and response and treatment are given in Table 12. In short, the combined table fails to show the benefit of treatment because Center 2 has

Table 10. A Hypothetical Example of Simpson's Paradox.

	Center 1		Center 2	
	Treatment (%)	Control (%)	Treatment (%)	Control (%)
Success	1600 (62)	800 (57)	2400 (44)	400 (40)
Failure	1000 (38)	600 (43)	3000 (56)	600 (60)

Table 11. Simpson's Paradox Realized: Centers Combined.

	Treatment	Control
Success	4000	1200
Failure	4000	1200

Table 12. Simpson's Paradox Explained.

	Center 1	Center 2
Treatment	2600	5400
Control	1400	1000

	Center 1	Center 2
Success	2400	2800
Failure	1600	3600

both poorer results and a higher proportion of treated patients than Center 1. The odds ratio relating center and response is 1.9, whereas the odds ratio relating center and treatment group is 0.34. Thus, the collapsed table is misleading because Center 2, where results were less favorable in both treated patients and controls, contributed a higher proportion of treated patients than Center 1. This imbalance dragged down the success rate in the combined treated group more than in the control group, so that treatment no longer seemed to be effective.

This example demonstrates the dangers of ignoring variables that affect the relationship between categorical variables of interest. (It uses contingency tables, but analogs exist for other kinds of data.) When examining the association between two categorical variables, one should generally explore the mediating effects of additional factors before presenting a two-variable contingency table.

Volume 349 of the *Journal* contains no contingency tables of more than two variables, because many *Journal* papers report the results of randomized clinical trials. Simpson's Paradox is unlikely to appear when a variable is assigned at random, because serious imbalance in the ratio of treated to control subjects is unlikely. Thus, misleading inferences about treatment are not likely to be created in RCT data by collapsing over other variables. Inferences for effects other than (randomized) treatment must still be analyzed cautiously. Randomization that is stratified and blocked (that is, forced to produce nearly equal numbers per treatment within each stratum) ensures that there is little association between treatment assignment and the stratification factors, and guarantees that misleading results will be avoided when collapsing over these factors. This is one of the reasons why the randomization in large clinical trials is often stratified by center and gender.

SIMPLE STRATIFIED ANALYSES

We have shown how collapsing over important factors can lead the analyst astray (Simpson's Paradox). Interest often focuses on obtaining an overall estimate of the association between two binary variables by stratifying by one or more other variables. These methods assume that the underlying association between the two variables is the same in each of the strata, and aim at getting a more-stable estimate of this common (underlying) association. Various measures of association such as relative risks and risk differences can be combined in this way, but the customary methods estimate a common odds ratio. The Mantel-Haenszel estimate[9] has some advantages. This analysis estimates the odds ratio as a weighted average of the odds ratios within the strata, giving more weight to strata with larger sample sizes (and hence smaller variances). The Mantel-Haenszel estimate requires the strong assumption that each stratum has the same odds ratio; but if it is (approximately) true, it allows pooling of many small strata, no one of which may be large enough to support some conclusion. Before using this method, it is a good idea to check whether the data are compatible with this assumption, and tests for homogeneity are available in many statistical software packages. Analyses usually include confidence intervals for the estimated common odds ratio and the Mantel-Haenszel test of whether the true common odds ratio is consistent with 1.

Many Original Articles in volume 349 of the *Journal* use the Mantel-Haenszel estimate and test. For example, Moses et al.[10] presented the results of a clinical trial comparing sirolimus-eluting stents versus standard stents in patients with stenosis in a native coronary artery. The article reports that the rate of failure of the target vessel was reduced from 21% with a standard stent to 8.6% with a sirolimus-eluting stent. Although the Mantel-Haenszel estimate was not presented in the article, a Mantel-Haenszel test was used to demonstrate a highly statistically significant association between type of stent and failure, stratified by study center ($p < 0.001$). Randomization was stratified by center, so there should not be an association between type of stent and center, and one can arrive at a valid estimate of the common odds ratio by collapsing over center.

REGRESSION METHODS FOR CATEGORICAL DATA

As discussed in Chapter 10, regression may be used to examine the effects of one or several factors or covariates on a continuous outcome variable. Categorical outcome variables have their own body of regression methods, with many similarities to ordinary regression as well as some special features. Unified treatments often include them among "generalized linear models." More-readily available software has led to increasing applications in the medical literature. The most common method is logistic regression, which allows investigators to examine the relation between a dichotomous response variable and a number of continuous or categorical predictors or covariates.

In mathematical notation $x_1, x_2, \ldots, x_k$ are values of a set of k covariates, and $P(x_1, x_2, \ldots, x_k)$ is the probability of a positive response when the covariates have the specific values $x_1, x_2, \ldots, x_k$. Logistic regression relates the logarithm of the odds of a positive response to a linear function of the covariates:

$$\log_e \left[\frac{P(x_1, x_2, \ldots, x_k)}{1 - P(x_1, x_2, \ldots, x_k)} \right] = \alpha + \beta_1 x_1 + \beta_2 x_2 + \cdots + \beta_k x_k.$$

The covariates can be either categorical variables such as gender or continuous variables such as age. The log-odds, $\log_e(P/(1 - P))$, known as the *logit transformation*, is widely used and has many useful features, chief of which is that it holds, at least approximately, for many kinds of medical and biologic data.

Figure 1 shows the relation between a single continuous covariate (x) and the probability of response when the probability is logistic with $\alpha = 0$ and $\beta = 1$. The relation is symmetric, in the sense that the logit of $1 - P$ is the negative of the logit of P. Also, the change in x corresponding to a given change in P is larger when P is near 0 or 1 than when P is near 0.5. Conversely, the change in P corresponding to a given change in x is largest toward the center of the curve.

When the logistic regression involves only one predictor, x_1, the coefficient β_1 can be interpreted directly as the log-odds ratio when the predictor is an indicator variable (i.e., its values are 0 or 1) or as an increase in the log-odds per unit change for a continuous variable. When additional predictors are present, each β; is interpreted as a log-odds ratio, adjusted for the contributions of these other variables (in the data at hand).

In the study of allergic reactions after use of a sulfonamide nonantibiotic (Table 5) Strom et al.[4] found a strong association between prior hypersensitivity after antibiotics and allergic reaction within 30 days after receipt of a sulfonamide nonantibiotic; the odds ratio was estimated to be 6.6, and the relative risk was estimated to be 6.1. Although these results demonstrate a strong

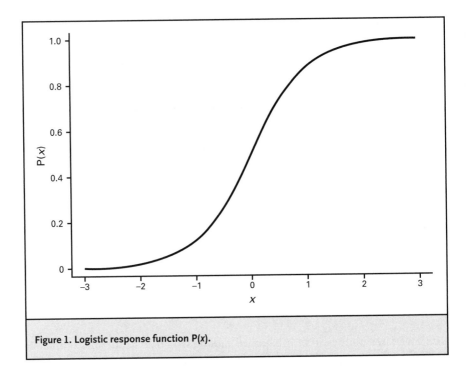

Figure 1. Logistic response function P(x).

association, they might reflect contributions from confounding factors such as sex, age at outcome, and a history of asthma. Strom et al. used logistic regression to adjust for differences in age at outcome, gender, history of asthma, use of drugs for asthma, and use of corticosteroids. The adjusted odds ratio was 2.8. Although still significantly different from 1 (the 95% confidence interval did not overlap 1), this was substantially lower than the unadjusted odds ratio of 6.6. Thus, the covariates accounted for some, but not all, of the association between prior hypersensitivity and allergic reaction within 30 days. As discussed earlier for unadjusted analyses, the adjusted odds ratio can be used as an estimate of the adjusted relative risk when the response is rare. Strom et al. interpreted these adjusted odds ratios as adjusted relative risk estimates, which was reasonable given the rarity of the response.

Logistic regression is often used to develop predictive models for a binary event. Brennan et al.[11] discuss the prognostic value of myeloperoxidase, a biomarker for inflammation, as a prognostic marker of acute coronary syndromes in patients with chest pain. The authors used logistic regression to estimate the prognostic value of this marker. They categorized the level of myeloperoxidase at baseline according to whether the patient was in the first, second, third, or fourth quartile of the population. The odds ratios of a major cardiac event within 30 days, relative to the lowest quartile, were estimated to be 1.7, 3.2, and 4.7 for the second, third, and fourth quartile of baseline myeloperoxidase level, respectively. These estimates were almost unchanged when they were adjusted for multiple demographic factors including C-reactive protein level, sex, and age.

Researchers commonly evaluate the logistic model on the same data set they used to fit that model. Such an approach provides an overly optimistic assessment of the model's predictive ability. Various strategies can avoid this bias. One approach splits the data at random into a "training set" and a "test set," fits the logistic regression model to the training set data, and evaluates the resulting model on the test set data. Another approach for unbiased assessment of predictive accuracy is leave-one-out cross-validation, usually based on splitting the data into 10 to 20 subsets, leaving out each subset in turn when fitting the model, and applying each of these models to the corresponding "left-out" observations. Neither of these approaches was reported for the myeloperoxidase study, so its assessments of predictive ability may be overly optimistic.

Logistic regression is a very useful tool in the analysis of data from case-control studies because investigators can estimate adjusted odds ratios. A case-control study of BRCA1 or BRCA2 mutations and the risk of ovarian cancer provides an illustrative example.[6] Table 6 shows the relationship between BRCA1/BRCA2 mutation and the risk of ovarian cancer. Particularly for a case-control study, cases may differ from controls on many factors, which could introduce a spurious relationship or hide a real one. To avoid this potential problem, the investigators used logistic regression analysis in the BRCA1/BRCA2 case-control study to adjust for age, ethnic background, history of breast or ovarian cancer, and a history of gynecologic surgery. The adjusted odds ratio, which approximates the adjusted relative risk, was 24.0, close to the unadjusted odds ratio (or relative risk) of 23.2 presented earlier. Thus, there was no evidence that the other factors influenced the relationship between BRCA1/BRCA2 mutation and the risk of breast cancer.

Overall, the wide availability of statistical software with sophisticated methods for the analysis of categorical data has led to more-elaborate models and more-sensitive analyses than in decades past, but both readers and authors need to know about the potential problems.

REFERENCES

1. Hylek EM, Go AS, Chang Y, et al. Effect of intensity of oral anticoagulation on stroke severity and mortality in atrial fibrillation. N Engl J Med 2003; 349:1019–26.

2. Fudala PJ, Bridge PT, Herbert S, et al. Office-based treatment of opiate addiction with sublingual-tablet formulation of buprenorphine and naloxone. N Engl J Med 2003; 349:949–58.

3. Schreiber MD, Gin-Mestan K, Marks JD, et al. Inhaled nitric oxide in premature infants with the respiratory distress syndrome. N Engl J Med 2003; 349:2099–107.

4. Strom BL, Schinnar R, Apter AJ, et al. Absence of cross-reactivity between sulfonamide antibiotics and sulfonamide nonantibiotics. N Engl J Med 2003; 349:1628–35.

5. Fleiss JL, Levin B, Paik MC. Statistical methods for rates and proportions. 3rd ed. Hoboken, New Jersey: John Wiley, 2003.

6. Modan B, Hartge P, Hirsh-Yechezkel G, et al. Parity, oral contraceptives, and the risk of ovarian cancer among carriers and noncarriers of a BRCA1 or BRCA2 mutation. N Eng J Med 2001; 345:235–40.

7. Regamey N, Tamm M, Wernli M, et al. Transmission of human herpesvirus 8 infection from renal-transplant donors to recipients. N Engl J Med 1998; 339:1358–63.

8. Agresti A. Categorical data analysis. 2nd ed. New York: John Wiley, 2002.

9. Mantel N, Haenszel W. Statistical aspects of the analysis of data from retrospective studies of disease. J Natl Cancer Inst 1959; 22:719–48.

10. Moses JW, Leon MB, Popma JJ, et al. Sirolimus-eluting stents versus standard stents in patients with stenosis in a native coronary artery. N Eng J Med 2003; 349:1315–23.

11. Brennan ML, Penn MS, Van Lente F, et al. Prognostic value of myeloperoxidase in patients with chest pain. N Engl J Med 2003; 349:1595–604.

Analyzing Data from Ordered Categories

LINCOLN E. MOSES, PH.D., JOHN D. EMERSON, PH.D.,

AND HOSSEIN HOSSEINI, PH.D.

Revised by the editors

ABSTRACT   Clinical investigations often involve data in the form of ordered categories—e.g., "worse," "unchanged," "improved," "much improved." Comparison of two groups when the data are of this kind should not be done by the chi-squared test, which wastes information and is insensitive in this context. The Wilcoxon–Mann–Whitney test provides a proper analysis. Alternatively, scores may be assigned to the categories in order, and the *t*-test applied. We demonstrate both approaches here.

Sometimes data in ordered categories are reduced to a 2×2 table by collapsing the high categories into one category and the low categories into another. This practice is inefficient; moreover, it entails avoidable subjectivity in the choice of the cutting point that defines the two super-categories. The Wilcoxon–Mann–Whitney procedure (or the *t*-test with use of ordered scores) is preferable.

The clinical investigator must at times rely on quantitative information that is intrinsically imprecise. The clinical response (worse, unchanged, improved) is such a variable; the response can be qualitatively ordered, but it often cannot be expressed on a precise numerical scale. Input variables of the same sort arise, too; stage of disease (I, II, III, IV) is an example. Effective ways to analyze such information are gaining in use. Sometimes inefficient methods of analysis are applied; this is equivalent to ignoring part of the data. This chapter points out ways to go wrong, but its primary emphasis is on methods that use such information efficiently, particularly for comparing two groups of observations expressed in an ordered classification. A randomized controlled clinical trial comparing two combination drug treatments for advanced Hodgkin's disease offers an illustration. If the response is three levels of tumor remission (complete, partial, none), then the methods described here are well suited to the analysis of the 2×3 table of counts.

The central feature of a set of ordered categories is that they express in increasing or decreasing order the extent or the degree of intensity or complexity of some observable phenomenon. Each class used has a definite place in the order of the set of classes; if numbers are used, as on a four-point scale, they exhibit the order, but it may not be obvious just how they are to be interpreted numerically. Pain scored at 4+ is more severe than that scored at 2+, but is it twice as severe?

Inappropriate analysis of such data (for example, reducing them to a two-point scale indicating presence or absence) can sacrifice much of the information in the data—information that has been obtained with considerable effort and expense, and perhaps patients' cooperation. Often, ordered categories are the best available way to capture important information, such as the stage of disease or the severity of symptoms. Efficient statistical methods for analyzing such data have considerable value.

Some medically important categorical variables are not ordered; ABO blood types are an example. Chapter 12 of this book[1] considers the analysis of unordered categorical variables. This chapter does not deal with the analysis of such data, but with problems in which the categories have a natural ordering. We assume also that over the range of data under consideration, "more" is either always better than "less," or always worse. This condition generally applies to variables such as degree of recovery, remission, or level of physical functioning. But there are some variables, such as levels of arousal (described by such terms as torpid, normal, and hyperactive) or trust in strangers (from too trusting to overly suspicious), that are optimal at intermediate values and for which "more" is not always better (or always worse) than "less." The methods described in this chapter may not be suitable for analyzing such data. This chapter also does not address the analysis of tables in which the entries are measurements.

A SUITABLE METHOD OF ANALYSIS

The Wilcoxon or Mann–Whitney test is appropriate for comparing two sets of results that are combined and then scored in terms of an ordered classification.[2] In 1945 Wilcoxon[3] reported a method for comparing two samples, taking account of only the relative order of the observations. He merged the two samples into a single rank order from smallest to largest and devised a test that compared the average ranks of the two samples in that ordering. He made use of the fact that large observations produce larger ranks, so that if one of the treatments tends to produce larger observations than the other, its average rank will be large. Thus, comparison of the average ranks in the two samples could replace comparison of the average values, as in the ordinary t-test. In addition to its uses described in this book, the Wilcoxon test is well suited to comparing two sets of precisely ordered measurements; it gives a nonparametric analysis that parallels the two-sample t-test.

Soon after Wilcoxon's method appeared, Mann and Whitney[4] devised the "U-test," a different version of Wilcoxon's test. The two forms are exactly equivalent; sometimes one is more convenient to use, and sometimes the other is. The computations for the two forms of the test are different, and lead to consulting different tables, although a knowledgeable person can easily deduce one table from the other. The Mann–Whitney form of the test compares each individual in the first group with each individual in the second group, recording how many times this comparison favors the individual from the second group. This chapter uses the Mann–Whitney form of the calculations because of their greater convenience for the $2 \times k$ table.

Kirkpatrick and Alling[5] applied the Mann–Whitney test in a clever way to assess the results of a randomized clinical trial dealing with the treatment of chronic oral candidiasis. Every subject was scored for his or her treatment response two to seven days after treatment was completed, as shown in Table 1. This scoring scheme captures two kinds of outcomes and combines them in such a way that the larger of any two scores connotes the poorer outcome; these scores define an ordered classification. (If any of the subjects in the study had had no improvement but negative laboratory tests, or an absence of clinical findings but positive laboratory tests, it would not have been obvious how to put their results into an ordered classification; but since only the four outcomes shown did occur, the investigators were able to use this ordered classification to analyze their data.) The authors presented the data reproduced in Table 2.

Table 1. Scoring System for Outcomes of Treatment for Chronic Oral Candidiasis.*

Clinical Findings	Laboratory Findings	Score
Absent	Negative	1
Improved	Negative	2
Improved	Positive	3
Unimproved	Positive	4

*From Kirkpatrick and Alling.[5]

Visual inspection of the tables suggests that the treatment led to predominantly smaller scores—i.e., to more-favorable outcomes. The Mann–Whitney test offers strong statistical support for this observation.

In the example, each of the 10 patients receiving treatment is compared with each of the 10 control patients, for a total of 100 comparisons. (If the sample sizes had been 15 and 20, there would have been $15 \times 20 = 300$ comparisons.) If the two treatments were equivalent in their effects, about half of such pairwise comparisons should favor the control group, and half the treatment group.

In the instance before us, the outcome is far from being half and half, as we shall see by doing the counting. Some pairs favor the placebo, some the treatment, and in some the two are tied; the frequencies of these three situations must add up to 100, the total number of pairs. The data provide six pairs in which a subject from the treatment group is tied with a subject from the placebo group; these six pairs are the ones comprising the placebo-group subject who was scored 1 and each of the six treatment-group subjects who also were scored 1 (if two placebo-group subjects had been scored 1, we would have had $2 \times 6 = 12$ ties from the pairings of the 1s). The data in the example provide four pairs in which the subject from the placebo group has a better (lower) score than the subject from the treatment group; these are the pairs involving the placebo-group subject who was scored 1, the three treatment-group subjects who were scored 2, and the one treatment-group subject who was scored 3. We have found six tied pairs and four pairs favoring the placebo; the remaining 90 ($= 100 - 6 - 4$) pairs must favor the treatment. This is readily confirmed: All 10 subjects who received treatment have scores of less than 4, and when each of those 10 is paired with each of the 9 placebo-group subjects who were scored 4, we have 90 pairs in which the treatment-group subject has the better score.

Table 2. Outcomes after Two to Seven Days of Treatment in 20 Patients with Chronic Oral Candidiasis.*

Treatment	Outcome Category				
	1	2	3	4	Total
Clotrimazole	6	3	1	0	10
Placebo	1	0	0	9	10

*Data from Kirkpatrick and Alling.[5] Data in columns represent the number of participants in each outcome category.

To summarize the results of this counting, in 90 pairs the treatment was better, and in 6 it was tied with the placebo; we credit half the ties to the treatment, as if it had been superior, and the other half to the placebo. Our summary statistic is then $90 + 3 = 93$. This statistic was named U by Mann and Whitney.[4] In general, U is calculated as we have done, by counting the pairs favoring one of the groups and adding half the tied pairs.

The calculated value of U allows us to do two useful things. First, we can construct an informative descriptive statistic, as follows: divide U by the total number of pairs—100 in our example. This ratio is the proportion of pairs favoring the treatment, and for the data in Table 2 we get $93/100 = 0.93$. The ratio estimates the probability that a subject chosen at random (from a group like those used in this randomized trial) and given the treatment will have a better outcome than will a subject similarly chosen and given the placebo. This index offers a numerical estimate in answer to the question "For this population, what is the probability of a better response to treatment than to placebo?" (In this question, we must understand that the "better" of two tied observations is to be determined by the flip of a coin.) The ratio cannot address the question "How much better?" This question may not even make sense when the scale is ordinal.

In a second use of U, we can assess statistical significance. In these data a value of about 50 would be expected for U if the placebo and treatment were equivalent in effect. Is the observed value of 93 convincingly different from 50? Computer programs[6, 7] allow us to answer the question. The exact two-sided significance level is 0.00041, and we conclude with a high degree of confidence that the treatment, clotrimazole, is superior to the placebo in producing more-favorable outcomes.

If the two sample sizes, m and n, are both large, the value of U is computed as we have done. The descriptive interpretation of U/mn continues to hold, but significance can be assessed without recourse to special computer programs, by the use of a normal approximation. With equivalent treatments, U is nearly normally distributed, with a mean of $mn/2$ (50 in this example) and with a standard deviation that is calculated approximately by

$$\sigma = \sqrt{mn(m + n + 1)/12}$$

(13.23 for this example). When some of the ranks are tied, as in this example, the approximation can be improved by multiplying σ by a *correction factor for ties* (0.930 for the example); we refer to Armitage et al.[2] for the algebraic details of the correction. We then express U as a departure from its mean ($mn/2$), measured in units of the corrected standard deviation (σ_U), obtaining

$$z = \frac{U - mn/2}{\sigma_U} = \frac{93 - 50}{(13.23)(0.930)} = 3.50.$$

From tables of the normal distribution we find that 3.50 corresponds to a two-sided significance level of 0.0005. Again, we conclude with a high degree of confidence that clotrimazole is superior to the placebo.

Considerable numerical investigation of the normal approximation shows that a clear indication of significance or nonsignificance can be relied on, provided that each sample comprises at least 10 observations and that no one category contains more than half the combined set of observations. If the normal approximation gives a result near the threshold of significance, it is wise to compute the exact p-value with an appropriate computer program. Emerson and Moses[8] give further recommendations on the use of exact methods for carrying out calculations for Mann–Whitney.

APPROXIMATE METHODS OF ANALYSIS

An alternative way to analyze data comparing two samples scored in ordered categories is to assign ordered numerical values to those categories and then compute the two sample averages, comparing them by means of the two-sample t-test. This procedure has advantages and drawbacks. We include it for completeness, but available software for applying the Mann–Whitney test with exact significance levels has made it obsolete. The main advantage is the familiarity of the t-test, although computing it from data presented in the format of Table 2 may seem strange at first. A clear example is given in Snedecor and Cochran.[9] The primary drawback is that the choice of numerical values for the ordered categories has an essential arbitrariness, so that different analyses of a set of ordered data may generate different p-values and thus lead to different conclusions.

This drawback is mitigated by two considerations, however. First, in any particular data set, the Mann–Whitney test can be shown necessarily to yield essentially the same result as that obtained from the t-test when some set of ordered scores (chosen for that data set) is used. Second, t-tests using different sets of ordered scores for a given data set ordinarily produce similar results.[9] From these two principles it follows that the t-test will serve as an approximation of the Mann–Whitney test.

To illustrate how the choice of scores may have very little effect (so long as the order is not disturbed), let us again consider the data presented in Table 2. If the results are analyzed by computing the t-statistic with numerical scores (1, 2, 3, and 4 or 1, 2, 8, and 9) for the four outcome categories, then the results are as follows: $t = 5.88$ with a p-value of 0.000014, and $t = 5.89$ with a p-value of 0.000014, respectively. The agreement is close. Both these values of t (with 18 degrees of freedom) give two-sided p-values that are considerably smaller than the exact value, 0.00041. Two points are illustrated rather sharply: changing the scores had little effect, and the evaluation of significance is qualitatively in accord with that of the Mann–Whitney result (clotrimazole being judged definitely better than the placebo), but the numerical agreement is not exact.

A second and inferior approximate method of treating such ordered data is to collapse the set of categories into only two. The imposition of such a coarse dichotomy on data that are intrinsically more fine-grained gives an appearance of simplicity but nearly always at a cost in information; the cost can be great, though it is not always so.

With the data in Table 2 we could reduce the ordered categories to a dichotomy without violating the order, by dividing them into two groups at the boundary between 1 and 2, between 2 and 3, or between 3 and 4. These three approaches yield the reduced data shown in Table 3.

Not only does collapsing the table waste data; it also forces us to be arbitrary in choosing where to divide the ordered categories. We can, as before, compute U/mn and estimate the probability that treatment will be better than placebo. Its values for A, B, and C in Table 3 are 0.75, 0.90, and 0.95, respectively. This kind of variation suggests a danger of imposing a dichotomy—that the choice of where to divide the categories may reflect the investigator's wish to maximize (or minimize) the appearance of difference between the two samples. To some extent, this same danger may be feared in the assignment of scores to the ordered categories, but the danger is greater in the case of dichotomization because that is an extreme instance of assigning scores. Imposing a dichotomy is equivalent to defining all the scores for categories on either side of the cutting point as being equal to each other. The Mann–Whitney approach has the property of using exactly the information about order—and nothing else—in the analysis.

Table 3. The Three Possible Dichotomized Versions of the Data in Table 2.

	A		B		C	
Treatment	1	2–4	1, 2	3, 4	1–3	4
Clotrimazole	6	4	9	1	10	0
Placebo	1	9	1	9	1	9

In summary, we have discussed two kinds of approximate analysis. One, the use of the t-statistic, is usually not objectionable; the other, collapsing the categories into a dichotomy, has important drawbacks.

At this point it is worth reviewing the advantages of the U statistic. First, it is applicable to very small samples (e.g., $m = 3$, $n = 5$), to which we would apply the t-test at our peril. Second, it yields a descriptive statistic that is much more valuable than is widely known; that statistic, U/mn, does not depend on the units of measurement. (Indeed, we have applied it where there are no units of measurement, only an underlying order.) The value of U/mn is interpretable directly in terms of the probability that one treatment will be more effective than the other in individual application to subjects of the kind used in the study furnishing the data. Third, the computation of U/mn is simple, once the data are arranged in order. Many standard computer packages include the Mann–Whitney test and report a p-value, suitable when m and n are not small, that is based on the normal approximation. However, advances in computing and in algorithms for implementing exact statistical methods now make the exact Wilcoxon–Mann–Whitney procedure available. Several microcomputer statistics packages incorporate exact methods; we have used StatXact.[10]

ORDERED INPUT VARIABLES

In the preceding two sections we have shown how to compare the responses of two groups, expressed in an ordered classification. But ordered classifications arise in medicine not only as outcomes but also as input variables. Examples of ordered input variables include the extent of disease in entering patients, their socioeconomic status, the elapsed interval before the initiation of treatment, and the patients' nutritional status. Woodward et al.[11] studied the ability of magnetic resonance imaging (MRI) to predict neurodevelopmental outcomes in 167 very premature infants. Table 4 shows the resulting four categories of white-matter abnormalities in the infants' brains and the presence of any neurodevelopmental impairment at age two years (corrected for prematurity). These data have columns bearing a natural and meaningful order, but they describe a condition, not a response; the outcomes correspond to "any impairment" or "no impairment"—that is, to the row variable. Here our attention naturally fastens on the percentage with impairment in each of the four columns. Before, when columns represented outcomes, we compared the rows. (In using the t-test we looked at two means, one for each row.)

Table 4. Presence of Any Neurodevelopmental Impairment at Age Two Years in Very Preterm Infants Classified According to the Extent of Their White-Matter Abnormality*

Neurodevelopmental Impairment	White-Matter Abnormality			
	None	Mild	Moderate	Severe
Any	7	22	14	4
None	40	63	15	2

*Data from Woodward et al.[11]

So this problem, with ordered columns corresponding to levels of an input variable, has a different structure. We naturally attend to the trend we see, in which the percentage with impairment increases as the white-matter abnormality becomes more severe. Is this trend statistically significant?

Answering this question is made easy by a pleasant, surprising mathematical fact: We can assess the significance of such a trend in a table with two rows by exactly the same methods presented earlier. This statement is formally justified by Armitage,[12] who shows that Kendall's rank-correlation coefficient (a measure of correlation that is based only on ranks and is suitable for testing trend) reduces to U when there are two rows. Furthermore, although it is far from obvious, it can be proved that the ordinary correlation coefficient, in which numerical scores are used for the columns and there are only two rows, yields as a test statistic the very t-statistic that we have already described. Though we do not pursue these issues here, they justify our using the statistical methods already described.

We have, then, two ways to test the trend of the percentage having impairment (for example) with regard to an ordered characteristic of treatment (intensity, duration) or of subject material (nutritional status, stage of disease). The first method is to apply the U test. This will do for assessing significance, but the descriptive interpretation of U is less direct than before. U now estimates the probability that if one impaired patient and one unimpaired patient are drawn randomly from the population that this sample represents, then the impaired patient will be the one with the more severe abnormality on MRI scanning. Alternatively, one can, as before, assign numbers to the columns and apply the t-test to the two rows. This will also do for assessing approximate significance; with the score for each column used to define the severity of abnormality in the column, the difference between the row averages serves as an estimate of the average difference in severity of abnormality between impaired and unimpaired children.

We now apply these two methods, using U and t, to the data in Table 4. The value of U is 3736. If there were no association between impairment and severity of white-matter abnormality, U would have an expected value of

$$\frac{47 \times 120}{2} = 2820.$$

The value of σ_U, corrected for ties, is 257.6; so the significance is assessed, with the aid of the normal approximation, in terms of

$$z = \frac{3736 - 2820}{257.6} = 3.56,$$

which corresponds to a two-sided p-value of 0.00038. (The exact p-value is 0.00034.) The value of U found from Table 4 is large enough that we can conclude with near certainty that the trend of increasing impairment with more severe abnormality is not an artifact of chance.

Before turning from this example, we pause to show the weakness of analyzing data with ordered categories using the usual chi-squared test for the $2 \times k$ table. The chi-squared statistic for the impairment-abnormality data, 14.51, is significant at 0.0023 with three degrees of freedom. Notice first that this p-value is considerably less critical than the two-sided p-value of 0.00038 that was attained by using U; the difference is not damaging here, but the lesser sensitivity of chi-squared for identifying trends is evident, and it can be decisive in some data sets. The underlying principle remains: The chi-squared statistic takes no account of the order.

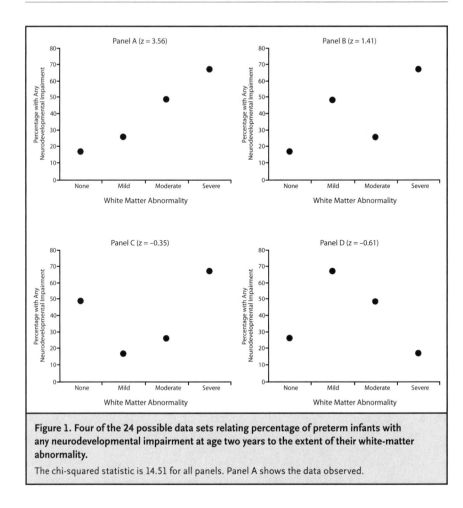

Figure 1. Four of the 24 possible data sets relating percentage of preterm infants with any neurodevelopmental impairment at age two years to the extent of their white-matter abnormality.

The chi-squared statistic is 14.51 for all panels. Panel A shows the data observed.

Panel A of Figure 1 plots the data from Table 4 as the percentage of patients with impairment at each of the four levels of MRI abnormality. The trend is clear. Now, if Table 4 had contained frequencies of presence and absence of impairment that were the same, but were differently associated with abnormality status, then other dispositions of the four percentages 0.15, 0.26, 0.48, and 0.67 would have resulted. The figure shows the actual association and three other possibilities. They have very different trends and very different values for z based on the Mann–Whitney test, but chi-squared is the same for all. When trend is the issue, then order matters, and the chi-squared test is inappropriate. Using a version of Fisher's exact test for a $2 \times k$ table is not a remedy; it too fails to take ordering into account and so has the same conceptual drawbacks as the chi-squared test.

SUMMARY AND RECOMMENDATIONS

Ordered classifications are often used in medicine to indicate individual responses to treatment. Both intended effects (e.g., improvement, lack of change, or deterioration) and side effects (e.g., whether they are absent, slight, moderate, or severe) are often scored in ordered classifications. Ordered variables often define the categories for contingency tables that undergo statistical analysis.

Comparing two groups in which the data come in this form is naturally and readily done by the Mann–Whitney U statistic. This statistic is easy to compute, and it provides a direct estimate of the probability that a patient will do better if treated with method A rather than with method B. The p-values are accurate even in very small samples, and a normal approximation for Mann–Whitney is often suitable.

A satisfactory alternative method when neither sample is very small is to apply numerical values to the categories and compare the two groups by means of a t-test. It is generally not satisfactory to collapse the ordered categories into only two so as to apply methods for comparing two proportions. Data are wasted by doing this.

Either U or t also applies when the rows give two possible outcomes (live or die, conceive or do not conceive) and the columns correspond to some ordered input variable, such as the stage of disease or the intensity of treatment. Now the issue is to assess any trend in the percentage of patients responding favorably, across the ordered input variable. It is a happy mathematical accident that this kind of problem can be treated by the methods natural to the first problem.

In contexts in which reasonable interpretation of the data should take the order of categories into account, it is a mistake to use the chi-squared statistic, which has often been adopted for tables with two rows and more than two columns, as the tool of analysis. That statistic completely ignores the order of the columns. As a consequence, the chi-squared test is not as responsive to trends that are truly present; the Mann–Whitney test or the t-test is more likely to find that a trend is statistically significant. For contingency tables with ordered variables on two margins and for tables with three or more rows and three or more columns in which at least one variable is ordered, special techniques are available,[13] and investigators should probably seek the assistance of a professional statistician.

For an analysis of a two-way contingency table, adequate information should be reported in order to allow independent verification of the analysis. The authors should clearly identify the table of frequencies analyzed; whether the data were collapsed and, if so, in what way; what test statistic was employed; the p-value of the test; and whether the p-value is one-sided or two-sided.

The adoption of suitable statistical methods, together with adequate reporting of the methods used and the results obtained, can enhance the credibility and value of the published report of a scientific investigation. The high costs of medical investigation, whether measured in time, effort, or money, mandate our careful attention to these issues.

ACKNOWLEDGMENTS

We are indebted to John Bailar, Graham Colditz, Katherine Godfrey, Katherine Taylor Halvorsen, Robert Lew, Thomas Louis, Frederick Mosteller, and John Williamson, all members of the Study Group for Statistical Methods in the Biomedical Sciences, who assisted us in reviewing articles published in Volume 306 of the *Journal*; to Cyrus Mehta and David Tritchler; and to Cleo Youtz, who provided useful suggestions on an earlier version of the manuscript. The editors are grateful to Elizabeth Apgar and Tanya Burton for help with the revisions for the third edition.

REFERENCES

1. Albert PS. Analysis of categorical data in medical studies. [Chapter 12 of this book.]

2. Armitage P, Berry G, Matthews JNS. Statistical methods in medical research. 4th ed. New York: John Wiley, 2001.

3. Wilcoxon F. Individual comparisons by ranking methods. Biometrics 1945; 1:80–3.

4. Mann HB, Whitney DR. On a test of whether one of two random variables is stochastically larger than the other. Ann Math Stat 1947; 18:50–60.

5. Kirkpatrick CH, Alling DW. Treatment of chronic oral candidiasis with clotrimazole troches: a controlled clinical trial. N Engl J Med 1978; 299:1201–3.

6. Klotz J, Teng J. One-way layout for counts and the exact enumeration of the Kruskal-Wallis H distribution with ties. J Am Stat Assoc 1977; 72:165–9.

7. Mehta CR, Patel NR, Tsiatis AA. Exact significance testing to establish treatment equivalence with ordered categorical data. Biometrics 1984; 40:819–25.

8. Emerson JD, Moses LE. A note on the Wilcoxon–Mann–Whitney test for $2 \times k$ ordered tables. Biometrics 1985; 41:303–9.

9. Snedecor GW, Cochran WG. Statistical methods. 8th ed. Ames, Iowa: Iowa State University Press, 1989.

10. Cytel Inc. StatXact 8. Cambridge, Mass.: 2007.

11. Woodward LJ, Anderson PJ, Austin NC, et al. Neonatal MRI to predict neurodevelopmental outcomes in preterm infants. N Engl J Med 2006; 355:685–94.

12. Armitage P. Tests for linear trends on proportions and frequencies. Biometrics 1955; 11:375–86.

13. Agresti A. Analysis of ordinal categorical data. New York: John Wiley, 1984.

Communicating Results

CHAPTER 14

∽

Guidelines for Statistical Reporting in Articles for Medical Journals: Amplifications and Explanations

JOHN C. BAILAR III, M.D., PH.D., AND

FREDERICK MOSTELLER, PH.D.

ABSTRACT   The Uniform Requirements for Manuscripts Submitted to Biomedical Journals, which are updated about once every two years, include guidelines for presenting statistical aspects of scientific research. The guidelines are intended to aid authors in reporting statistical aspects of their work in ways that are clear and helpful to readers. We examine these guidelines for statistics and the presentation of results using specific statements and our responses to them. Although the information presented relates to manuscript preparation, it will also help investigators make critical decisions about research approaches and protocols, and it will help readers understand why certain aspects are important and why they are presented as they are.

In 1979 the group now known as the International Committee of Medical Journal Editors (ICMJE) first published a set of uniform requirements for preparing manuscripts (URMs) to be submitted to their journals. These uniform requirements have been adopted by over 500 biomedical journals and are now revised and updated at intervals of about 12–24 months. These guidelines have surely improved the quality of submitted manuscripts; they have the added advantage that authors need not learn many different styles or rework a disapproved manuscript before submitting it to another journal. In the 1988 revision the Committee added guidelines for presenting and writing about statistical aspects of research, and these guidelines are updated with the rest of the document.[1] They aim to assist authors in reporting statistical aspects of their research in ways that will be helpful to editors, reviewers, and readers. This chapter, updated from our 1988 article,[2] is based on the October 2008 posting of the URMs (at www.icmje.org).

Authors can consult numerous guidelines for preparing precise and complete reports of various types of biomedical research studies. These guidelines are also valuable when studies are first designed. For example, the CONSORT guidelines for the reporting of clinical trials (available at www.consort-statement. org/?o=1011) are widely used. The EQUATOR Network (www.equator-network. org/index.aspx?o=1015) maintains a reasonable compendium of promulgated guidelines for reporting of experimental studies, observational studies, diagnostic test studies, economic valuations, and other specific types of studies.

In this chapter we present our interpretation of the statistical guidance offered by the ICMJE in the form of 14 statements from their guidelines with amplification and explanation of some of the reasoning behind them. The statements are identified by the section in the ICMJE guidelines where they appear. We include three additional points (numbers 5–7 below) that are prominent in the CONSORT guidelines for reporting clinical trials, but apply to other kinds of work as well. We believe that these three points may be helpful to readers and will be acceptable to editors of medical journals unless their Instructions to Authors say otherwise. Our text focuses on manuscript preparation, but it should also be helpful at earlier stages when critical decisions about research approaches and protocols are made. We also provide references to general statistical texts. The International Committee is not responsible for these amplifications; we have tried, however, to present the spirit of the Committee's decisions as well as our own views.

1. Describe your selection of the observational or experimental participants (patients or laboratory animals, including controls) clearly, including eligibility and exclusion criteria and a description of the source population. (IV. A. 6. a)

Reasons for and methods of selecting patients or other study units should always be reported, and, if the selection is likely to matter, the reasons should be reported in detail. The full range of potentially eligible subjects, or the scope of the study, should be precisely stated in terms that readers can interpret. It is not enough to say that the natural history of a condition has been seen in "100 consecutive patients." How do these patients compare with what is already known about the condition in terms of age, sex, and other factors? Are patients from an area or population that might be special? Are patients from an "unselected" series with an initial diagnosis, or do they include referral patients (who may be weighted with less serious or more serious problems, or otherwise atypical)? In comparing outcomes for patients who underwent surgery to outcomes for patients treated medically, were the groups in similar physical condition initially? What about probable cases not proved? Many other questions will arise in specific instances. Sometimes information is obvious (for example, the investigator studied patients from one hospital because that is where he or she practices). Other questions about scope need answers. (Why begin on 1 January 2000? Why include only patients admitted through the emergency room?) Authors should try to imagine themselves as readers who know nothing about the study.

Although every statistically sound study has such scope criteria to determine the breadth of the population considered by the investigator, many also include detailed eligibility criteria. Medical examples include the possible exclusion of patients outside a specified age range, those previously treated, and those who refuse randomization or are too ill to answer questions.

Which criteria are used to establish scope (i.e., inclusion criteria), and which are used to establish eligibility (i.e., exclusion criteria) may be uncertain, although both must be reported. Scope criteria push study boundaries outward, toward the full range of patients or other study units that might be considered as subjects, whereas eligibility rules narrow the scope by removing units that cannot be studied, that may give unreliable results, that are likely to be atypical (for example, at the extremes of age), that cannot be studied for ethical reasons (for example, pregnant women in some drug studies, or persons already treated in some way), or that are otherwise not appropriate for individual study.

The first goal in reporting on selection of subjects for an investigation is to state both scope and eligibility so that another knowledgeable investigator, facing the same group of patients or other study units, would make nearly the same decisions about including patients in the study.

The second goal is to provide readers with a solid link between the patients or cases studied and the population for which inferences will be made. Both scope and eligibility constraints can introduce substantial bias when results are generalized to other subjects, and readers need enough information to make their own assessment of this potential. Thus, reasons for each eligibility criterion should either be obvious (e.g., limited to women in a study of childbearing) or clearly stated. The two critical elements in setting the base for generalization are first to document each exclusion under the eligibility criteria with the reasons for that exclusion; and second, to present an accounting (often in a table) of the difference between patients falling within the scope of the study and those actually studied. The article should also say how patients who are excluded for more than one reason are handled; common approaches are to show specific combinations or to use a priority sequence. Such information helps the reader better understand how the study group is related to the population it came from, and also helps to ensure that all omissions are accounted for. It should be so stated if no subject was ineligible for more than one reason.

Scope and eligibility criteria should be set forth in a written protocol before work is started. If they evolved during the course of the study, specific information on the changes should be given. Were some eligibility criteria added at the end to deal with some problems not foreseen? For example, a written protocol might call for the study of "all" patients, but if only 5% of patients were female (or male), they might be set aside at this point—especially if they are thought to differ from male patients in ways relevant to the subject of the study. For the manuscript it is useful to provide an illustration that shows the details of patient enrollment; one proposed method of presenting these data is given in the CONSORT statement.

2. Describe statistical methods with enough detail to enable a knowledgeable reader with access to the original data to verify the reported results. (IV.A.6.c)

Authors should report which statistical methods they used, and why. In many instances, they should also report why other methods were not used, although this is rarely done.

The statistical methods should include a clear statement of the primary scientific question that the study was designed to answer, an explanation of the methods used to compute the sample size studied, and, for treatment trials, whether pre-defined stopping rules were to be applied to the study by an independent data safety and monitoring board. The Methods section must identify the primary outcome on which the trial was powered, the pre-specified secondary outcomes, and analyses that were post-hoc, and thus exploratory in nature.

The authors have an obligation to communicate clearly the strengths and weaknesses in study design in enough detail to give readers a clear and accurate impression of the reliability of the data, as well as any threats to the validity of findings and interpretations.

It is essential that people with the appropriate statistical expertise be involved at the time the study is conceived, during the drafting of the study protocol and statistical plan, and in the analysis and interpretation of the data. The manuscript should provide adequate detail so that the educated reader can appreciate the statistical issues that confronted the investigators in trying to tackle their scientific problem and why the form of the study provides an adequate solution to this problem. Whatever statistical task is defined, it is inappropriate, and indeed unethical, to try several methods and report only those results that suit the investigator. If overlapping methods are used, the results need not be presented separately when they largely agree, but authors should state which additional approaches were tried, and that they did agree. Of course, results that do not agree also should be given, and investigators may sometimes find that such disagreements arise from important and unexpected aspects of their findings.

Units should always be specified in text, tables, and figures, although not necessarily every time a number appears if the unit is clear to the reader. Often, careful choice of units of measurement can help clarify and unify the study question, biological hypotheses, and statistical analysis. Careful reporting of units can also help to avoid serious misunderstanding. Are quantities in milligrams or millimoles? Are rates per 10,000 or per 100,000? Does a figure show the number of patients, the number of myocardial infarcts among those patients (including repeat infarcts), or the number of admissions to a given hospital (including readmissions)? Research investigators often use abbreviated language that is clear to their colleagues, but they may have to make a special effort to ensure that such usage will not confuse nonspecialists, or even other experts. Precision of interpretation by the educated but not closely informed reader should be the goal.

3. References for the design of the study and statistical methods should be to standard works when possible (with pages stated). (IV.A.6.c)

An original paper on study design or methods can have great value for a few readers, but often does little to explain the method and its implications or the byways of calculation or meaning that may have emerged since the method was first reported. Standard works such as textbooks or review papers will usually give a clearer exposition, put the method in a larger context, and give helpful examples. The notation will be the current standard, and the explanation will orient readers to the general use of the method rather than the specific and sometimes peculiar use first reported. For example, it would be hard to recognize a student's t-distribution in his original paper; indeed, t was not even mentioned. Exceptions to the general advice about using textbooks, review papers, or other standard works occur where the original exposition is best for communication and where it is the only one available.

Where should statistical methods be described? This is a matter of individual journal and author styles. Our preference is to describe all methods in the Methods section, and to state in the Results and Discussion sections which methods were used at each point where they are relevant.

There must be adequate detail for the interested reader to replicate the approach, even if it is not likely that any will do so. Statements such as "statistical methods included analysis of variance, factor analysis, and regression, as well as tests of significance," when divorced from the outcomes or reasons for their use, give the reader little help. On the other hand, if the only method was the use of chi-squared tests with Yates's correction for 2×2 contingency tables, that fact might be sufficiently informative. Although the general statistical methods may be grouped, when reporting individual results, it is prudent to refer to the test used to obtain the result reported.

4. For reports of randomized, controlled trials, authors should refer to the CONSORT statement. (IV.A.1.b)

Here we focus on randomization. The CONSORT statement requires (among many other things) an explanation of the "Method used to generate the random allocation sequence" as well as "Details of any restriction [of randomization] (e.g. blocking, stratification)."

The reporting of randomization needs special attention for two reasons. First, some authors incorrectly use random as a synonym for haphazard. To prevent misunderstanding, tell readers how the randomization was done (such as a coin toss, table of random numbers, cards in sealed envelopes, telephone call to a central location after a patient is firmly enrolled). Readers will then know that a random mechanism was in fact applied, and they can also judge the likelihood that it was subject to bias or abuse (such as peeking at cards). Second, randomization can enter in many ways. For example, a sample may be selected from a larger population at random, or study patients may be randomly allocated to treatments, or treated patients may be randomly given one or another test. Thus, it is not enough just to say that a study was randomized. The many possible roles of randomization can be dealt with by careful reporting to ensure there is no ambiguity.

Even with randomization, imbalances can occur, and these may need attention in the analysis and interpretation of the data. Stratification or matching may be used in combination with randomization to increase the similarity between the treated and control groups, and should be reported. Sometimes an assessment of the efficacy of stratification or matching in overcoming the imbalance is feasible; if so, the assessment should be done and reported.

If the randomization was blocked (for example, by arranging that each successive group of six patients includes a random three assigned to one treatment and three to another), reasons for blocking and the blocking factors should be given. Blocking should ordinarily affect statistical analysis, and authors should say how they used blocking in their analysis or why they did not.

5. **[Report w]hether or not participants, those administering the interventions, and those assessing the outcomes were blinded to group assignment. (CONSORT 11(a))**

Blinding, sometimes called *masking*, is the concealment of certain information from patients or members of the research team during phases of a study. Blinding can be used to good effect to reduce bias, but because it can be applied in various ways, a research report should be explicit about who was blinded to what. An unadorned statement that a study was blind or double-blind is rarely enough.

Patients may be blinded to treatment, or to the time of treatment change in a crossover study, or to the time that certain observations are made, or to preliminary findings regarding their progress. A decision to admit a patient to a study may be made blind to that patient's specific circumstances, and a decision that a patient randomized to treatment was not eligible may be made blind to the assigned treatment. The observer who classifies clinical outcomes may be blinded to the treatment, as may be the pathologist who interprets specimens or the technician who measures a chemical substance. These and other efforts to prevent bias by blinding should be reported in enough detail for readers to understand what was done.

The effectiveness of blinding, both to the patients and to the study physicians, should also be discussed in any situation where the person who is blinded may learn or guess the concealed information, such as by side effects or changes in laboratory values that may accompany one treatment but not another. Such discoveries are particularly important for observations reported by patients themselves and for third-party observations of endpoints with a subjective component, such as level of patient activity.

A particularly critical aspect of blinding is whether the decision to admit a patient to a study was made before (or otherwise entirely and demonstrably independent of) any decision about choice of treatment to be used or offered. Where random allocation to treatments is used, the timing of randomization in relation to the decision to admit a patient should always be stated.

6. [Report a]ll important adverse events or side effects in each intervention group. (CONSORT 19)

Any intervention, or treatment, has some likelihood of causing unintended effects, whether the study is of a cell culture, a person, an ecologic community, or a hospital management system. Side effects may be good (quitting smoking reduces the risk of heart disease as well as the risk of lung cancer) or bad (drug toxicity). Side effects may be foreseen or unexpected. In most studies side effects will be of substantial interest to readers. Does a drug cause so much nausea that patients will not take it? If we stock an ecologic area with one species, what will happen to a predator? Does a new system for scheduling the purchase of hospital supplies at lower overall cost change the likelihood that some item will be exhausted before the replacement stock arrives?

Unwanted and unexpected effects should be sought at least as assiduously as beneficial effects, and they should be reported objectively and in detail. Treatment failure often gives the most useful information from a study. If no adverse effects can be found, the report should say so, with an explanation of what was done to find them. Because adverse events may occur beyond the pre-specified duration of the study, investigators should clearly state when the database for accrual of adverse events was closed; at minimum, the time for accrual of these data must encompass the time given for the accrual of salutory treatment events.

Statistical tests for adverse effects are likely to be uninformative, because such effects will generally be much less common than the endpoint the investigators are trying to change, so that statistical power is low. A further problem is that the number of possible adverse outcomes is generally many times larger than the number of beneficial effects sought (most often just one), so that one or more false positives should often be expected. Statistical tests should generally be reported, but their interpretation will often include such matters as historical observations about the frequency of some adverse outcome, the biologic plausibility of a link between treatment and the adverse outcome, results in trials of similar agents or procedures, and any special characteristics of patients among whom it appears. In short, the interpretation of data about adverse effects is both important and difficult.

7. [F]or each group report the numbers of participants randomly assigned, receiving intended treatment, completing the study protocol, and analyzed for the primary outcome. (CONSORT 13(a))

When the sample size for a table, graph, or text statement differs from that for a study as a whole, the difference should be explained. The methods for dealing with missing data because of patient drop-out should be clearly delineated in the description of the statistical methods. If some study units are omitted (for example, patients who did not return for six-month follow-up), the reduced number should be reconciled with the number eligible or expected by readers. Reporting of losses is often easiest in tables, where entries such as "patients lost," "samples contaminated," "not eligible," or "not available" (for example, no 15-meter sample from a lake with a maximum depth of 10 meters) can account for each study unit.

Loss of patients to follow-up, including losses or exclusions for noncompliance, should generally be discussed in depth because of the likelihood that patients lost are atypical in critical ways. Have patients not returned for examination because they are well? Because they are still sick and have sought other medical care? Because they are dead? Because they do not wish to burden a physician with a bad outcome? Failures to discuss both reasons for loss (or other termination of follow-up) and the nature and success of efforts to trace lost patients are common and serious. Similarly, issues of noncompliance (reasons, as well as numbers) are often slighted by authors.

8. Specify the computer software used. (IV.A.6.c)

General-purpose computer programs should be specified, because such programs are sometimes found to have errors. Readers may also wish to know about these programs for their own use. In contrast, programs written for a specific task need not be documented, because readers should already be alert to the likelihood of errors in ad hoc or privately developed programs, and because they will not be able to use the same programs for their own work. Because errors may be discovered, then corrected, it is best to report both the general program and the specific version used. If study-specific software was developed, the authors have an obligation to share the software with interested and qualified investigators who wish to replicate the work; a clear statement of availability should be included in the "statistical methods" section of the article.

9. Define statistical terms, abbreviations, and most symbols. (IV.A.6.c)

Although many statistical terms such as mean, median, and standard deviation of the observations have clear, widely adopted definitions, various fields of endeavor often use the same symbols for different entities. Authors have extra difficulty when they need to distinguish between the true but unknown value of a quantity (a parameter such as a population mean, often symbolized by the Greek letter μ) and a sample mean (often written as $\bar{x}$).

We usually take for granted the mathematical symbols =, +, −, and /, as well as the usual symbols for inequalities (greater than or less than); we do the same for powers such as x^3, and for the trigonometric and logarithmic abbreviations such as sin, cos, tan, and log, although it is essential to report the base for logarithms. Typography for ordinary multiplication varies, but is rarely a problem. Generally, symbols such as r for the correlation coefficient should be defined. The symbols n and N are often used for sample size, though it is not always clear to the reader what subjects have been excluded, if any.

The meaning of terms such as reliability and validity is much less standard, and such terms should always be defined when they are used in a statistical sense.

One difficulty with an expression such as $a \pm b$, even when a is a sample mean, is that b has many possibilities. The commonest ambiguity is not knowing whether b represents the standard deviation of individual observations or the standard error of the statistic designated by a or the half-width of a confidence interval for a. And no single choice is best in all situations. If the measure of variability is used only to test the size of its associated statistic, as for example whether a correlation coefficient differs from 0, then use the standard error. If the measure of variability needs to be combined with other such measures, the standard deviation of single observations is often more useful.

The same difficulty occurs with technical terms. A danger is that a special local language will become so ingrained in a particular research organization that its practitioners find it difficult to understand that their use of words is not widespread. Nearly every laboratory has special words that need to be defined or eliminated in reports of findings.

When one or two observations, terms, or symbols are not defined, readers may be able to struggle along. When several remain uncertain, readers may have to give up because the possibilities are too numerous.

A well-established convention is that mathematical symbols should be printed in italics. This practice has many advantages, including the reduction of ambiguity when the same character is commonly used to designate both a physical quantity and a mathematical or statistical quantity.

10. When possible, quantify findings and present them with appropriate indicators of measurement error or uncertainty (such as confidence intervals). (IV.A.6.c)

Readers have many reasons for studying a research report. One is to find out how a particular treatment does in its own right, not just in comparison with another treatment. At minimum, readers should be offered the mean and the standard deviation for every appropriate outcome variable in absolute units, not relative to another outcome. Investigators have to choose a way to report their findings that clearly communicates both the point estimate of an effect and a measure of the certainty of a finding. The most useful ways give information about the actual outcomes, such as means and standard deviations as well as confidence intervals. Reporting a test of significance alone—without this additional information—is not acceptable,[3, 4] but results of a significance test in the context of other information about an outcome may be satisfactory. In independent samples, information about means, standard deviations, and sample sizes can often be readily converted to a significance test and thus into a p-value, but the reverse is not true.

When significance levels (p-values) are appropriate, statements such as $p = 0.03$ are often reported to show that the difference seen or some other departure from a standard (a null hypothesis) had little probability of occurring if chance alone was the cause. Exact p-values rather than statements like "$p < 0.05$" or "p is not significant" should be reported where possible so that readers can compare the calculated value of p with their own choice of a critical value. In addition, other investigators may need exact values of p if they are to combine results of separate studies.

Make clear whether a reported standard deviation is for the distribution of single observations, for the distribution of means (standard errors), or for the distribution of some other statistic such as the difference between two means. If the standard deviation for single observations is given, together with sample sizes, then in independent samples the reader can compute the other standard deviations.

Each statistical test of data implies both a specific null hypothesis about those data (such as "The 60-day survival rate in Group A equals that in Group B," so that the difference is zero) and a specific set of alternative hypotheses (such as "The survival rate is different in Group B," which allows for a range of values, in either direction, for the difference). It is critical that both the null hypothesis and the alternative(s) be clearly stated. Clear reporting will not only help readers, it is also likely to reduce the frequency of abuse of p-values.

It is critical also that authors specify how and when they developed each null hypothesis in relation to their consideration of the data. Statistical theory and acceptable clinical research practice require that null hypotheses be fully developed before the data are examined—indeed, before even the briefest view of preliminary results. Otherwise, p-values cannot be interpreted as meaningful probabilities.

Authors should always specify whether they are using two-tail or one-tail tests; one-tail tests should be vanishingly rare.

11. When data are summarized, often in the Results section, give numeric results not only as derivatives (for example, percentages) but also as the absolute numbers from which the derivatives were calculated, and specify the statistical methods used to analyze them. (IV.A.7)

The basic observational units should be clearly specified, along with any study features that might cause basic observations to be correlated. A study of changes in blood pressure over time might take measurements from 5 patients at each of 7 times—35 measurements in all. But the relevant sample size for one or another purpose may be 5 (patients), or 7 (times), or 35 (patients at different times). In a meta-analysis of such work[5] the whole study may count as only a single observation.

Similarly, a study in several institutions of rates of infection after surgery may be considered to have a sample size of 3 hospitals, 15 surgeons, 600 patients, or 3000 days of observation after surgery.

Choice of the basic unit of observation determines the proper method of analysis. This choice is critical, and may require an informed understanding of statistics as well as the subject matter. The analysis and reporting of correlated observations, such as the water samples and the infection rates described above, raise difficult issues of statistical analysis that often require expert statistical help.

A different kind of problem arises from ambiguity in reporting ratios, proportions, and percentages, where the denominator is often not specified and may be unclear to readers. It is critical to report absolute differences before reporting relative differences.

Whatever the investigators adopt as their basic unit of observation, relationships to and possible correlations with other units must be discussed. Such internal relationships can sometimes be used to strengthen an analysis (when a major source of difference is balanced or held constant), and sometimes they weaken the analysis (by obscuring a critical limitation on effective sample size). Complicated data structures need special attention in study reporting, not just in study design, performance, and analysis.

12. Avoid relying solely on statistical hypothesis testing, such as p-values, which fail to convey important information about effect size. (IV.A.6.c)

Summaries of primary data, including confidence intervals, offer a more informative way to deal with the significance test than does a simple p-value. Confidence intervals for a single mean or a proportion provide information about both magnitude and its variability. Confidence intervals on a difference of means or proportions provide information about the size of an effect and its uncertainty, but not about component means, so these should also be given.

A significance test of observed data, generally to determine whether the (unknown) means of two populations differ, usually winds up with a score that is either referred to a table (such as a t-, normal-, or F-table) or calculated within a program, which can hide even more of the underlying statistical story.

Authors need a lively appreciation of the fact that an incorrect null hypothesis is not the only source of statistical significance or of confidence bounds that exclude "no effect." Although confidence intervals offer appraisals of variability and uncertainty, in some studies, such as certain large epidemiologic and demographic studies, biases are often greater threats to the validity of inferences than ordinary random variability (expressed in the standard deviation). Coding or typing errors may exaggerate the number of deaths from a cause, nonresponse to treatment may be selective (those patients more ill being less likely to respond), and so on. And, of course, even when the null hypothesis is true, sheer luck will produce low p-values and significant confidence intervals with the stated frequency.

13. Restrict tables and figures to those needed to explain the argument of the paper and to assess supporting data. (IV.A.7)

Authors have an understandable wish to tell readers everything they have learned or surmised from their data, but economy is much prized by scientific readers as well as editors. A basic point is that economy in writing and exposition gives an article its best chance of being read. Although many tables may help support the same basic point and might be appropriate in a monograph, an article generally requires only enough information to make its point—the mathematician's concept of "necessary and sufficient."

Exceptions may occur. Sometimes a study generates data that have consequences beyond the article. For example, if information about certain biological or physical constants is obtained, it should be retained in the article. An author should inform the editor of this situation in a cover letter. Sometimes such data need to be preserved, but not in the article itself. Many journals now allow or even encourage authors to put supplemental material in an Internet-based data repository provided with the article; such arrangements are often mentioned in a journal's instructions to authors.

14. Tables capture information concisely and display it efficiently; they also provide information at any desired level of detail and precision. (IV.A.10)

The presentation of tables often receives less attention than it needs. Little scientific investigation has been done in the field of tabular presentation, but there seems to be much value in some rules proposed by Ehrenberg[6]:

Give marginal (row and column) averages to provide a visual focus. Order the rows and columns of the table by the marginal averages or some other measure of size or another logical order (keeping to the same order if there are many similar tables). Put figures to be compared into columns rather than rows (with larger numbers on top if possible). Round to two effective (significant) digits. Use layout to guide the eye and facilitate comparisons. In the text give brief summaries to lead the reader in the main patterns and exceptions.

These rules, which we have adapted slightly for the present setting, do not replace judgment. For example, the logical order for rows or columns may be alphabetical order by label of category. Ehrenberg discusses the advantages of two-digit numbers for short-term memory and suggests modifications guided by the data.

To show the effects of Ehrenberg's rules, we present an extended example. We chose Table 1 from the National Halothane Study[7] showing death rates observed in a pool of four high-death-rate operations (exploratory laparotomy, craniotomy, heart with pump, large bowel). Our primary interest is in a comparison of death rates among anesthetic groups, with only a secondary interest in effect of physical status as measured by the code for anesthetic risk, which is used to improve anesthetic comparisons.

Table 1. Death Rates in Proportions for High-Death-Rate Operations by Anesthetic Risk Levels.[7]

Anesthetic Risk Code	Anesthetic				
	Halothane	Nitrous Oxide	Cyclopropane	Ether	Other
Unknown	0.11369	0.08682	0.08147	0.06148	0.09957
Risk 1	0.02454	0.02452	0.01634	0.01355	0.03358
Risk 2	0.05471	0.06893	0.04941	0.03812	0.05859
Risk 3	0.12471	0.16599	0.18187	0.11453	0.15306
Risk 4	0.15892	0.23140	0.18582	0.17919	0.35531
Risk 5	0.04665	0.06759	0.05725	0.04898	0.07606
Risk 6	0.22143	0.12996	0.17615	0.16008	0.17741
Risk 7	0.44164	0.43689	0.36689	0.62121	0.43348

Table 1 is obviously "busy" with five-digit numbers. In Table 2 we have rounded these to two decimal places and converted the death rates to percentages; this eliminated both decimal points and leading zeros.

Because of our interest in anesthetics we put anesthetics into rows, ordered according to a weighted average of death percentages for that anesthetic from highest to lowest. We have not included the weights.

The averages for anesthetic risk led us to rearrange the risk columns according to a weighted average death rate. The risk code is not a graded assessment of risk, and the death rates do not follow a regular progression. Risk 1 has the best and Risk 2 the second best prognosis, and Risk 5 is nearly as low as Risk 2 because it represents Risk 2 patients with an emergency. Similarly Risk 6 is a mixture of Risk 3 and Risk 4 patients with an emergency. The Unknown Risk patients take a place between Moderate Complications with an emergency (Risk 5) and Severe Complications (Risk 3). In Table 2 entries generally rise from left to right and rise from bottom to top.

The text summarizing the table might read as follows, "The table shows that the overall weighted percentage of deaths in these high-death-rate operations is 9.3%. When the risk levels are arranged according to the average death rate for the risk, each anesthetic leads to a nearly monotonic increase in death rate according to risk, the order being Codes 1, 2, 5, Unknown, 3, 6, 4, and 7. The last five groups have sharply higher death rates, with Risk 7 (moribund) giving 42.4%.

"Looking down columns, the death rates do not change much from one anesthetic group to another, though Other (a collection of many anesthetics) has the highest rate, not surprising because the anesthetist is probably avoiding the standard anesthetics because of some complication in the patient. Ether has the lowest rate, but from other data we know it is seldom used at some institutions and rarely in these high-risk operations. In the four low-risk-code (1, 2, 5, Unknown) patients, Halothane, Cyclopropane, and Nitrous Oxide have similar rates for these high-death-rate operations."

The rearrangements and the simplifications have led to a much more understandable table than the original. Although Ehrenberg's recommendations need not be slavishly followed, they can improve the readers' understanding. There is further discussion of presenting tables in Chapter 16, Writing about Numbers.

Table 2. Death Rates in Percentages for High-Death-Rate Operations by Anesthetics Versus Anesthetic Risk Levels.[7]

| Anesthetic Group | Anesthetic Risk Code | | | | | | | | |
	1	2	5	Unknown	3	6	4	7	Weighted Average
Other	3	6	8	10	15	18	36	43	11.7
Nitrous oxide	2	7	7	9	17	13	23	44	10.3
Cyclopropane	2	5	6	8	18	18	19	37	9.8
Halothane	2	5	5	11	12	22	16	44	8.7
Ether	1	4	5	6	11	16	18	62	6.1
Weighted average	2.2	5.5	5.7	9.6	14.6	17.4	20.6	42.4	9.3

Tables (and figures) are often poorly labeled. Consider the title and subtitles, head (across the top), stub (down the side), and footnotes. It is generally best to keep the title fairly "clean" and to put only essential information in the head and stub (including units used). This leaves the footnotes to do the heavy lifting. The title, head, and stub should, however, tell the reader just what is in the table. Consider the reader who has only a photocopy of the table; if it cannot be understood, the labeling is inadequate.

15. Use graphs as an alternative to tables with many entries; do not duplicate data in graphs and tables. (IV.A.7)

Whether tables or graphs better present material is sometimes a vexing question. Some readers go blind when faced with a table of numbers; others have no idea how to read graphs. Unfortunately, these groups are not mutually exclusive, and some users of statistical data need to see quantitative findings in text. It is important to consider the entirety of the data presented to support or refute the hypotheses under test. Each application will require a different approach. One of the best ways to obtain insight into data presentation is to ask a colleague, familiar with the field but not the specific research, to read and critique the methods of data presentation used.

16. Avoid nontechnical uses of technical terms in statistics, such as "random" (which implies a randomizing device), "normal," "significant," "correlations," and "sample." (IV.A.7)

Many words in statistics, and in mathematics more generally, come from everyday language and yet have specialized meanings. When statistical reporting is an important part of a paper, the author should not use statistical terms in his/her everyday meanings.

The family of normal (or Gaussian) distributions refers to a collection of probability distributions described by a specific formula; it is not just any more-or-less bell-shaped curve. The distribution of usual or average values of some quantity found in practice is rarely normal in the statistical sense. Normal also has many other mathematical meanings, such as a line perpendicular to a plane. When we mix these meanings with the meaning of normal for a patient without disease, we have the makings of considerable confusion.

Significance and related words are used in statistics, and in scientific writing generally, to refer to the outcome of a formal test of a statistical hypothesis or test of significance (essentially the same thing). Significant means that the outcome of such a test fell outside a chosen, predetermined region. Careful statisticians and other scientists distinguish between statistical and medical or social significance. For example, a large enough sample might show statistically significant differences in averages on the order of one tenth of a degree in average body temperature of groups of humans. Such a difference might be regarded as of no biological or medical significance. In the other direction, a dietary program that reduces weight by an average of 5 kg might be regarded as important to health, and yet this finding may not be well established, as expressed by statistical significance. Although the 5 kg is important, the data do not support a firm conclusion that a difference has actually been achieved.

Association is a usefully vague word to express a relation between two or more variables without any implication of either causation or its absence from one variable to another. Correlation, a more technical term, refers to a specific way to measure association, and should not be used in writing about statistical findings except in referring to that measure.

Sample usually refers to an observation or a collection of observations gathered in a well-defined way. To describe a sample as having been drawn at random means that a randomizing device has been used to make the choice, not that some haphazard event has created the sample, such as the use of an unstructured set of patient referrals to create the investigator's control group.

17. Where scientifically appropriate, analyses of the data by such variables as age and sex should be included. (IV.A.7)

The ICMJE guidelines add, elsewhere, that the relevance of such variables as age and sex to the object of research is not always clear, so that authors should explain their use when they are included in a study report—for example, authors should explain why only participants of certain ages were included, or why women or previously treated patients were excluded. Chapter 15 explains some of the difficulties in the study of subgroups, and Chapter 12 shows how Simpson's pardox (which is rooted in subgroup comparisons) can mislead the investigator, but cautious interpretation can often be useful in understanding overall findings and in generating hypotheses for future study.

CONCLUSION

Overall, generally accepted guidelines such as these serve several important functions. They help to ensure that readers and users can learn how a paper may or may not suit their needs, they have at least some of the critical information that editors and reviewers need to evaluate a published paper, and they serve authors by providing a single template for submissions (or re-submissions) to the many leading journals that now accept the ICMJE recommendations. But guidelines are not laws and should not be a straitjacket; when there is a good and pressing reason for omitting some item, the author should ask the intended journal whether the omission would be acceptable.

REFERENCES

1. International Committee of Medical Journal Editors. Uniform requirements for manuscripts submitted to biomedical journals. Ann Intern Med 1988; 108:258–65.

2. Bailar JC III, Mosteller F. Guidelines for statistical reporting in articles for medical journals: amplifications and explanations. Ann Intern Med 1988; 108:266–73.

3. Simon R. Confidence intervals for reporting results of clinical trials. Ann Intern Med 1986; 105:429–35.

4. Rothman KJ. Significance questing. Ann Intern Med 1986; 105:445–7.

5. Louis TA, Fineberg HV, Mosteller F. Findings for public health from meta-analyses. Annu Rev Public Health 1985; 6:1–20.

6. Ehrenberg ASC. The problem of numeracy. Am Statistician 1981; 35:67–71.

7. Bunker JP, Forrest WH Jr, Mosteller F, Vandam LD. The national halothane study. Washington, DC: U.S. Government Printing Office, 1969.

ADDITIONAL REFERENCES

The following references may be helpful to readers who want to pursue these topics further.

1. Armitage P, Berry G, Matthews JNS. Statistical methods in medical research. 4th ed. New York: John Wiley, 2001.

2. Chow SC, Shao J, Wang H. Sample size calculations in clinical research. 2nd ed. Boca Raton, Florida: CRC Press, 2003.

3. Cochran WG. Planning and analysis of observational studies. New York: John Wiley, 1983.

4. Cochran WG. Sampling techniques. 3rd ed. New York: John Wiley, 1977.

5. Cohn V. News and numbers: a guide to reporting statistical claims and controversies in health and other fields. Ames, Iowa: Iowa State University Press, 1989.

6. Committee for Evaluating Medical Technologies in Clinical Use. Assessing medical technologies. Washington, DC: National Academy Press, 1985.

7. Fleiss JL, Levin B, Paik MC. Statistical methods for rates and proportions. 3rd ed. Hoboken, New Jersey: John Wiley, 2003.

8. Ingelfinger JA, Mosteller F, Thibodeau LA, Ware JH. Biostatistics in clinical medicine. 2nd ed. New York: Macmillan, 1987.

9. Lohr SL. Sampling: design and analysis. Pacific Grove, California: Duxbury Press, 1999.

10. Meinert CL. Clinical trials: designs, conduct, and analysis. New York: Oxford University Press, 1986.

11. Proschan MA, Lan KK, Wittes JT. Statistical monitoring of clinical trials. New York: Springer, 2006.

12. Robbins NB. Creating more effective graphs. Hoboken, New Jersey: John Wiley, 2005.

13. Rosenbaum PR. Observational studies. 2nd ed. New York: Springer, 2002.

14. Shapiro SH, Louis TA, eds. Clinical trials: issues and approaches. New York: Marcel Dekker, 1983.

15. Sackett DL, Haynes RB, Tugwell P. Clinical epidemiology: a basic science for clinical medicine. Boston: Little, Brown & Co., 1985.

16. Snedecor GW, Cochran WG. Statistical methods. 8th ed. Ames, Iowa: Iowa State University Press, 1989.

CHAPTER 15

☙

Reporting of Subgroup Analyses in Clinical Trials

RUI WANG, PH.D., STEPHEN W. LAGAKOS, PH.D.,

JAMES H. WARE, PH.D., DAVID J. HUNTER, M.B.B.S.,

AND JEFFREY M. DRAZEN, M.D.

ABSTRACT Medical research relies on clinical trials to assess therapeutic benefits. Because of the effort and cost involved in these studies, investigators frequently use analyses of subgroups of study participants to extract as much information as possible. Such analyses, which assess the heterogeneity of treatment effects in subgroups of patients, may provide useful information for the care of patients and for future research. However, subgroup analyses also introduce analytic challenges and can lead to overstated and misleading results.[1-7] This chapter outlines the challenges associated with conducting and reporting subgroup analyses, and it sets forth guidelines for their use. Although this chapter focuses on the reporting of clinical trials, many of the issues discussed also apply to observational studies.

SUBGROUP ANALYSES AND RELATED CONCEPTS

Subgroup Analysis

By "subgroup analysis" we mean any evaluation of, and often a comparison of, treatment effects for a specific endpoint in subgroups of patients defined by baseline characteristics. The endpoint may be a measure of treatment efficacy or safety. For a given endpoint, the treatment effect—a comparison between the treatment groups—is typically measured by a relative risk, odds ratio, or arithmetic difference. The research question usually posed is this: Do the treatment effects vary among the levels of a baseline factor?

A subgroup analysis is sometimes undertaken to assess treatment effects for a specific patient characteristic; this assessment is often listed as a primary or secondary study objective. For example, Sacks et al.[8] conducted a placebo-controlled trial in which the reduction in the incidence of coronary events with the use of pravastatin was examined in a diverse population of persons who had survived a myocardial infarction. In subgroup analyses the investigators further examined whether the efficacy of pravastatin relative to placebo in preventing coronary events varied according to the patients' baseline low-density lipoprotein (LDL) levels.

Subgroup analyses are also undertaken to investigate the consistency of the trial conclusions among different subpopulations defined by each of multiple baseline characteristics of the patients. For example, Jackson et al.[9] reported the outcomes of a study in which 36,282 postmenopausal women 50 to 79 years of age were randomly assigned to receive 1000 mg of elemental calcium with 400 IU of vitamin D_3 daily or placebo. Fractures, the primary outcome, were ascertained over an average follow-up period of 7.0 years; bone density was a secondary outcome. Overall, no treatment effect was found for the primary outcome—that is, the active treatment was not shown to prevent fractures. The effect of calcium plus vitamin D supplementation relative to placebo on the risk of each of four fracture outcomes was further analyzed for consistency in subgroups defined by 15 characteristics of the participants.

Heterogeneity and Statistical Interactions

The heterogeneity of treatment effects across the levels of a baseline variable refers to the circumstance in which the treatment effects vary across the levels of the baseline characteristic. Heterogeneity is sometimes further classified as being either *quantitative* or *qualitative*. In the first instance one treatment is always better than the other, but by various degrees, whereas in the second instance one treatment is better than the other for one subgroup of patients and worse than the other for another subgroup of patients. Such variation, also called *effect modification*, is typically expressed in a statistical model as an interaction term or terms between the treatment group and the baseline variable. The presence or absence of interaction is specific to the measure of the treatment effect.

The appropriate statistical method for assessing the heterogeneity of treatment effects among the levels of a baseline variable begins with a statistical test for interaction.[10-13] For example, Sacks et al.[8] showed the heterogeneity in pravastatin efficacy by reporting a statistically significant ($p = 0.03$) result of testing for the interaction between the treatment and baseline LDL level when the measure of the treatment effect was the relative risk. Many trials lack the power to detect heterogeneity in treatment effect; thus, the inability to find significant interactions does not show that the treatment effect seen overall necessarily applies to all subjects. A common mistake is to claim heterogeneity on the basis of separate tests of treatment effects within each of the levels of the baseline variable.[6, 7, 14] For example, testing the hypothesis that there is no treatment effect in women, and then testing it separately in men, does not address the question of whether treatment differences vary according to sex. Another common error is to claim heterogeneity on the basis of the observed treatment-effect sizes within each subgroup, ignoring the uncertainty of these estimates.

Multiplicity

It is common practice to conduct a subgroup analysis for each of several—and often many—baseline characteristics, for each of several endpoints, or for both. For example, the analysis by Jackson and colleagues[9] of the effect of calcium plus vitamin D supplementation relative to placebo on the risk of each of four fracture outcomes for 15 participant characteristics resulted in a total of 60 subgroup analyses.

When multiple subgroup analyses are performed, the probability of a false-positive finding can be substantial.[7] For example, if the null hypothesis is true for each of 10 independent tests for interaction at the 0.05 significance level, the chance of at least one false-positive result exceeds 40%. Thus, one must be cautious in the interpretation of such results. Several methods for addressing multiplicity use more-stringent criteria for statistical significance than the customary p < 0.05.[7, 15] A less formal approach for addressing multiplicity is to note the number of nominally significant interaction tests that would be expected to occur by chance alone. For example, after noting that 60 subgroup analyses were planned, Jackson et al.[9] pointed out that "[up] to three statistically significant interaction tests (p < 0.05) would be expected on the basis of chance alone," and then they incorporated this consideration in their interpretation of the results.

Prespecified Analysis Versus Post-Hoc Analysis

A prespecified subgroup analysis is one that is planned and documented before any examination of the data, preferably in the study protocol. This analysis includes specification of the endpoint, the baseline characteristic, and the statistical method used to test for an interaction. For example, the Heart Outcomes Prevention Evaluation 2 investigators[16] conducted a study involving 5522 patients with vascular disease or diabetes to assess the effect of homocysteine lowering with folic acid and B vitamins on the risk of a major cardiovascular event. The primary outcome was a composite of death from cardiovascular causes, myocardial infarction, and stroke. In the Methods section of their article the authors noted that "[p]respecified subgroup analyses involving Cox models were used to evaluate outcomes in patients from regions with folate fortification of food and regions without folate fortification, according to the baseline plasma homocysteine level and the baseline serum creatinine level." Post-hoc analyses refer to those in which the hypotheses being tested are not specified before any examination of the data. Such analyses are of particular concern because it is often unclear how many were undertaken and whether some were motivated by inspection of the data. However, both prespecified and post-hoc subgroup analyses are subject to inflated false-positive rates arising from multiple testing. Investigators should avoid the tendency to prespecify many subgroup analyses in the mistaken belief that these analyses are free of the multiplicity problem.

SUBGROUP ANALYSES IN THE *JOURNAL*— ASSESSMENT OF REPORTING PRACTICES

As part of internal quality-control activities at the *Journal*, we assessed the completeness and quality of subgroup analyses reported in the *Journal* during the period from July 1, 2005 through June 30, 2006. A detailed description of the study methods can be found in the Supplementary Appendix, available with the full text of this article at www.nejm.org. In this report we describe the clarity and completeness of subgroup-analysis reporting, evaluate the authors' interpretation and justification of the results of subgroup analyses, and recommend guidelines for reporting subgroup analyses.

Among the original articles published in the *Journal* during the period from July 1, 2005 through June 30, 2006, a total of 95 articles reported primary outcome results from randomized clinical trials. Among these 95 articles, 93 reported results from one clinical trial; the remaining two articles reported results from two trials. Thus, results from 97 trials were reported, from which subgroup analyses were reported for 59 trials (61%). Table 1 summarizes the characteristics of the trials. We found that larger trials and multicenter trials were significantly more likely to report subgroup analyses than smaller trials and single-center trials, respectively. With the use of multivariate logistic-regression models, when ranked according to the number of participants enrolled in a trial and compared with trials with the fewest participants, the odds ratio for reporting subgroup analyses for the second quartile was 1.38 (95% confidence interval [CI], 0.45 to 4.20), for the third quartile was 1.98 (95% CI, 0.62 to 6.24), and for the fourth quartile was 8.90 (95% CI, 2.10 to 37.78) ($p = 0.02$, trend test). The odds ratio for reporting subgroup analyses in multicenter trials as compared with single-center trials was 4.33 (95% CI, 1.56 to 12.16).

Among the 59 trials that reported subgroup analyses, these analyses were mentioned in the Methods section for 21 trials (36%), in the Results section for 57 trials (97%), and in the Discussion section for 37 trials (63%); subgroup analyses were reported in both the text and a figure or table for 39 trials (66%). Other characteristics of the reports are shown in Figure 1. In general, we are

Variable	Trials Reporting Subgroup Analyses	*p*-Value	
	No. of Trials/ Total No. (%)	Univariate Odds Ratio	Multivariate Odds Ratio
No. of subjects		0.002[†]	0.02[†]
≤218	11/25 (44)		
219–429	13/25 (52)		
430–1012	14/23 (61)		
>1012	21/24 (88)		
Superiority trial		0.25	0.89
Yes	53/84 (63)		
No	6/13 (46)		
Trial sites		0.005	0.05
Single-center	7/21 (33)		
Multicenter	52/76 (68)		
Type of disease studied		0.18	0.37
Cardiovascular	16/20 (80)		
Infectious	2/7 (29)		
Oncologic	9/11 (82)		
Respiratory	7/10 (70)		
Pediatric	5/10 (50)		
Psychiatric or neurologic	6/10 (60)		
Metabolic, endocrine, or gastrointestinal	5/10 (50)		
Gynecologic	3/6 (50)		
Other	6/13 (46)		
Statistically significant primary endpoint		0.24	0.38
Yes	35/62 (56)		
No	24/35 (69)		

Table 1. Characteristics and Predictors of Reporting Subgroup Analyses in 97 Clinical Trials.*

*A total of 59 trials reported subgroup analyses.

[†]*p*-values were determined with the use of trend tests.

unable to determine the number of subgroup analyses conducted; we attempted to count the number of subgroup analyses reported in the article and found that this number was unclear in nine articles (15%). For example, Lees et al.[17] reported, "We explored analyses of numerous other subgroups to assess the effect of baseline prognostic factors or coexisting conditions on the treatment effect but found no evidence of nominal significance for any biologically likely

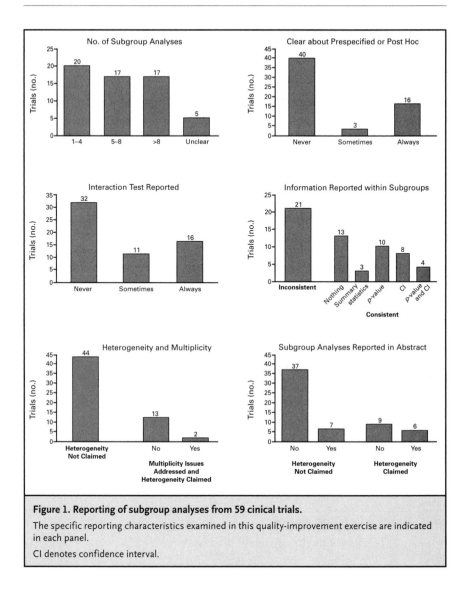

Figure 1. Reporting of subgroup analyses from 59 cinical trials.

The specific reporting characteristics examined in this quality-improvement exercise are indicated in each panel.

CI denotes confidence interval.

factor." For four of these nine articles, we were able to determine that at least eight subgroup analyses were reported. In 40 trials (68%) it was unclear whether any of the subgroup analyses were prespecified or post-hoc, and in three others (5%) it was unclear whether some were prespecified or post-hoc. Interaction tests were reported to have been used to assess the heterogeneity of treatment effects for all subgroup analyses in only 16 trials (27%), and they were reported to be used for some, but not all, subgroup analyses in 11 trials (19%).

We assessed whether information was provided about treatment effects within the levels of each subgroup variable (Fig. 1). In 25 trials (42%) information about treatment effects was reported consistently for all of the reported subgroup analyses, and in 13 trials (22%) nothing was reported. Investigators in 15 trials (25%), all using superiority designs,[10] claimed heterogeneity of treatment effects between at least one subject subgroup and the overall study population (see Table 1 of the Supplementary Appendix). For 4 of these 15 trials this claim was based on a nominally significant interaction test, and for 4 others it was based on within-subgroup comparisons only. In the remaining seven trials significant results of interaction tests were reported for some but not all subgroup analyses. When heterogeneity in the treatment effect was reported, for two trials (13%), investigators offered caution about multiplicity, and for four trials (27%) investigators noted the heterogeneity in the Abstract section.

ANALYSIS OF OUR FINDINGS AND GUIDELINES
FOR REPORTING SUBGROUPS

In the one-year period studied, the reporting of subgroup analyses was neither uniform nor complete. Because the design of future clinical trials can depend on the results of subgroup analyses, uniformity in reporting would strengthen the foundation on which such research is built. Furthermore, uniformity of reporting will be of value in the interval between recognition of a potential subgroup effect and the availability of adequate data on which to base clinical decisions.

Problems in the reporting of subgroup analyses are not new.[1-6, 18] Assmann et al.[2] reported shortcomings of subgroup analyses in a review of the results of 50 trials published in 1997 in four leading medical journals. More recently, Hernández et al.[4] reviewed the results of 63 cardiovascular trials published in 2002 and 2004 and noted the same problems. To improve the quality of reports of parallel-group randomized trials, the Consolidated Standards of Reporting Trials statement was proposed in the mid-1990s and revised in 2001.[19] Although there has been considerable discussion of the potential problems associated with subgroup analysis and recommendations on when and how subgroup analyses should be conducted and reported,[19, 20] our analysis of recent articles shows that problems and ambiguities persist in articles published in the *Journal*. For example, we found that in about two thirds of the published trials, it was unclear whether any of the reported subgroup analyses were prespecified or post-hoc. In more than half of the trials it was unclear whether interaction tests were used, and in about one third of the trials within-level results were not presented in a consistent way.

When properly planned, reported, and interpreted, subgroup analyses can provide valuable information. With the availability of Web supplements, the opportunity exists to present more-detailed information about the results of a trial.

The purpose of the guidelines (see box) is to encourage more clear and complete reporting of subgroup analyses. In some settings a trial is conducted with a subgroup analysis as one of the primary objectives. These guidelines are directly applicable to the reporting of subgroup analyses in the primary publication of a clinical trial when the subgroup analyses are not among the primary objectives. In other settings, including observational studies, we encourage complete and thorough reporting of the subgroup analyses in the spirit of the guidelines listed.

The editors and statistical consultants of the *Journal* consider these guidelines to be important in the reporting of subgroup analyses. The goal is to provide transparency in the statistical methods used in order to increase the clarity and completeness of the information reported. As always, these are guidelines and not rules; additions and exemptions can be made as long as there is a clear case for such action.

In the Abstract:	Present subgroup results in the Abstract only if the subgroup analyses were based on a primary study outcome, if they were prespecified, and if they were interpreted in light of the totality of prespecified subgroup analyses undertaken.
In the Methods section:	Indicate the number of prespecified subgroup analyses that were performed and the number of prespecified subgroup analyses that are reported. Distinguish a specific subgroup analysis of special interest, such as that in the article by Sacks et al.,[8] from the multiple subgroup analyses typically done to assess the consistency of a treatment effect among various patient characteristics, such as those in the article by Jackson et al.[9] For each reported analysis indicate the endpoint that was assessed and the statistical method that was used to assess the heterogeneity of treatment differences.
	Indicate the number of post-hoc subgroup analyses that were performed and the number of post-hoc subgroup analyses that are reported. For each reported analysis indicate the endpoint that was assessed and the statistical method used to assess the heterogeneity of treatment differences. Detailed descriptions may require a supplementary appendix.
	Indicate the potential effect on type I errors (false positives) from multiple subgroup analyses and how this effect is addressed. If formal adjustments for multiplicity were used, describe them; if no formal adjustment was made, indicate the magnitude of the problem informally, as done by Jackson et al.[9]
In the Results section:	When possible, base analyses of the heterogeneity of treatment effects on tests for interaction, and present them along with effect estimates (including confidence intervals) within each level of each baseline covariate analyzed. A forest plot[21, 22] is an effective method for presenting this information.
In the Discussion section:	Avoid overinterpretation of subgroup differences. Be properly cautious in appraising their credibility, acknowledge the limitations, and provide supporting or contradictory data from other studies, if any.

Guidelines for Reporting Subgroup Analyses

ACKNOWLEDGMENTS

We thank Doug Altman, John Bailar, Colin Begg, Mohan Beltangady, Marc Buyse, David DeMets, Stephen Evans, Thomas Fleming, David Harrington, Joe Heyse, David Hoaglin, Michael Hughes, John Ioannidis, Curtis Meinert, James Neaton, Robert O'Neill, Ross Prentice, Stuart Pocock, Robert Temple, Janet Wittes, and Marvin Zelen for their helpful comments.

REFERENCES

1. Yusuf S, Wittes J, Probstfield J, Tyroler HA. Analysis and interpretation of treatment effects in subgroups of patients in randomized clinical trials. JAMA 1991; 266:93–8.

2. Assmann SF, Pocock SJ, Enos LE, Kasten LE. Subgroup analysis and other (mis)uses of baseline data in clinical trials. Lancet 2000; 355:1064–9.

3. Pocock SJ, Assmann SF, Enos LE, Kasten LE. Subgroup analysis, covariate adjustment and baseline comparisons in clinical trial reporting: current practice and problems. Stat Med 2002; 21:2917–30.

4. Hernández A, Boersma E, Murray G, et al. Subgroup analyses in therapeutic cardiovascular clinical trials: are most of them misleading? Am Heart J 2006; 151:257–64.

5. Parker AB, Naylor CD. Subgroups, treatment effects, and baseline risks: some lessons from major cardiovascular trials. Am Heart J 2000; 139:952–61.

6. Rothwell PM. Subgroup analysis in randomised controlled trials: importance, indications, and interpretation. Lancet 2005; 365:176–86.

7. Lagakos SW. The challenge of subgroup analyses—reporting without distorting. N Engl J Med 2006; 354:1667–9. [Erratum, N Engl J Med 2006; 355:533.]

8. Sacks FM, Pfeffer MA, Moye LA, et al. The effect of pravastatin on coronary events after myocardial infarction in patients with average cholesterol levels. N Engl J Med 1996; 335:1001–9.

9. Jackson RD, LaCroix AZ, Gass M, et al. Calcium plus vitamin D supplementation and the risk of fractures. N Engl J Med 2006; 354:669–83. [Erratum, N Engl J Med 2006; 354:1102.]

10. Pocock SJ. Clinical trials: a practical approach. Chichester, England: John Wiley, 1983.

11. Halperin M, Ware JH, Byar DP, et al. Testing for interaction in an I×J×K contingency table. Biometrika 1977; 64:271–5.

12. Simon R. Patient subsets and variation in therapeutic efficacy. Br J Clin Pharmacol 1982; 14:473–82.

13. Gail M, Simon R. Testing for qualitative interactions between treatment effects and patient subsets. Biometrics 1985; 41:361–72.

14. Brookes ST, Whitely E, Egger M, et al. Subgroup analyses in randomized trials: risks of subgroup-specific analyses; power and sample size for the interaction test. J Clin Epidemiol 2004; 57:229–36.

15. Bailar JC III, Mosteller F, eds. Medical uses of statistics. 2nd ed. Boston, MA: NEJM Books, 1992.

16. Lonn E, Yusuf S, Arnold MJ, et al. Homocysteine lowering with folic acid and B vitamins in vascular disease. N Engl J Med 2006; 354:1567–77. [Erratum, N Engl J Med 2006; 355:746.]

17. Lees KR, Zivin JA, Ashwood T, et al. NXY-059 for acute ischemic stroke. N Engl J Med 2006; 354:588–600.

18.   Al-Marzouki S, Roberts I, Marshall T, Evans S. The effect of scientific misconduct on the results of clinical trials: a Delphi survey. Contemp Clin Trials 2005; 26:331–7.

19.   Moher D, Schulz KF, Altman DG, et al. The CONSORT Statement: revised recommendations for improving the quality of reports of parallel-group randomized trials. (Accessed November 1, 2007, at http://www.consort-statement.org/.)

20.   International Conference on Harmonisation (ICH). Guidance for industry: E9 statistical principles for clinical trials. Rockville, MD: Food and Drug Administration, September 1998. (Accessed November 1, 2007, at http://www.fda.gov/cder/guidance/ICH_E9-fnl.PDF.)

21.   Cuzick J. Forest plots and the interpretation of subgroups. Lancet 2005; 365:1308.

22.   Wactawski-Wende J, Kotchen JM, Anderson GL, et al. Calcium plus vitamin D supplementation and the risk of colorectal cancer. N Engl J Med 2006; 354:684–96.

Writing about Numbers

FREDERICK MOSTELLER, PH.D., MARGARET PERKINS, M.A.,

AND STEPHEN MORRISSEY, PH.D.*

ABSTRACT   In writing about numbers, as in other tasks in scientific writing, there are no absolute rules, and good practice depends on what sort of document is being prepared. The goals of writing the truth and communicating well with the reader may be at odds with considerations of length and the interests of the audience, as well as with ground rules of journals or editors. This chapter provides advice, with examples, on writing about numbers in the biomedical literature.

Because authors need to decide whether to provide numerical data primarily in text or in tables, this chapter discusses first the allocation of numbers. Then it gives advice on issues that arise more often in the text, makes a few suggestions about numbers in tables, and ends with some remarks about symbols.

NUMBERS IN TABLES OR TEXT?

Among the problems facing authors is how to allocate numbers to tables and text. The Uniform Requirements for Manuscripts Submitted to Biomedical Journals (at www.icmje.org) advise (in IV.A.7. Results), "Do not repeat all the data in the tables or illustrations in the text; emphasize or summarize only the most important observations. . . . Use graphs as an alternative to tables with many entries." Space in print journals is at a premium. In writing reports and text-books and in publishing online, authors may have more room to maneuver.

The availability of alternative ways to report and store data—such as providing complete data in large online-only files and making data sets available more generally through online data repositories—has made completeness a more achievable goal. The writer must still analyze and interpret the data and organize their presentation, but extensive data can be made available in their entirety. For a smaller document that may summarize the data and that is more

---

*Frederick Mosteller died in 2006. Margaret Perkins and Stephen Morrissey updated and revised the chapter for this edition.

likely to be read, however, decisions about the reporting of numerical data may be even more challenging and important than they were in the past.

For large collections of numerical values, tables are usually the best way to organize the numbers for the reader. If the table will be printed and read on paper, selection of a subset of data may be necessary, to fit the table on printed pages. Very large tables to be posted online may have fewer constraints on length; this option may be ideal for data that readers will want to download for their own analyses but are unlikely to read. For tables that are to be read online, however, space considerations are similar to those for tables that will appear on a printed page; readers are no more able to cope with a vast table in one medium than in another. It is often useful to provide tabular data in a computational spreadsheet format for on-line posting, so that readers can manipulate the data.

In a document that readers will refer to repeatedly—for example, a consensus document that outlines diagnostic criteria and guidelines for treatment—even a small number of numerical data points may warrant display in a table or figure. There readers can easily find and use them, and if the document is published online, the reader may be able to download and store it for even easier access.

Readers differ in their attitudes toward numbers. Some, almost like sponges, can sop up numbers from tables and interpret them readily. Others like to have the numbers in the text, and still others go snow-blind when collections of numbers appear in one place. They like numbers to be explained one at a time and to be few and far between. Thus, although the distribution of numbers should be guided by the logic of the writing and the requirements of documentation, it should also be influenced by the audience's preferences and customs.

Whatever the reasons for writing, include the message of the table in the text. Even the spongelike readers may not get the message the author wants to convey from reading the table, because tables often have several messages.

To help the reader understand a table, an explanation of the source or meaning of a number or a group of numbers may be necessary. This may be especially true when the rows and columns have headings that are severely abbreviated. Such explanations should be given in footnotes to the table; a table that can be understood on its own, without reference to the text, is more useful to readers, especially if it will be published online and downloaded for use apart from the text. For example, if the table uses a rating scale, the range and sign of the scale should be included in a footnote.

NUMBERS IN THE TEXT

Although some manuals of style[1-3] go into detail about handling numbers in the text, the rules have many exceptions. Some manuals are oriented more toward the humanities or journalistic writing than toward scientific or technical writing. Again, clarity and ease of reading are goals that should override style sheets, though editors can often cleverly revise manuscripts to meet style rules. Some specific issues are taken up below.

Using Words or Numerals

The choice between words and numerals affects readability. Just as a page full of abbreviations may be taxing to read, a page full of numbers may look impenetrable. Words are generally less daunting to some readers. On the other hand, rendering large numbers as words takes space, and it can make comparison of values difficult.

Some journals and style manuals have a rule that numbers smaller than 10 should be written out in words and larger ones should be given in Arabic numerals. Or they may recommend writing out isolated two-digit numbers as well. Such rules are satisfactory when the numbers are unimportant in themselves or when nothing is to be gained by following other rules. Those rules, however, do not recognize the various possibilities.

If a number is the first word in a sentence, some journals allow use of an Arabic numeral, and others (still in the majority) require writing it out in words. When other rules come into play, as discussed below, it is better to recast the sentence to avoid having the number at the beginning.

To say "Three physicians met before the operation" can be satisfactory whether the exact number matters or not; it is sometimes simpler to give a concrete number than a vague one. Saying that "A few physicians met before the operation" is equally informative if we do not care whether two or seven met, but only that a small group did. When accuracy is possible, it is usually preferable to vagueness. The reader who gets the impression that the author cannot keep track of or count small numbers may conclude that the author is equally incapable of dealing with larger numbers.

The use of numerals signals to the reader that exact values matter. Numerals are easy to spot in text, so their use facilitates calculation and comparison. Rules that specify a number-of-digits threshold for words versus numerals tend to lose sight of this (e.g., "of 83 patients, eight died"). If the exact number matters, and especially if numbers are to be compared, numerals are typically the better choice.

Exhaustion and Checking

When data are sorted into categories, the author reassures the reader that all cases have been accounted for by using the principle of exhaustion. Sometimes this requires an "all other" category, or something of the sort.

Consider the following passage: "The results of clinical follow-up were available for 341 patients (99.1%). At 30 days, 6 of 135 patients who had been referred from the field had died (4.4%), as had 12 of 209 patients (5.7%) who had been referred from emergency departments."[4] This example, taken on its own, illustrates what happens when the exhaustion principle is not satisfied; the patients in the two referral categories add up to more than the 341 patients mentioned (i.e., 135 + 209 = 344). The reader has just been reminded that 341 is only 99.1% of the total, however, and the careful reader may remember that the total number of patients given elsewhere in the article is 344. This momentary difficulty might have been avoided with "The results of clinical follow-up were available for 341 of the 344 patients (99.1%)." Reminding the reader of the total makes the passage easier to understand.

Large Numbers and Precision

Although scientific journals encourage precise writing, numbers with many distinct digits can lose readers in details when they need primarily to grasp the magnitude. Rounding tends to emphasize the order of magnitude, as does the use of scientific notation. For example, "Nearly 1 million patients were admitted to this class of hospitals in 2008" may be preferable to "This class of hospitals admitted 969,537 patients in 2008." Unfortunately, the author may need to include the actual number in the text, if it is not included in a table, as well as to make sure the reader understands that the number is about a million. In such a case, it is necessary to mention the round number in discussing the magnitude after the precise number has been given. More generally, the author must decide whether to emphasize precision, magnitude, or both. Avoid using precise numbers for estimates. For example, you may calculate that 314,587 heart attacks attributable to a drug side effect may occur in the coming year, but it makes sense to report this estimate only to one or two significant figures (e.g., about 300,000).

Relative and Absolute Differences

In discussing differences and change, it is important to be aware of the distinction between relative differences and absolute differences and to indicate them clearly. An increase in the differential count of band forms from 4% to 6% represents a relative increase of 50%, but it is an absolute increase of 2 percentage points. Similarly, in clear writing, a 5% increase in a hematocrit of 60% results in a hematocrit of 63%, whereas a 5-percentage-point increase results in a hematocrit of 65%.

Numbers Close Together

Putting unrelated numbers side by side confuses the reader, at least temporarily. For example, the sentence "In 2008, 969,537 patients were admitted to this class of hospitals" dazzles the reader because the numbers seem to run together. Perhaps worse examples are the sentences "For $375, 125 women were vaccinated" and "This group of patients with leukemia had an average white-cell count of 257, 112 lymphocytes and 145 other types." Such sentences should be recast to eliminate even momentary confusion.

Parallelism and Similarity

In describing parallel or similar groups, maintain order and similarity of statement to keep the reader oriented. For example, "Among the 30 patients receiving treatment A, 8 contracted pneumonia and 1 of these died; and among the 28 patients receiving treatment B, 4 contracted pneumonia and 2 of these died" is better than "Among the 30 patients receiving treatment A, 8 contracted pneumonia and 1 died, and also 2 died who received treatment B, of whom there were 28 in all, 4 suffering from pneumonia." In the following example the first sentence establishes the order of elements and the second sentence maintains it; this helps the reader to compare the assignment of patients in two trials. "In the European trial, 680 patients were screened, and 612 were randomly assigned to study groups to receive treatment (411 to the dronedarone group and 201 to the placebo group). In the non-European trial, 731 patients were screened, and 625 were randomly assigned to receive treatment (417 to the dronedarone group and 208 to the placebo group)."[5]

Be sure that numbers to be compared are presented in the same way—words or numerals. Either, and even both, can be useful in special circumstances, but keep related numbers alike. For example, write "Among the 78 patients, 14 had fever and 3 had jaundice," not "Seventy-eight patients included 14 with fever and three with jaundice."

When numbers are to be compared, Arabic numerals should be preferred to words. For example, "Among 78 patients, 8 contracted pneumonia" is preferable to "Among 78 patients, eight contracted pneumonia" and also to "Among seventy-eight patients, 8 contracted pneumonia." The first version suggests that 78 and 8 are to be compared and, without saying so, that about 10% contracted pneumonia.

Complications arise when two sets of numbers must be treated simultaneously. Often the numbers in one set act as labels, whereas in the other set the size of the numbers counts. In this circumstance, it may be useful to present one set in numerals and the other in words. For example, either "The three groups of patients included 15 in the one-dose group, 12 in the two-dose group, and 27 in the three-dose group" or "The one-, two-, and three-dose groups included 15, 12, and 27 patients, respectively" is more readable than "In the study, 15 received 1 dose, 12 received 2, and 27 received 3."

Factors and -Fold

For increases or decreases from a starting value, express the change in a way that is clear to the reader. For example, if you write that a rate of 100 per hour increased by a factor of 4, will the reader know whether the new rate is 400 or 500 per hour? It is important to make clear whether you are comparing the initial rate with the new rate or with the amount of increase; in such cases it may be best to be more specific, perhaps by writing that the rate of 100 per hour increased by a factor of four, to 400 per hour, or that the new rate, 400 per hour, was four times the baseline rate, avoiding the word "increase" altogether.

Similarly, a "four-fold increase" is used by some writers to describe a new value that is four times as great as the baseline (e.g., 100 times 4, for a new value of 400) and by others to describe the amount of the increase (e.g., the initial 100 plus 400, for a new value of 500). Some writers use numerals with decimals for "fold increases" (e.g., "a 3.5-fold increase"), giving the appearance of greater precision, but the same concern applies. "Fold decreases" can be even more problematic; can you be sure that a reader will know that by a two-fold decrease you mean a decrease of 50%? Avoiding ambiguity by providing specific values for increases and decreases is typically the safest choice.

Ranges

When numerical values are spelled out in text, express ranges with words. For a range that is defined by two points, the word "to" is usually sufficient (e.g., "treatment typically requires three to five outpatient visits"). Some kinds of numerical ranges, however, require the word "through," to avoid ambiguity. For example, a study conducted from 2006 to 2008 might be a 2-year study or a 3-year study; a study conducted from 2006 through 2008 is likely to have been a 3-year study. It may be better to specify the months in which the study began and ended (e.g., "from July 2006 through December 2008").

For ranges of years used to name time periods, on the other hand, a dash may be used, as long as there is no ambiguity. The following example illustrates this use: "Cross-protection by the unmatched vaccine strain varies, but in the 2003–2004 and 2007–2008 seasons, the influenza A (H3N2) component of the vaccine provided suboptimal protection."[6] The reader immediately understands that two seasons are being compared, each defined according to the calendar years it spans.

A range of numerical values expressed as numerals may be indicated by a hyphen or a dash. To the reader, a hyphen or a dash means up to and including. This treatment of ranges is likely to be confusing if the range involves mathematical symbols or, especially, negative numbers. In such situations it is safer to use words, as in "from 2 to <10" or "from −11.6 to −7.8." In any event, the choice is between using a hyphen or a dash and using "from" and "to"; do not mix the two, as in "from 75–100."

NUMBERS IN TABLES

To discuss numbers in tables, we need the concept of significant figures. In the term "significant figures" the word "significant" refers to the degree of accuracy the number seems to give. The context is usually that of measurement.

The numbers (a) 23,000, (b) 230, (c) 2.3, and (d) 0.0023 all have two significant digits or figures—namely, 2 and 3. In scientific notation, they would be written as follows: (a) 2.3×10^4, (b) 2.3×10^2, (c) 2.3, and (d) 2.3×10^{-3}. In scientific and medical writing, zeros following the last nonzero digit are not ordinarily regarded as significant digits, unless the degree of accuracy is specified, and in a decimal fraction the opening zeros to the right of the decimal point do not count as significant figures. The exception is that in scientific notation it is understood that all digits in a coefficient are significant. Without scientific notation, one may need to emphasize the accuracy of a number such as 300 if exactly 300 is meant.

The number of significant figures gives a hint of the accuracy of the number. For example, 98.2° has three significant digits and might be regarded as correct to within 0.05°. (One should not count heavily on this level of accuracy.) If, however, measurements were taken only to the nearest 10°, a report of 98.2° might mislead the reader about the accuracy of the number, and a one-significant-digit report of 100° might well be regarded as correct to within half a degree. Therefore, in these ambiguous circumstances, the author should tell the reader what degree of accuracy is intended, as nearly as possible.

In scientific notation, 2.3×10^4 equals 23,000, and writing the coefficient as 2.3 suggests that the coefficient is correct to within 0.05, whereas 2.30×10^4 suggests that the coefficient 2.30 is correct to within 0.005. In Table 1, from a case-control study of risk of statin-induced myopathy, the p-values have two significant digits.

Tables have two main, not mutually exclusive, purposes: to record and preserve the numbers for later reference or analysis, and to communicate a message for immediate comprehension and use. If the data are especially valuable for their accuracy or extent, then the purpose may be to preserve the numbers; very large tables of numerical data are often preserved online rather than in print,

Table 1. Genomic Regions Associated with Myopathy in the Genomewide Association Study.*

Chromosome	SNP	Position	p-Value for Trend (1 df)	p-Value for Genotypic Test (2 df)	Risk Allele	Other Allele	Risk-Allele Frequency		p-Value for Hardy–Weinberg Equilibrium among Controls
							Cases	Controls	
12p12	rs4363657	21259989	4.1×10^{-9}	2.5×10^{-8}	C	T	0.46	0.13	1.8×10^{-1}
1p12	rs2490197	118656353	2.6×10^{-5}	1.4×10^{-4}	A	G	0.39	0.18	7.3×10^{-1}
	rs6665507	118661127	2.7×10^{-5}	1.5×10^{-4}	T	C	0.39	0.19	7.3×10^{-1}
	rs10494209	118664994	3.4×10^{-5}	1.8×10^{-4}	A	C	0.39	0.19	7.3×10^{-1}
	rs6428744	118726966	3.6×10^{-5}	1.1×10^{-4}	T	C	0.48	0.26	4.1×10^{-1}
2p11	rs404892	76157421	1.9×10^{-1}	4.0×10^{-5}	T	C	0.54	0.47	6.0×10^{-5}

*Adapted from the SEARCH Collaborative Group.[7] SNP denotes single-nucleotide polymorphism.

Table 2. Antibiotic Use.*

Antibiotic	SDD		SOD		Standard Care
	No. of Defined Daily Doses	Percent Change (vs. Standard Care)	No. of Defined Daily Doses	Percent Change (vs. Standard Care)	No. of Defined Daily Doses
Penicillins	9,767	−27.8	12,805	−5.3	13,523
Carbapenems	724	−45.7	995	−25.4	1,334
Cephalosporins	8,473	+86.6	3,935	−13.3	4,541
Quinolones	2,637	−31.4	3,291	−14.4	3,846
Lincosamides	473	−11.6	553	+3.4	535
Other antibiotics	7,589	−23.4	8,720	−12.0	9,909
All systemic antibiotics	29,663	−11.9	30,299	−10.1	33,688

*Adapted from de Smet et al.[8] SDD denotes selective digestive tract decontamination, and SOD selective oropharyngeal decontamination.

and they may be downloaded for analysis rather than read. In tables of physical constants, normal laboratory values, or population censuses, for example, a great number of significant digits may be given for the benefit of a future user. In such cases, it is wise to keep as many digits as the data afford or the future user may wish. To preserve numbers because of their accuracy or extent, storage online in an appendix or a data repository may be advisable.

Instead of recording or preserving numbers, many scientific tables communicate messages that the authors wish to deliver. For this purpose, the rule should be to use as few digits as will still deliver the message; the fewer the digits, the more comprehensible the numbers. Readers who are daunted by one six-digit number may find whole tables of them incomprehensible, but most readers are able to compare one- or two-digit numbers.

In some instances, showing both numerical data and their deviation from a standard communicates the message better than the data would alone. In Table 2, numbers of doses of antibiotics among intensive-care patients receiving specific infection-prevention treatments are compared with numbers of doses among patients receiving standard care; the two Percent Change columns show how much the specific treatments vary from standard care. This way of presenting the data simplifies the comparisons; because the authors have already done the calculations and provided the differences as positive and negative values, it is easy to spot large and small differences and their direction.

The discussion above emphasizes understanding numbers within an article. When the numbers are to be used again in secondary analyses, a high degree of accuracy in the primary numbers can be very useful. Consequently, statistics on improvements in therapy, such as percentage survival, average length of hospital stay, and test statistics such as t and chi-squared, should be given accurately (usually to three significant figures), and significance levels should, when possible, be given to two significant figures, rather than merely reported as $p < 0.05$ or $p > 0.05$, for example.

A good deal of folklore and personal experience suggest that when numbers are to be compared, they are better understood when lined up vertically instead of horizontally. Table 3 illustrates this principle, using data from a retrospective study of in vitro fertilization (IVF) treatment at a large center. If, however, the columns after the first had given only the percentages, the results for the cycles would have been easier to compare. Note that reading across is difficult, not only because the numbers are farther apart, but also because of uncertainty that the eye is following the appropriate row, and in this example because each entry gives two types of information (a number and a percentage). Empty rows can aid the eye in reading across, but they weaken the vertical comparisons. Very light shading can be useful in leading the eye across rows and, in more complex tables, in grouping data.

Table 3. Cycle Outcomes in Various In Vitro Fertilization Procedures. [*]

Cycle	No. in Cohort	Oocyte-Retrieval Procedures[†]	Embryo-Transfer Procedures[†]	Pregnancies[†]	Live Births[†]	Deliveries[‡] Singleton	Deliveries[‡] Twin	Deliveries[‡] Triplet
	no.				no. (%)			
1	6164	5360 (87.0)	4825 (78.3)	2025 (32.9)	1511 (24.5)	1046 (69.2)	439 (29.1)	26 (1.7)
2	3837	3450 (89.9)	3142 (81.9)	1115 (29.1)	784 (20.4)	563 (71.8)	207 (26.4)	14 (1.8)
3	2228	2019 (90.6)	1839 (82.5)	673 (30.2)	475 (21.3)	343 (72.2)	125 (26.3)	7 (1.5)
4	1170	1078 (92.1)	993 (84.9)	337 (28.8)	221 (18.9)	160 (72.4)	55 (24.9)	6 (2.7)
5	573	527 (92.0)	483 (84.3)	157 (27.4)	99 (17.3)	78 (78.8)	19 (19.2)	2 (2.0)
6	276	255 (92.4)	235 (85.1)	58 (21.0)	36 (13.0)	27 (75.0)	9 (25.0)	0

[*]Adapted from Malizia et al.[9]

[†]The denominator is the number of women in the cycle cohort. (All patients without a live birth in an IVF cycle were eligible for the subsequent cycle, but some did not return for treatment.)

[‡]The denominator is the number of live births in the cycle.

Although using fewer digits promotes understanding, greater precision and more digits may be required for comparison of numerical values within the table. (Calculation is a different matter, not treated here.)

In Table 4, Section A shows attractive uniformity, but it leans more toward preserving the data than toward making them comprehensible. As Section B illustrates, the same table with the decimals rounded off (or dropped, if preferred) is more readable. In reducing the number of digits for ease of comprehension, it may not matter whether the later digits are dropped or rounded off; dropping them may be more convenient. When rounding, a good rule is to round to the nearest number, or if rounding a 5, to the nearest even number. Round 95.1 to 95, but 95.5 to 96 and 94.5 to 94. In this table, rounding makes the similarities within and among cohorts more apparent, and it makes vertical comparisons among age groups easier. Note also that the age groups listed have neither gaps nor overlaps.

Like the totals in the text, the totals in tables should check. Unless individuals can belong to more than one category, percentages should add up to nearly 100. Because of rounding, the percentages will often not add up to exactly 100, except when one is dealing with two categories. Keeping more decimal places does not solve this problem.[11] It is customary to add a footnote stating that, because of rounding, the percentages do not add up to 100. When an author gives, without comment, many columns of percentages based on frequencies, each adding up to exactly 100, the reader has reason to suspect that the author has "fudged" the numbers a bit in a manner that has not been described (except for such special sample sizes as 2, 4, 5, 10, 20, 25, and 50, where two-digit percentages always do add up to 100). For scientific writing, the numbers should not be manipulated in this way. In nonscientific writing, the failure of the percentages to add up to 100 may be a distraction that prevents the reader from paying attention to the main points of the discussion, and so the recommendation does not apply. For intellectual honesty, a footnote might state that the percentages have been adjusted to add up to 100. Chapter 14 has a further discussion of presenting tables; see especially the National Halothane Study example.

SYMBOLS

Unfortunately no single set of symbols covers all occasions, and various symbols customarily mean different things in different contexts. Still, for general use in statistical writing, the lists in Table 5 may be helpful. Whatever notation is chosen, conventional or not, the definitions of any letters should be specified. The reader should not have to guess that n is the sample size or that π is the usual 3.14.

Table 4. Baseline Age of Study Patients Undergoing Coronary-Artery Bypass Grafting (CABG), According to Cohort.*

Age	Primary Cohort		Highly Selected Cohort		Instrumental-Variable Subcohort (90% vs. 10%)†	
	Aprotinin (N = 33,517)	Aminocaproic Acid (N = 44,682)	Aprotinin (N = 4799)	Aminocaproic Acid (N = 4799)	Aprotinin (N = 15,228)	Aminocaproic Acid (N = 10,556)
Section A				percent of patients		
18–24 yr	0	0	0	0	0	0
25–34 yr	0.2	0.2	0.2	0.2	0.2	0.2
35–44 yr	2.4	3.0	2.7	2.5	2.4	3.1
45–54 yr	12.4	13.9	12.9	13.1	12.4	13.6
55–64 yr	25.9	27.9	26.3	25.8	26.1	28.2
65–74 yr	32.4	32.1	31.3	31.6	32.7	32.2
≥75 yr	26.7	23.0	26.6	26.8	26.2	22.7
Section B						
18–24 yr	0	0	0	0	0	0
25–34 yr	0	0	0	0	0	0
35–44 yr	2	3	3	2	2	3
45–54 yr	12	14	13	13	12	14
55–64 yr	26	28	26	26	26	28
65–74 yr	32	32	31	32	33	32
≥75 yr	27	23	27	27	26	23

*Adapted from Schneeweiss et al.[10]

†In this subcohort, CABG was performed by surgeons who used aprotinin in 90% or more of their patients or by those who used aprotinin in 10% or fewer of their patients.

In the physical sciences and in mathematics, it is an international convention to use italic letters for variables such as p for probability, t for time, and x for the ubiquitous unknown of algebra. Roman letters are used for the abbreviations for functions such as cos for cosine or log for logarithm or ln for natural logarithm (logarithm to the base e).

Some symbols that cause relatively little trouble are $=$, meaning "equals" or sometimes "which equals"; $\neq$, meaning "does not equal"; $\doteq$ or $\approx$, meaning "approximately equal"; and $\equiv$, usually meaning "equal by definition." Thus, if we define the circumference (C) of a circle in terms of the radius (r), we could say "$C = 2\pi r$, where $\pi = 3.14$."

More trouble comes from the inequality signs, $>$ and $<$. These symbols mean "greater than" and "less than," respectively. For example, $3 > 2$ and $-10 < 2$. In the correct sequence $0.2 < p < 0.5$, the interpretation is that p exceeds 0.2 and is exceeded by 0.5, and therefore it is in the interval from 0.2 to 0.5. Some writers think these symbols are a frame and write incorrectly that $0.2 < p > 0.5$. If this expression means anything, it means that p exceeds 0.2 and that it also exceeds 0.5, and so the latter part of the statement would have conveyed all the information. In text, it is preferable to write out expressions such as "greater than" instead of using $>$ as an abbreviation, though parenthetical remarks such as "$(r > 0.87)$" can be used.

In some physics works, $<x>$ has been used to mean the average value of x. In statistics it is more usual to indicate averages by putting a bar over a symbol, so that $\bar{x}$ is the average of the x values and $\overline{\log x}$ is the average of the logarithms of the x values.

Most publications prefer unstacked fractions and equations (that is, those that fit on a single line of text) because they take up less space. An equation that is stacked usually requires the addition of fences (parentheses, brackets, or braces) when it is unstacked, to avoid a change in meaning. For example,

$$\frac{a+b}{c} \neq a + b/c = a + \frac{b}{c}.$$

Instead, use

$$\frac{a+b}{c} = (a+b)/c.$$

Unstacking requires care and knowledge, and often more effort, than simply inserting the solidus ($/$, also called a virgule) between the numerator and the denominator.

A related complication applies to the use of the square-root symbol $\sqrt{}$. In $\sqrt{a+b}$ the horizontal bar or vinculum actually serves as a pair of parentheses; it groups $a + b$. Without it, $\sqrt{a}+b$ might mean $b + \sqrt{a}$ or it might mean $\sqrt{a+b}$. Nevertheless, the square-root sign without the vinculum is often used in mathematical

Table 5. Symbols Commonly Used in Statistical Writing.

English Alphabet

a, b, c, d	often stand for constants, especially c because it is the first letter of "constant"; also, b is often used for coefficients in a regression equation.
e	may be reserved for the base of the natural logarithms, 2.71828…; also used for errors.
f	used both for mathematical function and for frequency.
F	special statistic used in the analysis of variance; also often a cumulative distribution function.
g, h	a mathematical function.
i, j	often used for an integer, but sometimes for an imaginary number.
k	an integer or a constant (first letter of German word "Konstant").
l, o	often avoided because of confusion with 1 and 0 (one and zero).
m	an integer.
n, N	an integer, especially a sample size (n) or a population size (N).
p, P	a probability.
q	a probability, usually the complement ($q = 1 - p$) of some probability, p.
r, s, t, T	integers; each also has a common technical meaning: r, a sample correlation coefficient; s, a sample standard deviation; t, a special statistic called Student's t, after the pseudonym of William S. Gosset (t is also often used to indicate time); T, a generalized t-statistic for higher dimensions called Hotelling's T.
u, v	variables.
w	often used for weighting.
x, y, z	usually variables; z is sometimes a variable with zero mean and unit standard deviation.

Greek Alphabet

α	the significance level of a statistical test, also called the probability of a Type I error.
β	the power of a statistical test is $1 - \beta$, and β is the probability of accepting the null hypothesis when it is false (called a Type II error); also a coefficient in a regression equation.
δ, Δ	a difference.
ε	usually a small number.
θ	a parameter to be estimated.
κ	a statistical measure of association in a contingency table (table of counts).
λ	often the mean of a Poisson distribution.
μ	a population mean.
ν	a frequency, or a raw moment.
π, Π	3.14… ; more often a true probability, or proportion; $\prod_{i=1}^{n}$ indicates a product.
σ	a population standard deviation.
Σ	a summation operator.
τ	a measure of association.
ϕ, Φ	a mathematical function, sometimes the Gaussian (normal) density function and cumulative distribution function.
ρ	a population correlation coefficient.
χ	when squared, the distribution for a statistic measuring goodness of fit (X^2), among other things.
ψ	a mathematical function.

writing, even though it may be unclear how far the radical extends. For example, a coefficient in the probability density function of the Gaussian distribution involves $\sqrt{2\pi\sigma^2}$, which could be written as $\sqrt{2\pi}\sigma$ or as $\sigma\sqrt{2\pi}$. Some authors write instead $\sqrt{2\pi}\sigma$, which is satisfactory for those who know that the radical applies only to 2π but not for those unfamiliar with the formula. Apparently, the radical without the vinculum is like words for Humpty Dumpty in *Through the Looking Glass*: it means what the author intends it to mean.

One way out of this difficulty, though not an attractive one, is to use fractional exponents. In the examples above, $\sqrt{a+b}$ could be replaced by $(a + b)^{1/2}$; $\sqrt{2\pi\sigma^2}$ could be replaced by $(2\pi\sigma^2)^{1/2}$, by $(2\pi)^{1/2}\sigma$, or even by $\sigma(2\pi)^{1/2}$.

ACKNOWLEDGMENTS

John Bailar, David Dorer, Karen Falkner, Katherine Godfrey, Colin Goodall, David Hoaglin, Edward Huth, Lois Kellerman, Philip Lavori, Robert Lew, Lillian Lin, Thomas Louis, Marjorie Olson, Kay Patterson, Marcia Polansky, and Kerr White contributed helpful discussion and comments on Frederick Mosteller's manuscript for the original version of this chapter.

REFERENCES

1. Chicago manual of style. 15th ed. Chicago: University of Chicago Press, 2003.

2. AMA manual of style: A guide for authors and editors. 10th ed. New York: Oxford, 2007.

3. Scientific style and format: The CSE manual for authors, editors, and publishers. 7th ed. Reston, VA: Council of Science Editors, 2006.

4. Le May MR, So DY, Dionne R, et al. A citywide protocol for primary PCI in ST-segment elevation myocardial infarction. N Engl J Med 2008; 358:231–40.

5. Singh BN, Connolly SJ, Crijns HJ, et al. Dronedarone for maintenance of sinus rhythm in atrial fibrillation or flutter. N Engl J Med 2007; 357:987–99.

6. Glezen WP. Prevention and treatment of seasonal influenza. N Engl J Med 2008; 359:2579–85.

7. The SEARCH Collaborative Group. *SLCO1B1* variants and statin-induced myopathy—a genomewide study. N Engl J Med 2008; 359:789–99.

8. de Smet AM, Kluytmans JA, Cooper BS, et al. Decontamination of the digestive tract and oropharynx in ICU patients. N Engl J Med 2009; 360:20–31.

9. Malizia BA, Hacker MR, Penzias AS. Cumulative live-birth rates after in vitro fertilization. N Engl J Med 2009; 360:236–43.

10. Schneeweiss S, Seeger JD, Landon J, Walker AM. Aprotinin during coronary-artery bypass grafting and risk of death. N Engl J Med 2008; 358:771–83.

11. Mosteller F, Youtz C, Zahn D. The distribution of sums of rounded percentages. Demography 1967; 4:850–8.

Specialized Methods

Combining Results from Independent Studies: Systematic Reviews and Meta-Analysis in Clinical Research

MICHAEL A. STOTO, PH.D.

ABSTRACT   Systematic review and meta-analysis are tools that provide a logical framework for synthesizing the results of independent scientific studies bearing on a clinical or public health issue. Systematic reviews identify, analyze, and present available data and offer the potential to identify areas of agreement, clarify the nature and causes of disagreement, establish what is known prior to further research, identify areas needing more research, and frame results so they can be translated into practice and policy. When meta-analysis is appropriate, it can substantially increase statistical power and resolve issues relating to conflicting results among many small studies.

Like all statistical tools, however, meta-analysis can be abused, and indeed some systematic reviews, and especially meta-analyses, that have used these tools have been controversial. In some cases the issue itself is contentious, and any analysis would be controversial. For other issues the best available evidence is simply not very good, and no analysis can resolve the uncertainty and provide clarity. In other instances, however, analysts have not used the most appropriate methods, or may have intentionally biased the results.

For systematic review and meta-analysis to live up to their promise, it is at least as important for readers to understand the methods and pitfalls as it is for authors to give proper attention to best practices in research synthesis, including judicious use of formal meta-analysis and the careful exploration of study quality and heterogeneity. The expertise needed for doing a systematic review includes both clinical and technical (statistical) understanding, and the amount of effort required is similar to that for a standard research paper.

E vidence-based medicine requires that practitioners use the most relevant research results in a rapidly growing medical literature, whose sheer volume makes the task time-consuming. *Systematic reviews* employ a set of procedures developed to provide a logical framework for the science of research synthesis—the systematic and objective review of the results of independent scientific studies bearing on a common clinical issue. Within this general framework, the statistical tool of *meta-analysis* involves the quantitative analysis of a collection of statistical results from individual studies for the purpose of integrating the findings into a common measure of effect. Systematic review and meta-analysis are increasingly popular in clinical research, and the results of this research are widely used as the basis for evidence-based medicine, practice recommendations, and policy decisions.

The methods of systematic review were introduced into clinical medicine in the 1980s, largely by the British clinical researcher Archie Cochrane, one of the strongest advocates for randomized clinical trials (RCTs). He was suggesting by 1979 that the results of these trials be systematically summarized. The systematic review methods were further developed in the 1990s, drawing on statistical tools for meta-analysis from the social and behavioral sciences. The support of the U.S. Agency for Health Care Policy and Research (now the Agency for Healthcare Research and Quality [AHRQ]) through a network of Patient Outcome Research Teams (PORTs) at academic medical centers, was especially influential in the development and dissemination of methods for research synthesis and meta-analysis. In the 21st century the Cochrane Collaboration, a global network of clinical researchers that develops methods for systematic reviews and works collaboratively to carry them out and publish the results, plays an important leadership role in the field. In the United States, AHRQ's network of Evidence-based Practice Centers plays a similar role.

Systematic reviews, and meta-analyses in particular, are increasingly popular. Figure 1 displays the number of meta-analyses recorded between 1995 and 2007 in MEDLINE. In a decade, the number has almost quadrupled. The enthusiasm reflected in these numbers, however, is tempered by skepticism by some and complete aversion by others. The title of Shapiro's paper—"Meta-analysis shmeta-analysis"—makes his views clear.[1] In 1997, for instance, Bailar wrote in *The New England Journal of Medicine*[2] that

> In my own review of selected meta-analyses,[3] problems were so frequent and so serious, including bias on the part of the meta-analyst, that it was difficult to trust the overall "best estimates" that the method often produces. On present evidence, we can generally accept the results of a well-done meta-analysis as a way to present the results of disparate studies on a common scale... but any attempt to reduce the results to a single value, with confidence bounds, is likely to lead to conclusions that are wrong, perhaps seriously so. I still prefer conventional narrative reviews of the literature, a type of summary familiar to readers of the countless review articles on important medical issues.[2]

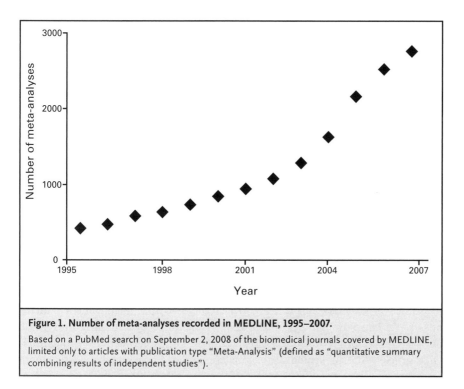

Figure 1. Number of meta-analyses recorded in MEDLINE, 1995–2007.
Based on a PubMed search on September 2, 2008 of the biomedical journals covered by MEDLINE, limited only to articles with publication type "Meta-Analysis" (defined as "quantitative summary combining results of independent studies").

Although there are clearly problems with meta-analyses in the published literature, consider the alternative—unsystematic review of existing evidence. The narrative reviews that typically appear in the introduction of new research results or as review articles rely on the judgment of the reviewer in selecting and weighting the relevance of results from diverse studies, and it is often difficult to gauge the comprehensiveness of the review and impossible to verify its conclusions. Oxman and Guyatt, for instance, noted that "experts, on average, write reviews of inferior quality; that the greater the expertise, the more likely the quality is to be poor; and that the poor quality may be related to the strength of the prior opinions and the amount of time they spend preparing a review article."[4]

In 2005 Chalmers wrote in *The Lancet* that it "is unscientific and unethical to embark on new research without first analysing systematically what can be learned from existing research; . . . it is impossible for consumers of research results to assess what contribution a new study has made unless its results have been set systematically in the context of an up-to-date review of the totality of the relevant evidence."[5] Noting that "Unnecessary . . . clinical research injures volunteers and patients as surely as any other form of bad medicine, as well as wasting resources and abusing the trust placed in investigators by their trial participants," Young and Horton announced a policy that *The Lancet* will require authors of clinical trials "to include a clear summary of previous research findings, and to explain how their trial's findings affect this summary."[6]

Like all statistical tools and research methods, the validity of the results and conclusions from systematic reviews and meta-analyses depends on proper use of the appropriate tools. Pitfalls include not using proper methods, misinterpreting results, and focusing on summarizing many studies in a single number when the studies differ in design, populations, and methods. This chapter aims to enable the reader to judge the quality of published systematic reviews and meta-analyses and the relevance of their results to clinical decision-making.

SYSTEMATIC REVIEWS IN
THE NEW ENGLAND JOURNAL OF MEDICINE

Although averaging only about one per year, the systematic reviews and meta-analyses published in the *Journal* illustrate the breadth of current practice of research synthesis, perhaps tending toward more-sophisticated statistical methods. Table 1 lists the ten systematic reviews identified by searching for "meta" or "systematic review" in title or abstract of all issues between 1993 and 2005. Only articles that presented an original or updated meta-analysis either as a primary focus or a major component of the research publication were included. Table 1 also summarizes key methodological aspects of each paper, including publication bias, input study quality, statistical methods, and heterogeneity, each of which is discussed below.

Three of the systematic reviews summarize RCTs of interventions to treat cancer (radiotherapy and surgery in early breast cancer,[7] adjuvant chemotherapy for resected colon cancer in elderly patients,[8] and prophylactic cranial irradiation for patients with small-cell lung cancer in complete remission[9]). Three more reviews summarize the effects of a broader range of interventions (cesarean sections and the risk of vertical transmission of HIV,[10] effect of increasing soy protein intake on serum lipids,[11] and the efficacy of placebos[12]).The other systematic reviews summarize observational epidemiological studies. One deals with the relationship between coronary heart disease and passive smoking[13] and one with evaluating the predictive value of C-reactive protein in general populations.[14] The final two examine the association between silicone breast implants and the risk of connective-tissue diseases[15] and mutations in the HRAS1 minisatellite locus and the risk of cancer.[16]

To illustrate the range of systematic reviews currently used in the medical literature, consider the following examples. He and colleagues[13] conducted a meta-analysis of the risk of coronary heart disease associated with passive

Table 1. Key Characteristics of Systematic Reviews and Meta-Analyses Published in *The New England Journal of Medicine*, 1993 to 2005.

Author, Date	Topic	Publication Bias	Study Quality	Statistical Methods	Heterogeneity
Krontiris, 1993[16] (MA included along with new original results)	Mutations in the HRAS1 mini-satellite locus and the risk of cancer (observational)	No evidence of publication bias by funnel plot or analysis of non-significant studies	Sensitivity analysis by study quality measures	FE analysis of log OR; RE analysis of differences in probability of rare alleles	Chi-squared tests indicate no evidence of heterogeneity in subgroups tested
Anderson, 1995[11]	Effect of increasing soy protein intake on serum lipids (RCTs)	NA	NA	RE analysis of net change and mean difference in lipid concentration	Subgroup analysis by initial serum cholesterol; hierarchical linear predictive models with study- and individual-level data
Early Breast Cancer Trialists' Collaborative Group, 1995[7]	Efficacy of radiotherapy and surgery in early breast cancer (RCTs)	NA	NA	FE analysis of proportional hazard rate for mortality	Chi-squared tests indicate no evidence of heterogeneity in subgroups tested
He, 1999[13]	Passive smoking and the risk of CHD (observational)	No evidence of publication bias by funnel plot or Kendall's tau	Sensitivity analysis by type of study	FE analysis of log of matched or adjusted OR (identical to RE)	Linear regression to test dose-response relation
Aupérin, 1999[9]	Efficacy of prophylactic cranial irradiation for patients with small-cell lung cancer in complete remission (RCTs)	NA	NA	FE analysis of proportional hazard rate for mortality calculated from individual-level data	Chi-squared test indicates no evidence of heterogeneity

Abbreviations: MA, meta-analysis; NA, not applicable; FE, fixed-effects model; RE, random-effects model

Table 1. Key Characteristics of Systematic Reviews and Meta-Analyses Published in *The New England Journal of Medicine*, 1993 to 2005 (*continued*).

International Perinatal HIV Group, 1999[10]	Mode of delivery and the risk of vertical transmission of HIV (RCTs)	NA	NA	FE and RE analysis of OR; pooled analysis of individual-level data (indicator variables for study not significant)	Chi-squared test indicates no evidence of heterogeneity
Janowsky, 2000[15]	Silicone breast implants and the risk of connective-tissue diseases (observational)	NA	Stratified analysis by study quality measures	FE analysis of unadjusted and adjusted log OR or RR	Chi-squared test indicates no evidence of heterogeneity once outliers are removed
Hrobjartsson, 2001[12]	Efficacy of placebo compared to no treatment (RCTs)	No evidence of publication bias by funnel plot	Sensitivity analysis by study quality measures	RE analysis of RR or standardized mean difference	Chi-squared or F tests; pre-planned subgroup analyses by type of placebo and outcome
Sargent, 2001[8]	Efficacy of adjuvant chemotherapy for resected colon cancer in elderly patients (RCTs)	NA	NA	MA of hazard rates (method not stated); pooled analysis of individual-level data (no indication whether study-level variables were included in the model)	Between-study heterogeneity not significant (method not stated)
Danesh, 2004[14] (Updated MA included along with new original results)	Predictive value of C-reactive protein in the prediction of CHD in general populations (observational)	Extreme findings in early, smaller studies may be due to publication bias	NA	FE analysis of adjusted log OR for CHD	Chi-squared test indicates heterogeneity not associated with subgroups tested

Abbreviations: MA, meta-analysis; NA, not applicable; FE, fixed-effects model; RE, random-effects model smoking among nonsmokers. They identified 18 epidemiologic (10 cohort and 8 case–control) studies that met pre-stated inclusion criteria. The results are presented in a *forest plot*, in which each study is represented by one line, as the trees in a forest. Summarizing study-level measures of association, they found that nonsmokers exposed to environmental smoke had a relative risk of coronary heart disease of 1.25 (95% confidence interval, 1.17 to 1.32) as compared with nonsmokers not exposed to smoke (see Figure 2). Passive smoking was consistently and significantly associated with an increased relative risk of coronary heart disease in cohort studies and case–control studies, in men and women, and in those exposed to smoking at home or in the workplace. A dose-response relation was identified, with respective relative risks of 1.23 and 1.31 for nonsmokers who were exposed to the smoke of 1 to 19 cigarettes per day and those who were exposed to the smoke of 20 or more cigarettes per day, as compared with nonsmokers not exposed to smoke ($p = 0.006$ for linear trend).

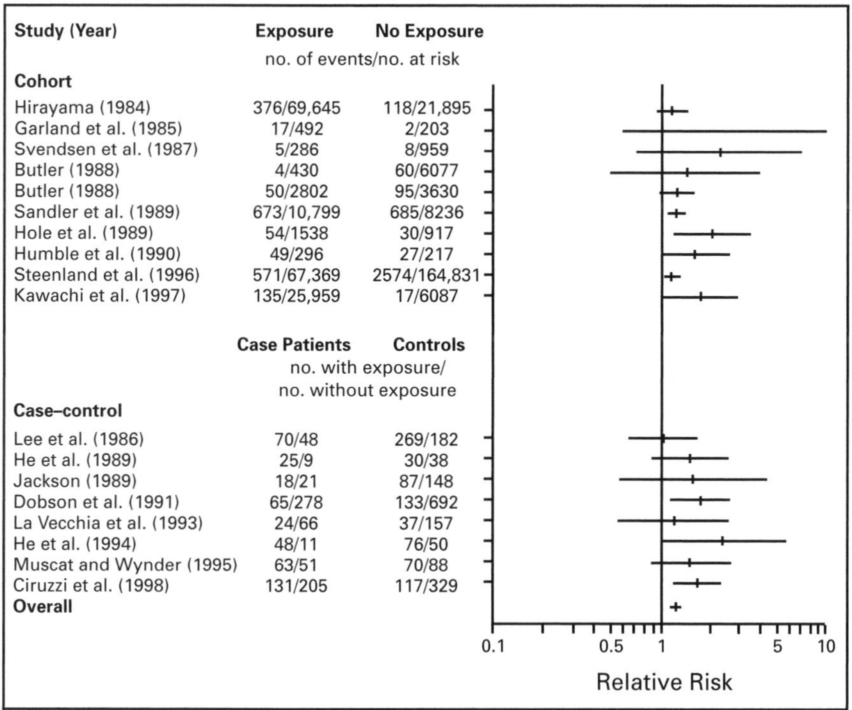

Study (Year)	Exposure	No Exposure	
	no. of events/no. at risk		
Cohort			
Hirayama (1984)	376/69,645	118/21,895	
Garland et al. (1985)	17/492	2/203	
Svendsen et al. (1987)	5/286	8/959	
Butler (1988)	4/430	60/6077	
Butler (1988)	50/2802	95/3630	
Sandler et al. (1989)	673/10,799	685/8236	
Hole et al. (1989)	54/1538	30/917	
Humble et al. (1990)	49/296	27/217	
Steenland et al. (1996)	571/67,369	2574/164,831	
Kawachi et al. (1997)	135/25,959	17/6087	
	Case Patients	**Controls**	
	no. with exposure/		
	no. without exposure		
Case–control			
Lee et al. (1986)	70/48	269/182	
He et al. (1989)	25/9	30/38	
Jackson (1989)	18/21	87/148	
Dobson et al. (1991)	65/278	133/692	
La Vecchia et al. (1993)	24/66	37/157	
He et al. (1994)	48/11	76/50	
Muscat and Wynder (1995)	63/51	70/88	
Ciruzzi et al. (1998)	131/205	117/329	
Overall			

Relative Risk scale: 0.1, 0.5, 1, 5, 10

Figure 2. Forest plot and meta-analyses summarizing the relative risk of coronary heart disease associated with passive smoking.

The relative risk in the study by Garland et al. was 14.9.

Source: He et al., 1999.[13]

From this analysis the authors concluded that passive smoking is associated with an increase in the risk of coronary heart disease.

In his critique of the study, Bailar mentioned the possibility of publication bias, the quality of the original studies (including the potential for bias), and heterogeneity of the results from these studies.[17] These important issues for all meta-analyses are discussed in detail below. Bailar also noted that the 25% increase in risk that He and colleagues found is roughly one-third to one-fourth of the risk associated with direct smoking, making the magnitude of the meta-analysis result seem implausible. (Bailar questioned the size of the relationship, not its existence.) Howard and Thun[18] addressed this question by using linear regression to describe the relationship between daily cigarette use and CHD mortality. Assuming that involuntary smokers had been exposed to the equivalent of 0.75 cigarettes per day, the authors found that the expected CHD mortality ratio ranged from 1.13 to 1.47 across the seven studies they examined, with an overall average of 1.32. The authors of the 2006 Surgeon General's report on involuntary smoking[19] updated He and colleagues' meta-analyses[13] and found similar results, and addressed the issues of publication bias, quality of studies, and heterogeneity, but did not find that they undercut the results of the meta-analysis. The Surgeon General's report also endorsed the Howard and Thun analysis,[18] and concluded that "[t]he evidence is sufficient to infer a causal relationship between exposure to secondhand smoke and increased risks of coronary heart disease . . . mortality among both men and women" and that the "pooled relative risks from meta-analyses indicate a 25 to 30% increase in the risk of coronary heart disease from exposure to secondhand smoke."[19]

The International Perinatal HIV Group[10] used a systematic review to evaluate the relation between elective cesarean section and vertical transmission of HIV-1. Their analysis (Figure 3) included 15 prospective cohort studies with at least 100 mother–child pairs. Going beyond the typical meta-analysis, the authors obtained the original patient-level data from the studies and applied a common set of inclusion and exclusion criteria to select a comparable group of individuals from each study. Using a statistical model similar to those used in a multi-institutional study, after adjusting for receipt of antiretroviral therapy, maternal stage of disease, and infant birth weight, the authors found that elective cesarean section decreased the likelihood of vertical transmission of HIV-1 by approximately 50% as compared with other modes of delivery (adjusted odds ratio, 0.43; 95% confidence interval, 0.33 to 0.56). The authors concluded that elective cesarean section reduces the risk of transmission of HIV-1 from mother to child independently of the effects of other treatments.

Because the randomized trials of radiotherapy and surgery for early breast cancer may have been too small to detect differences in long-term survival and recurrence reliably, the Early Breast Cancer Trialists' Collaborative Group[7]

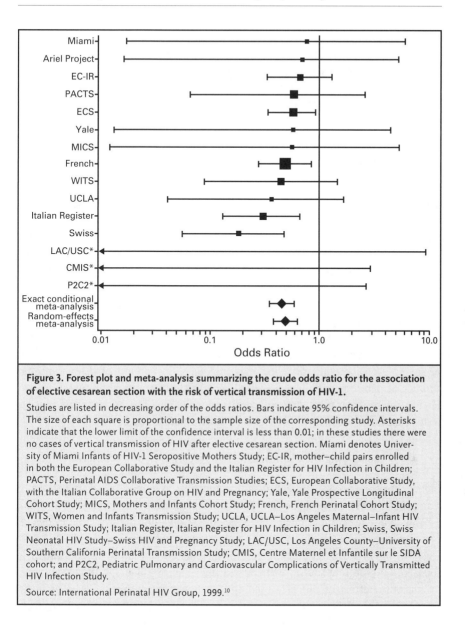

Figure 3. Forest plot and meta-analysis summarizing the crude odds ratio for the association of elective cesarean section with the risk of vertical transmission of HIV-1.

Studies are listed in decreasing order of the odds ratios. Bars indicate 95% confidence intervals. The size of each square is proportional to the sample size of the corresponding study. Asterisks indicate that the lower limit of the confidence interval is less than 0.01; in these studies there were no cases of vertical transmission of HIV after elective cesarean section. Miami denotes University of Miami Infants of HIV-1 Seropositive Mothers Study; EC-IR, mother–child pairs enrolled in both the European Collaborative Study and the Italian Register for HIV Infection in Children; PACTS, Perinatal AIDS Collaborative Transmission Studies; ECS, European Collaborative Study, with the Italian Collaborative Group on HIV and Pregnancy; Yale, Yale Prospective Longitudinal Cohort Study; MICS, Mothers and Infants Cohort Study; French, French Perinatal Cohort Study; WITS, Women and Infants Transmission Study; UCLA, UCLA–Los Angeles Maternal–Infant HIV Transmission Study; Italian Register, Italian Register for HIV Infection in Children; Swiss, Swiss Neonatal HIV Study–Swiss HIV and Pregnancy Study; LAC/USC, Los Angeles County–University of Southern California Perinatal Transmission Study; CMIS, Centre Maternel et Infantile sur le SIDA cohort; and P2C2, Pediatric Pulmonary and Cardiovascular Complications of Vertically Transmitted HIV Infection Study.

Source: International Perinatal HIV Group, 1999.[10]

performed a systematic review of 36 trials comparing radiotherapy plus surgery with the same type of surgery alone, 10 comparing more-extensive surgery with less-extensive surgery, and 18 comparing more-extensive surgery with less-extensive surgery plus radiotherapy. These studies included a total of over 28,000 women. The investigators found that the addition of radiotherapy to surgery resulted in a rate of local recurrence that was three times lower than the rate with surgery alone, but no significant difference in 10-year survival. Some of the therapies had substantially different effects on the rates of local recurrence—such as the reduced recurrence rate when radiotherapy was added to surgery—but they produced no definite differences in overall survival at 10 years (see Figure 4).

THE PRACTICE OF RESEARCH SYNTHESIS

If the results of systematic reviews and meta-analyses are to be both credible and useful, certain research practices must be carefully followed. Systematic reviews involve five discrete steps, each of which requires some important judgments. First, authors must identify the specific clinical or policy question to be addressed, and express it in terms of research results. Second, all relevant studies that have a bearing on that question must be identified and retrieved, and the necessary descriptive information and results extracted. The choice of articles is often the most critical decision that a meta-analyst makes, and it must be objective and reproducible. Third, the reviewer must evaluate the quality of individual studies, and decide whether some should be excluded or given less weight in the analysis. Fourth, the results must be analyzed and summarized. The summaries can be qualitative or quantitative, and may include a description of the nature and sources of heterogeneity in the results. Each of these points is discussed below. Finally, the reviewer must draw appropriate conclusions and present them in ways well suited to guide clinical practice and inform policy decisions.

Identifying the Clinical or Policy Question to Be Addressed

Identifying the specific clinical or policy question to be addressed in a research synthesis is often more difficult than one might expect. The choice must strike a balance between the clinical and policy questions and the available evidence. For instance, "What is the mortality reduction in colorectal cancer from yearly fecal occult blood screening in 40- to 45-year-old females?" is too narrowly focused, and too few studies will address this specific issue. On the other hand, "What is the effect of cancer screening on the general public?" is too broad to be meaningful. "What is the mortality reduction in colorectal cancer from fecal occult blood screening in adults?" strikes a good balance.[20]

Research syntheses can serve a variety of purposes, and should use methods suitable for the intended purpose. Systematic reviews aim to identify, analyze, and present the results of all relevant scientific studies bearing on a common clinical issue. In doing so, they may serve one or more of the following purposes:

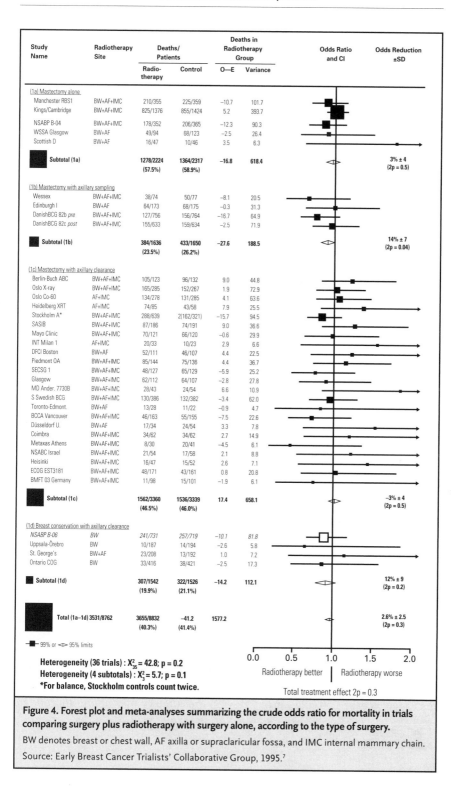

Figure 4. Forest plot and meta-analyses summarizing the crude odds ratio for mortality in trials comparing surgery plus radiotherapy with surgery alone, according to the type of surgery.

BW denotes breast or chest wall, AF axilla or supraclaricular fossa, and IMC internal mammary chain.

Source: Early Breast Cancer Trialists' Collaborative Group, 1995.[7]

- identify areas of agreement in the literature;
- clarify the nature and causes of disagreement;
- establish what is known, and not known, prior to further research;
- identify areas needing more research, or help to decide that no further research is needed;
- frame results so they can be translated into clinical practice and policy.

Meta-analysis, which uses statistical methods to prepare quantitative summaries of the results of individual papers, also offers the potential to:

- improve the precision of summary effect estimates relative to the individual studies;
- increase statistical power; and
- describe conflicting results in terms of differences in study methods, treatments, or outcomes.

Identifying Relevant Studies

Systematic reviews are fundamentally observational research, in which the reviewer has no control over the original research or its reporting. Moreover, choices about identifying and including original results face some of the same biases regarding availability of information as in all observational research, and good practice carefully addresses and minimizes them.

Identifying the relevant research begins with a systematic search of the literature. The ability to search the medical literature electronically has increased greatly in the last decade, and with PubMed and similar sources, many reviewers can now perform credible searches from their desks. For more complex questions, however, and in order to more effectively manage the results, a trained librarian's help is still important.

Even the most careful electronic search of a single source such as MEDLINE, however, generally misses some important research results. Good practice requires searching multiple sources. Some approaches are "snowball searching," that is, searching the reference lists of review papers and primary research articles identified early in the search; "hand searching" key journals, that is, reading the table of contents of the journals most likely to include relevant papers; consulting registries of clinical trials, where they exist; and contacting experts in the field.

Some analysts choose to limit their review to published reports, or studies published in peer-reviewed journals. Usually justified in terms of ensuring that the review is based on high-quality results, this strategy may not be appropriate in a fast-moving field when important studies have not yet been published or, for example, when clinical trials have been presented to the U.S. Food and Drug Administration (FDA) but not published. And, of course, peer review is not always a good indicator of study quality.

A careful research synthesis is guided by an *a priori* search protocol, identifying which databases will be searched and how, and clearly stating specific inclusion and exclusion criteria. Such a protocol provides for replicability, and offers readers an opportunity to evaluate the comprehensiveness of the search, verify the conclusions from a particular review, and consider the implications of using various criteria. An *a priori* protocol can help to protect the reviewer from unconscious bias in decisions about which results to include and the appearance of such bias to readers. From this perspective, the most defensible inclusion and exclusion criteria are based on relevance to the clinical question and the quality of the primary research articles.

Reliable and Unbiased Abstracting

Before the results can be analyzed, each primary study must be abstracted. Readers identify the key results from each study, along with the major study characteristics including measures of study quality, and enter them into a database or summary table. This step can be challenging because the authors of the original studies present their results in different ways, sometimes using a variety of metrics, depending on the original study design and objectives. Aspects of study design that are of interest to the meta-analyst may not have been clearly presented by the original authors, in some cases working years earlier with a different understanding of the scientific and clinical issues or with a different set of objectives and technical methods. The quality of the original studies is often difficult to judge as well. Despite these difficulties, the strength of the systematic review findings comes from abstracting this information in a reliable and unbiased way. To improve the quality of the data for the meta-analysis, researchers often use two or more readers and adopt some process to achieve consensus.

Assessing the Quality of Primary Studies

Before the analysis proceeds, a careful meta-analyst will evaluate the quality of the component studies. Quality measures can be used to decide whether some should be excluded from the analysis in a sensitivity analysis, or as the basis for an analysis stratified by quality. For example, some meta-analysts cite quality concerns to include only RCTs in their analyses of medical interventions. Beyond this, developing and applying appropriate quality measures can be challenging, as discussed below.

SYNTHESIZING THE RESULTS OF MULTIPLE STUDIES

Once assembled and assessed, the results of the studies in a systematic review must be analyzed and summarized. These analyses can be qualitative, perhaps in the form of a comparative evidence table. In a meta-analysis the summary is quantitative, sometimes in the form of a single summary statistic, or perhaps a quantitative description of the nature and source of heterogeneity in the results. Often research syntheses analyze the results in several different ways in order to tell a complete story.

Narrative Summaries

The simplest and most basic qualitative analysis is a narrative summary: the key characteristics of each study that meets the inclusion and exclusion criteria are described, along with the results, objectively and in a parallel fashion. Comments about the quality of each study may also be included. Such summaries are similar in many respects to those found in a typical review article, but they differ in three important ways. First, the studies described are the result of a systematic and unbiased selection process, not chosen to illustrate an author's point. Second, to the degree possible, narrative summaries focus on the same characteristics of the primary studies. This approach makes it easier for the reader to assess the studies and their contribution to the overall summary. Finally, narrative summaries typically include more information on the quality of the individual studies, and how flaws might lead the results to be biased in one direction or the other, than do standard review articles.

Evidence Tables

Evidence tables, one step beyond narrative summaries yet short of formal meta-analytic summaries, present the most important characteristics and results of a systematic review in parallel form. Depending on the systematic review, authors might choose to focus an evidence table on the study's population and publication date; its design, sample size, and quality; specific interventions or exposures studied, and how they were assessed and measured; specific outcomes studied, and how they were assessed and measured; and the primary results.

An evidence table is most useful when it includes the most salient characteristics of the studies, especially those that may lead to differences in the studies' results. Too much detail creates a risk of losing focus on the important ones. Janowsky and colleagues,[15] for instance, include an evidence table summarizing the case-control or cross-sectional studies of breast implants and connective-tissue diseases (see Table 2). The key characteristics that the authors chose

to emphasize were the location and year of the study, the category of connective-tissue disease studied, the number of cases and controls with and without
breast implants, the estimated odds ratio for association and its 95% confidence
interval, and the factors that were adjusted for in the analysis.

For some systematic reviews, it may not be appropriate to go beyond an evidence table (or even a narrative summary). If, for instance, the primary studies
share no common quantitative measures of results, or the studies are too heterogeneous, a formal meta-analysis is not appropriate. The systematic review,
however, will have made an important contribution through its systematic and
objective identification and assessment of the relevant studies and the abstraction
of salient characteristics and results in the evidence table, and it may indicate a
need for additional research, more detail on specific issues, or redirection along
different lines.

Statistical Models for Combining Data

The simplest way to combine the data from a series of similar primary studies
is to count the number that are "positive"—either because their results differ from the null value in the anticipated direction, or because they do so in
a statistically significant way. For instance, in the study of the relative risk of
coronary heart disease associated with passive smoking summarized in Figure
2,[13] all 18 studies had relative risks above 1.0, but according to the paper only 7
were significantly elevated in the sense that the 95% confidence interval did not
include RR = 1. On the face of it, this is useful information. The chance that all
18 studies would have relative risks greater than 1, assuming no relationship
and independence, is $1/(2^{18})$, which is approximately 4 per million. The problem
with such *vote counting*, as it is sometimes called, is that it uses the available data
inefficiently. Studies with sample sizes ranging from 102 to 232,200 each have
equal weight in this analysis.

One step beyond vote counting uses statistical methods to combine the
p-values from the individual studies into a single overall summary.[21] Such an
approach makes more efficient use of the available information, but does not
produce a quantitative estimate of the size of the effect. In the passive smoking
example, this approach would give a more precise test of the null hypothesis
that passive smoking is not associated with coronary heart disease, but not
an estimate of the elevated risk in those exposed to passive smoking. In some
systematic reviews, though, this approach is the best that can be done because
the original studies either do not present effect sizes such as RRs or present the
results in incompatible formats.

When the results of the studies in a systematic review are available in a consistent, quantitative form such as a relative risk or an odds ratio, a quantitative

Table 2. Evidence Table Summarizing Key Characteristics of Case–Control or Cross-Sectional Studies of Breast Implants and Connective-Tissue Diseases.

Study	Location and Year	Category	No. of Cases/No. with Breast Implants	No. of Controls/No. with Breast Implants	Odds Ratio (95% CI)*	Adjustment†
Burns et al.	Michigan, 1996	Scleroderma or systemic sclerosis	274/2	1184/14	0.95 (0.21–4.36)	Age, birth year, race
Dugowson et al.	Washington State, 1992	Rheumatoid arthritis	300/1	1456/12	0.41 (0.05–3.13)	Age
Englert et al.	Australia, 1996	Scleroderma or systemic sclerosis	286/3	253/4	1.00 (0.16–6.16)	Socioeconomic status, age, ethnicity
Goldman et al.‡	Atlanta, 1995	Rheumatoid arthritis and connective-tissue diseases	721/12	3508/138	0.52 (0.29–0.92)	Age at first visit to practice, income, time of first visit
		Rheumatoid arthritis	392/9		0.84 (0.41–1.62)	
		Systemic lupus erythematosus	180/1		0.14 (0.02–1.23)	
		Scleroderma or systemic sclerosis	64/0		—	
		Sjögren's syndrome	49/2		1.46 (0.36–6.39)	
		Dermatomyositis or polymyositis	36/0		—	
		Mixed connective-tissue disease	49/0		—	
Hennekens et al.§	United States, including Puerto Rico, 1996	Any connective-tissue disease	11,805/231	383,738/10,599	1.24 (1.08–1.41)	Age, birth year
		Rheumatoid arthritis	6429/107		1.18 (0.97–1.43)	
		Systemic lupus erythematosus	1593/32		1.15 (0.81–1.63)	
		Scleroderma or systemic sclerosis	324/10		1.84 (0.98–3.46)	
		Sjögren's syndrome	774/22		1.49 (0.97–2.28)	
		Dermatomyositis or polymyositis	747/20		1.52 (0.97–2.37)	
		Other connective-tissue diseases	3354/83		1.30 (1.05–1.62)	
Hochberg et al.	Baltimore; San Diego, Calif.; Pittsburgh, 1996	Scleroderma or systemic sclerosis	837/11	2507/31	1.07 (0.53–2.13)	Age, race, geographic site
Lacey et al.¶	Ohio, 1997	Scleroderma or systemic sclerosis	189/1	1043/10	1.01 (0.13–8.15)	Age, birth year

Table 2. Evidence Table Summarizing Key Characteristics of Case–Control or Cross-Sectional Studies of Breast Implants and Connective-Tissue Diseases *(continued).*

Laing et al.[¶]	Michigan, Ohio, 1996	Undifferentiated connective-tissue disease	205/3	2220/27	2.27 (0.67–7.71)	Age, birth year
Strom et al.	Philadelphia, 1994	Systematic lupus erythematosus	133/1	100/0	—	Age
Teel[‖]	Washington State, 1997	All connective-tissue diseases	427/6	1577/24	0.9 (0.4–2.3)	Age, year of diagnosis, race
		Systematic lupus erythematosus	191/2		0.8 (0.2–3.4)	
		Scleroderma or systemic sclerosis	55/0		—	
		Sjögren's syndrome	161/4		1.6 (0.5–4.7)	
		Dermatomyositis or polymyositis	17/0		—	
		Mixed connective-tissue disease	3/0		—	
Wolfe	Kansas, 1995	Rheumatoid arthritis	637/3	1134/4	1.35 (0.30–6.06)	Age

*CI denotes confidence interval.

[†]Adjustments were made for the variables listed.

[‡]This study was cross-sectional. "Mixed connective-tissue disease" was defined according to IDC-9 codes 710.9 and 711. Six of 12 cases of connective-tissue disease were diagnosed before implantation.

[§]This study was cross-sectional. "Any connective-tissue disease" included all definite connective-tissue diseases and "other connective-tissue diseases." "Other connective-tissue disease" included mixed connective-tissue disease.

[¶]"Undifferentiated connective-tissue disease" was defined according to ICD-9 code710.9. The diagnosis was assigned if the referring physician's diagnosis of the discharge code of Health Care Investment Analysts was undifferentiated connective-tissue disease or the patient had been given the diagnosis of scleroderma, but did not meet the criteria of the American College of Rheumatology; the patient did not meet the diagnostic criteria for another connective-tissue disease; and a minimum of two signs, symptoms, or laboratory values suggestive of a connective-tissue disease were documented.

[‖]The criteria for establishing a diagnosis of mixed connective-tissue disease were from the literature.

Source: Janowsky et al., 2000.[15]

meta-analysis becomes possible. In clinical studies with dichotomous outcomes, the most common measures or *metameters* are relative risks, risk differences, and odds ratios. With continuous measures, common metameters are differences in means or average differences. Survival studies that focus on time to event may be meta-analyzed via hazard rates or similar measures. All of these measures might be adjusted for confounders. Regardless of the way that the results are presented, quantitative meta-analysis is technically possible if a common metameter and an estimate of its standard error are available or can be calculated for a group of primary studies. Whether it is advisable to combine the data in this way, however, is a different question, and most of the art as well as the science of research synthesis focuses on this question.

Many statistical models, each with strengths and weaknesses, serve to combine the results of studies with a common metameter. The most basic distinction is between fixed-effects models and random-effects models. A *fixed-effects model* assumes that all studies estimate exactly the same effect except for sampling variation. A *random-effects model*, on the other hand, assumes that the available studies reflect a distribution of possible effects. Random-effects estimates are more "conservative" in the sense that they have wider confidence intervals that reflect the estimated variability among studies. Random-effects estimates default to the fixed-effects estimates if the estimated variance among studies is not greater than zero.

Statisticians disagree on which methods are appropriate. Some feel, for instance, that if the studies differ for reasons other than sampling variation (that is, they are heterogeneous), meta-analysis is simply not appropriate, so fixed-effects models are appropriate whenever meta-analysis itself is. Other statisticians recognize that variation among research reports in populations studied, implementation of interventions, measurement methods, and other factors is a fact of life; and as long as the studies are not too heterogeneous, random-effects meta-analysis is not only appropriate, but necessary. Ultimately, neither model uses assumptions that are strictly true, and the decision depends on which set of assumptions most closely reflects reality, and thus is likely to give the best estimates. This issue is covered further under the discussion of heterogeneity below.

One of the simplest fixed-effects models is sometimes referred to as the inverse-variance method.[22] The summary estimate is simply a weighted average of the individual study metameters, using weights that are inversely proportional to the metameter's variance. As illustrated in the "overall" line in Figure 2, He and colleagues[13] use this fixed-effects method to summarize the odds ratios from 10 cohort studies and 8 case-control studies. They note that the random-effects model yielded nearly identical results.

Other fixed-effects models such as those of Mantel and Haenszel[23] or Peto[24] tend to give similar results, but are more appropriate in certain circumstances.[25]

The Early Breast Cancer Trialists' Collaborative Group,[7] for instance, uses Peto's odds-ratio method.

The most common random-effects model is the one developed by DerSimonian and Laird.[26] This approach modifies the inverse-variance method by adding a term to the weights that allows for a distribution of possible study outcomes that goes beyond sampling variation. The International Perinatal HIV Group,[10] for instance, used both the DerSimonian and Laird method and a fixed-effects approach. Consistent with their findings of no statistically significant heterogeneity between studies, the two methods gave nearly identical results, as can be seen in Figure 3.

Another statistical model, meta-regression, is designed to represent the variation in the metameter in terms of study-level variables.[25] Reynolds and colleagues,[27] for instance, used this method to analyze the relationship between the risk of stroke and the amount of alcohol consumed, and found evidence of a quadratic relationship for both men and women. For women, the evidence suggests that for alcohol intake levels up to 40 grams per day, the relative risk of stroke is less than one (compared to zero consumption); that is, alcohol consumption may be mildly protective in women.

Adding more generality, various approaches use Bayesian statistical methods.[28] Typically, these methods must be tuned to the details of a clinical issue, and they require the input of a biostatistician expert in *Bayesian meta-analysis*.

In 1992 Lau and colleagues[29] introduced *cumulative meta-analysis* to illustrate how the evidence about a clinical or policy question develops over time. Figure 5 illustrates this approach using the results of 33 trials of intravenous streptokinase for acute myocardial infarction. Summarizing the first two studies published, and then the first three, and so on, adding one study at a time, until the most recently published study is included, the right-hand panel of Figure 5 shows how intravenous streptokinase could have been shown to be lifesaving in the early 1970s, two decades before Lau and colleagues' analysis was published. One might ask why it is relevant to know that a policy question could have been settled at some point in the past, since the best evidence for decision-making now is the most complete simple meta-analysis. When Jüni and colleagues[30] published a cumulative meta-analysis in 2004, showing that the FDA could have had strong evidence about the risk of myocardial infarction in patients taking COX-2 inhibitors four years earlier (see Figure 6), it called the efficacy of the FDA's drug safety apparatus into question.

On occasion, a systematic review includes a pooled analysis, using patient-level data from the available studies as if they were from one trial. The analysis could include an indicator variable to represent differences among studies, just as the analysis of a multi-site clinical trial might include such a variable for site. The International Perinatal HIV Group,[10] for instance, gathered individual-level data from all of the studies they identified. This allowed the authors to calculate

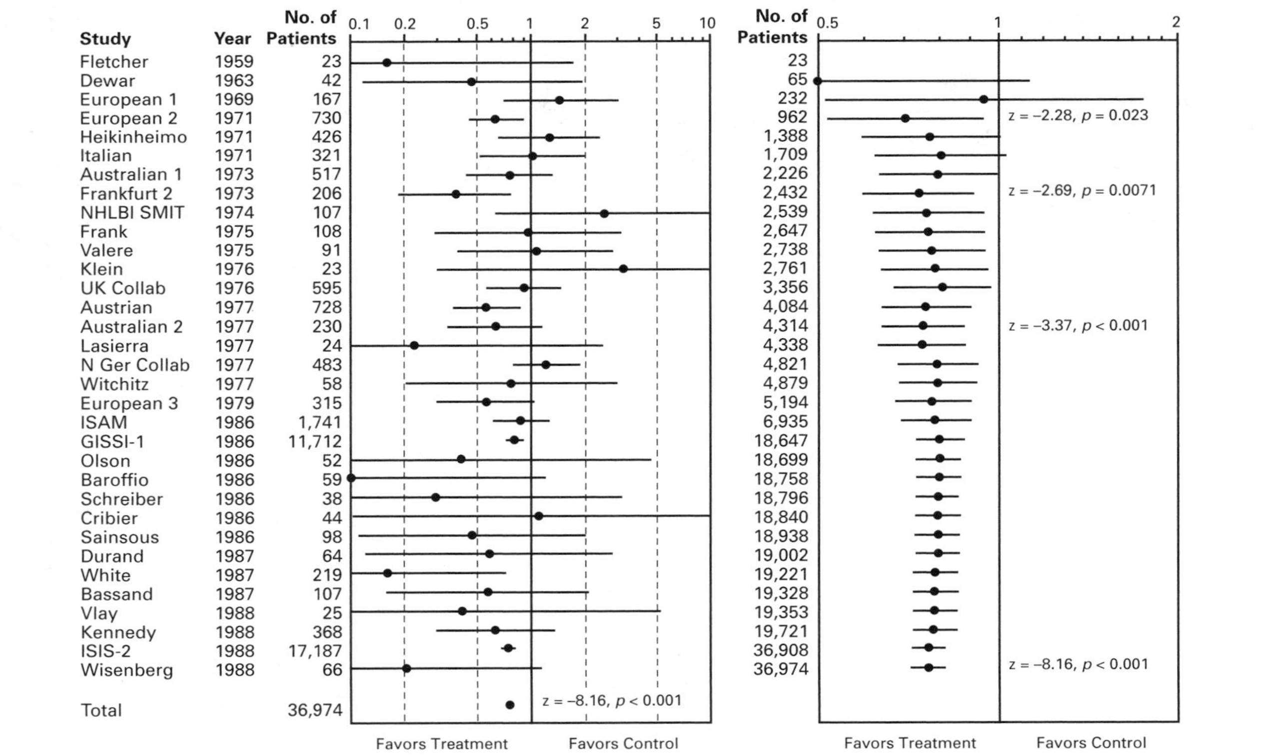

Figure 5. Conventional and cumulative meta-analysis of 33 trials of intravenous streptokinase for acute myocardial infarction.
The odds ratio and 95% confidence interval for an effect of treatment on mortality are shown on a logarithmic scale.

Source: Lau et al., 1992.[29]

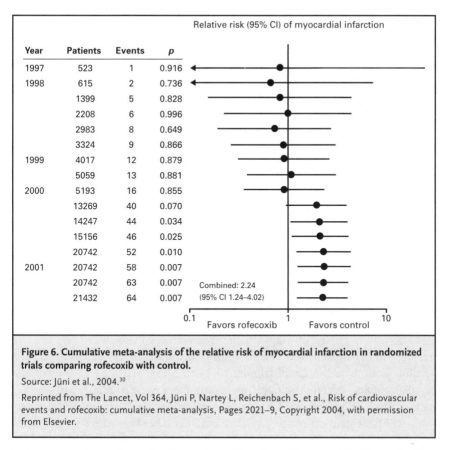

Relative risk (95% CI) of myocardial infarction

Year	Patients	Events	p
1997	523	1	0.916
1998	615	2	0.736
	1399	5	0.828
	2208	6	0.996
	2983	8	0.649
	3324	9	0.866
1999	4017	12	0.879
	5059	13	0.881
2000	5193	16	0.855
	13269	40	0.070
	14247	44	0.034
	15156	46	0.025
	20742	52	0.010
2001	20742	58	0.007
	20742	63	0.007
	21432	64	0.007

Combined: 2.24
(95% CI 1.24–4.02)

0.1   1   10
Favors rofecoxib   Favors control

Figure 6. Cumulative meta-analysis of the relative risk of myocardial infarction in randomized trials comparing rofecoxib with control.

Source: Jüni et al., 2004.[30]

Reprinted from The Lancet, Vol 364, Jüni P, Nartey L, Reichenbach S, et al., Risk of cardiovascular events and rofecoxib: cumulative meta-analysis, Pages 2021–9, Copyright 2004, with permission from Elsevier.

truly comparable odds ratios for analyses like those illustrated in Figure 3. Having the original data also made possible a pooled analysis of individual-level data to estimate the impact of receipt of antiviral therapy and other factors, yielding information beyond what would be available in a standard meta-analysis. Gathering all the original data in a form suitable for such a pooled analysis, however, can be difficult.

Drawing Clinical and Policy Conclusions

Overly enthusiastic interpretation of results of systematic reviews is common, perhaps because the authors feel that they have gathered and analyzed *all* of the relevant data on a clinical or policy question. Given the possible pitfalls, systematic reviews and especially meta-analyses must be interpreted with caution.

In particular, the following questions should be addressed in interpreting and drawing conclusions from a systematic review:

- How good is the quality of the studies that contribute to the summary result?
- Is there evidence of publication bias or other biases?
- How robust is the summary result? Is it sensitive to the choice of statistical models used, or to the inclusion or exclusion of studies?
- Is unexplained heterogeneity a problem?
- Are the patients studied representative of the patient population to which the results are being extrapolated?
- Can the results from clinical trials be extended to patients outside those studies?
- Does evidence about association in epidemiological studies suggest a causal relationship (that is, is there biological plausibility, evidence of a dose-response relationship, consistency and coherence, or other factors that epidemiologists use to assess causality)?

CONTROVERSIAL ISSUES IN SYSTEMATIC REVIEWS

The success or failure of a systematic review rests on many factors, but five issues have been extensively debated in the literature and are discussed in this section. Four issues—the possibility of publication bias, the quality of the original studies, heterogeneity in the results from these studies, and whether meta-analysis is appropriate for non-randomized studies—are important determinants of a systematic review's validity. Another issue is whether formal meta-analysis techniques should be used for observational studies in epidemiology or other fields.

Publication Bias

One common concern about meta-analyses is the possibility, or even likelihood, that some negative studies are not published and are unavailable for the analysis, thus biasing the results away from the null hypothesis. The term "publication bias" suggests that the problem arises when editors do not find such studies interesting enough to publish, but in some cases, authors might prejudge this outcome and simply not submit the results; this is known as the "file drawer problem." Some such studies may not even be completed if the investigator thinks that publication is unlikely. For these or other reasons, a body of research results is systematically missing from the literature available for a meta-analysis, and the calculated summary effect is biased compared to the summary of all studies that have been done. The existence of publication bias has been clearly documented,[31] but by its very nature it involves smaller, less-precise studies, which have relatively little weight in a meta-analysis, so the impact is limited.

Graphical tools such as funnel plots[32] and statistical tests[22, 33, 34] can help meta-analysts detect publication bias, and good practice requires the use of such techniques and exploration of the implications. It should be recalled, however, that statistical tests cannot distinguish publication bias from a real differential in the results by study size; nor can they detect intentional bias in publication, such as the suppression of unfavorable drug safety results. Six of the ten studies summarized in Table 1 do not address publication bias; three of them claim that they investigated it, but found no evidence to support bias. Danesh[14] suggested that extreme findings in early, smaller studies may be due to publication bias.

Publication bias reflects a much bigger problem related to the reward system in science and other pressures to publish (or not). Some journal editors note that the literature is not produced just for meta-analysts, and other users are already overwhelmed by the growing flood of articles that make little or no useful contribution other than to reduce the bias in a meta-analysis. On the other side, it seems likely that studies showing adverse effects or lack of efficacy of drugs that have already been marketed are sometimes suppressed. Perhaps results that would be useful to a handful of other scientists and would complete the record for meta-analysts could be transmitted as meeting abstracts or on the internet. Indeed, one way to identify and adjust for publication bias is to search registries of RCTs that have been funded, but perhaps not published. Similarly, some have proposed that pharmaceutical manufacturers be required to report the results of all trials that they undertake, not just those needed to make a case for a new indication.

Quality of Original Studies

One of the common criticisms of systematic reviews and meta-analyses is expressed in the phrase "garbage in, garbage out," and systematic reviews truly can mislead if they take an uncritical view of the evidence. Statistical meta-analyses can increase the precision of parameter estimates, but do nothing to reduce bias. Indeed, if all of the studies included have the same bias, a meta-analysis will simply provide a more precise estimate of that bias. Weakness in the original studies, however, is a problem with any kind of review, and the systematic approach adopted by experienced meta-analysts offers the opportunity to understand and minimize the impact of quality problems and perhaps correct for them.

The first step in addressing quality is to identify possible problems in the individual studies. In clinical trials, the most important dimensions of quality are randomization (whether done or not, or how well), masking or blinding of patients and clinicians, and completeness of follow-up. Observational studies in epidemiology are more varied, and generally have greater potential for bias because randomization was not used. In this setting, systematic reviews typically note the type of study (cohort, case-control, or other), whether groups differ only in exposure (or whether an adequate adjustment has been made), how outcomes were measured, and whether there is reasonable evidence of causation.

Systematic reviews sometimes use this information to create quality scores for the individual studies. For RCTs, Jadad and colleagues[35] have developed a generic quality score that is increasingly becoming a standard. The Jadad score focuses on randomization, blinding, and the description of withdrawals and dropouts. Because the quality problems vary more from one meta-analysis to another, epidemiological studies have no commonly agreed scoring system.

Some analysts use the quality score as a kind of weight in preparing a single parameter estimate, but this is not statistically justified. Alternatively, one could analyze subgroups of studies categorized by quality (e.g., high vs. low) or omit the lowest-quality studies to see whether quality is associated with differences in outcome. Some meta-analysts use specific dimensions of quality (study design, blinding, completeness of follow-up) judged to be the most important as the basis of subgroup or sensitivity analyses. However used, the question is the same: do the results of the meta-analysis depend on which studies are included in the analysis? If they do not, all can be kept in, and the results will be more precise. Otherwise, the summary should be based only on the highest-quality studies.

Heterogeneity

Heterogeneity in study results, which can be defined as differences greater than expected (by chance from sampling error or randomization) is common in meta-analysis, and must be assessed. It can arise from differences in populations studied, methods used, the treatment or exposure under study, or other factors. Heterogeneity is both a statistical issue and a clinical one: how much heterogeneity is there, what are the sources, and what level of differences is meaningful?

If the goal of a meta-analysis is to produce a more precise estimate of a single quantity such as effect of mastectomy and radiotherapy (alone and in combination) on breast cancer mortality,[7] heterogeneity is a problem because it suggests that the formulation of the question is wrong—there is no single number, but rather efficacy depends on other factors.

However, Berlin[36] and Colditz[37] note that the exploration of heterogeneity can be helpful in at least two respects. First, consistency reflects robustness. For instance, if case-control and cohort studies in a variety of populations, measuring exposure to passive smoking in different ways, find similar estimates of its effect on coronary heart disease,[13] it is less likely that the estimate is a result of bias in the original studies. Or if cesarean section has a similar effect on the risk of transmission of HIV in a variety of populations and birth settings,[10] it is more likely to be similarly effective in other populations and settings not reflected in the available studies.

Second, subgroup analysis and meta-regression[25] can be used to look for insights from differences in the results according to populations studied, treatment or exposure intensity and duration, and outcomes measured. For instance, in their study of the clinical benefits of placebos, Hrobjartsson and Gøtzsche[12] found no significant effects on objective or binary outcomes, but possible small benefits in studies with continuous subjective outcomes and for the treatment of pain. This subgroup is where the lack of double blinding would be most likely to bias the results, possibly explaining the finding.

However, because the number of possible subgroup and meta-regression analyses is often large compared to the number of available studies, Berlin[36] recommends that analyses of heterogeneity be done in an exploratory mode and the results interpreted with caution. Also, the results of such analyses are stronger if the primary potential sources of heterogeneity are identified *a priori*.

Meta-Analysis of Epidemiologic and Other Observational Studies

Because randomization and other approaches to improving the quality of clinical trials are simply not available in epidemiologic and other observational studies, systematic reviews of topics in which such studies provide the bulk of the evidence are inherently challenging. Moreover, since observational studies must capitalize on available exposed cohorts or series of cases, and often involve attempts to reconstruct historical exposures from extant data, the studies available to address most topics are typically heterogeneous. These factors have led some to question, and eventually reject, the validity of systematic review and especially meta-analysis for epidemiological and other observational studies.

For meta-analysis in particular, the available studies sometimes are simply too heterogeneous for any single summary estimate to have meaning. Indeed, if the answer depends on what population is studied, what and how much the subjects were exposed to, what outcomes are assessed, or what study designs are used, a standard meta-analysis is simply not valid and should not be used. Sometimes, however, as illustrated by the study of secondhand smoking and coronary heart disease discussed above,[13] the lack of heterogeneity in the face of different populations, study designs, and other factors provides evidence of the robustness of the results. Heterogeneity may allow subgroup analysis or meta-regression to learn from the differences. One cannot learn from heterogeneity, however, if the idea of meta-analysis is rejected out of hand.

Janowsky and colleagues,[15] for example, capitalize on heterogeneity in their meta-analysis of the association between breast implants and connective-tissue diseases. As illustrated in Table 2, the nine case-control studies and two cross-sectional studies included in their analysis differed with respect to populations studied, study design, definition of connective tissue disease, and adjustments for other factors. Table 3 demonstrates the effect of including and excluding various groups of studies on the estimate of the odds ratio for the association between breast implants and connective-tissue diseases. Together with similar analyses investigating the impact of different adjustments, this analysis allowed the authors to conclude that "there was no evidence of an association between breast implants in general, or silicone-gel–filled breast implants specifically, and any of the individual connective-tissue diseases, all definite connective-tissue diseases combined, or other autoimmune or rheumatic conditions."[15]

Table 3. Sensitivity Analysis Illustrating the Effect of Including and Excluding Various Groups of Studies on the Estimate of the Odds Ratio for the Association between Breast Implants and Connective-Tissue Diseases.

Disease and Studies Included in Analysis	No. of Studies	Summary Odds Ratio (95% CI)*	p-value for Homogeneity[†]
All connective-tissue diseases combined			
All studies	16	0.69 (0.62–0.78)	0.10
All studies, excluding Friis et al.	15	0.68 (0.60–0.77)	0.31
Rheumatoid arthritis	10	0.62 (0.52–0.73)	0.17
Systemic lupus erythematosus	8	0.63 (0.44–0.86)	0.24
Scleroderma or systemic sclerosis			
All studies	12	0.73 (0.46–1.10)	0.10
All studies, excluding Friis et al.	11	0.70 (0.44–1.08)	0.14
Sjögren's syndrome	8	1.10 (0.74–1.58)	0.56
Dermatomyositis or polymyositis	6	0.90 (0.55–1.39)	0.88
Other autoimmune or rheumatic conditions			
All studies	12	0.91 (0.79–1.04)	<0.001
All studies, excluding Friis et al. and Sánchez-Guerrero et al.	10	0.92 (0.77–1.10)	0.52

*Conditional maximum-likelihood estimates are presented, except for the categories of all connective-tissue diseases combined and rheumatoid arthritis, for which estimates by the Mantel–Haenszel method are shown. Exact confidence intervals (CIs) are presented, except for the categories of all connective-tissue diseases combined and rheumatoid arthritis, for which limits obtained with the methods of Robins, Breslow, and Greenland are shown.

[†]Exact p-values obtained by the method of Zelen are presented, except for the categories of all connective-tissues diseases combined, rheumatoid arthritis, and other autoimmune or rheumatic conditions, for which p-values obtained with the Breslow–Day chi-squared statistic are shown.

Source: Janowsky et al., 2005.[15]

Concerns about the validity of statistical meta-analysis should not dissuade one from using other systematic review tools, including a careful statement of the research question, systematic literature searching, and the objective review, critique, and abstraction of information from the studies identified. Narrative reviews or evidence tables based on this approach typically allow for a less-biased assessment of the evidence than standard review articles (in which the evidence is sometimes chosen to support a pre-conceived point). Stoto[38] describes how the Institute of Medicine has used such an approach to assess and synthesize the evidence on controversial topics.

CONCLUSIONS

Systematic review and meta-analysis can provide a framework for synthesizing the results of independent scientific studies bearing on a common clinical or public health issue. Systematic reviews identify, analyze, and present available data and offer the potential to identify areas of agreement, clarify the nature and causes of any disagreement, establish what is known prior to further research, identify areas needing more research, and frame results so they can be translated into practice and policy. When meta-analysis is appropriate, it can substantially increase statistical power and resolve issues relating to conflicting results among many small studies. Like all tools, however, meta-analysis can be abused, and indeed some systematic reviews, and especially meta-analyses, that have used these tools have been controversial.

For systematic reviews and meta-analyses to live up to their promise, authors must give proper attention to best practices in research synthesis, including judicious use of formal meta-analysis and the careful exploration of study quality and heterogeneity. As noted above, the skills needed for doing a systematic review include both clinical and technical (statistical) expertise, and the amount of effort required is similar to that for a standard research paper. Readers, for their part, must be wary of the pitfalls.

REFERENCES

1. Shapiro S. Meta-analysis shmeta-analysis. Am J Epidemiol 1994; 140:771–8.
2. Bailar JC III. The promise and problems of meta-analysis. N Engl J Med 1997; 337:559–61.
3. Bailar JC III. The practice of meta-analysis. J Clin Epidemiol 1995; 48:149–57.
4. Oxman A, Guyatt G. The science of reviewing research. In: Doing more good than harm: the evaluation of health care interventions. Annals of the New York Academy of Sciences, 1993; 703:125–34.
5. Chalmers I. Academia's failure to support systematic reviews (letter). Lancet 2005; 365:469.
6. Young C. Horton R. Putting clinical trials into context (editorial). Lancet 2005; 366:107–8.

7. Early Breast Cancer Trialists' Collaborative Group. Effects of radiotherapy and surgery in early breast cancer—an overview of the randomized trials. N Engl J Med 1995; 333:1444–55.

8. Sargent DJ, Goldberg RM, Jacobson SD, et al. A pooled analysis of adjuvant chemotherapy for resected colon cancer in elderly patients. N Engl J Med 2001; 345:1091–7.

9. Aupérin A, Arriagada R, Pignon J-P, et al., for the Prophylactic Cranial Irradiation Overview Collaborative Group. Prophylactic cranial irradiation for patients with small-cell lung cancer in complete remission. N Engl J Med 1999; 341:476–84.

10. International Perinatal HIV Group. The mode of delivery and the risk of vertical transmission of human immunodeficiency virus type 1—a meta-analysis of 15 prospective cohort studies. N Engl J Med 1999; 340:977–87.

11. Anderson JW, Johnstone BM, Cook-Newell ME. Meta-analysis of the effects of soy protein intake on serum lipids. N Engl J Med 1995; 333:276–82.

12. Hrobjartsson A, Gøtzsche PC. Is the placebo powerless?—an analysis of clinical trials comparing placebo with no treatment. N Engl J Med 2001; 344:1594–602.

13. He J, Vupputuri S, Allen K, et al. Passive smoking and the risk of coronary heart disease—a meta-analysis of epidemiologic studies. N Engl J Med 1999; 340:920–6.

14. Danesh J, Wheeler JG, Hirschfield GM, et al. C-reactive protein and other circulating markers of inflammation in the prediction of coronary heart disease. N Engl J Med 2004; 350:1387–97.

15. Janowsky EC, Kupper LL, Hulka BS. Meta-analyses of the relation between silicone breast implants and the risk of connective-tissue diseases. N Engl J Med 2000; 342:781–90.

16. Krontiris TG, Devlin B, Karp DD, et al. An Association between the risk of cancer and mutations in the HRAS1 minisatellite locus. N Engl J Med 1993; 329:517–23.

17. Bailar JC III. Passive smoking, coronary heart disease, and meta-analysis. N Engl J Med 1999; 340:958–9.

18. Howard G, Thun MJ. Why is environmental tobacco smoke more strongly associated with coronary heart disease than expected: a review of potential biases and experimental data. Environmental Health Perspectives 1999; 107(Suppl 6):853–8.

19. U.S. Department of Health and Human Services. The health consequences of involuntary exposure to tobacco smoke: a report of the surgeon general, 2006.

20. Glasziou P, Irwig L, Bain C, Colditz G. Systematic reviews in health care: a practical guide. Cambridge, UK: Cambridge University Press, 2001.

21. Fisher RA. Combining individual tests of significance. Am Statistician 1948; 2(5):30.

22. Egger M, Davey Smith G, Schneider M, Minder C. Bias in meta-analysis detected by a simple, graphical test. Br Med J 1997; 315:629–34.

23. Mantel N, Haenszel W. Statistical aspects of the analysis of data from retrospective studies of disease. J Natl Cancer Inst. 1959, 22:719–48.

24. Peto R, Pike MC, Armitage P, et al. Design and analysis of randomized clinical trials requiring prolonged observation of each patient. II. Analysis and examples. Br J Cancer 1977; 35:1–39.

25. Egger M, Davey Smith G, Altman D, eds. Systematic reviews in health care: meta-analysis in context. 2nd ed. London: BMJ Books, 2001.

26. DerSimonian R, Laird N. Meta-analysis in clinical trials. Control Clin Trials 1986; 7:177–88.

27. Reynolds K, Lewis LB, Nolen JD, et al. Alcohol consumption and risk of stroke: a meta-analysis. JAMA 2003; 289:579–88.

28. Normand S-L, Meta-analysis: formulating, evaluating, combining, and reporting. Stat Med 1999; 18:321–59.

29. Lau J, Antman EM, Jimenez-Silva J, et al. Cumulative meta-analysis of therapeutic trials for myocardial infarction. N Engl J Med 1992; 327:248–54.

30. Jüni P, Nartey L, Reichenbach S, et al. Risk of cardiovascular events and rofecoxib: cumulative meta-analysis. Lancet 2004; 364:2021–9.

31. Simes J. Publication bias: the case for an international registry of clinical trials. J Clin Oncol 1986; 4:1529–41.

32. Light R, Pillemer D. Summing up: the science of reviewing research. Cambridge, Mass.: Harvard University Press, 1984.

33. Begg CB, Mazumdar M. Operating characteristics of a rank correlation test for publication bias. Biometrics 1994; 50:1088–101.

34. Duval SJ, Tweedie RL. Trim and fill: a simple funnel-plot-based method of testing and adjusting for publication bias in meta-analysis. Biometrics 2000; 56:455–63.

35. Jadad AR, Moore RA, Carroll D, et al. Assessing the quality of reports of randomized clinical trials: is blinding necessary? Control Clin Trials 1996; 17:1–12.

36. Berlin JA. Invited commentary: Benefits of heterogeneity in meta-analysis of data from epidemiologic studies. Am J Epidemiol 1995; 142:383–7.

37. Colditz GA, Burdick E, Mosteller F. Heterogeneity in meta-analysis of data from epidemiologic studies: A commentary. Am J Epidemiol 1995; 142:371–82.

38. Stoto MA. Research synthesis for public health policy: experience of the Institute of Medicine. In: Meta-analysis in medicine and health policy. Stangl D, Berry D, eds. New York: Marcel Dekker, 2000:321–57.

CHAPTER 18

Biostatistics in Epidemiology:
Advanced Methods of Regression Analysis

MARK S. GOLDBERG, PH.D.

ABSTRACT   This chapter reviews some of the types of statistical analyses commonly used in epidemiological studies to investigate health states. The focus is on what the reader should know to understand the analysis of a study and its results. Topics include incidence cohort studies, case-control studies, longitudinal cohort studies, and cross-sectional studies. The discussion emphasizes regression methods and their ranges of application, underlying assumptions, and strengths and weaknesses, especially in the context of specific examples.

C hapter 7 discusses elementary principles of design in epidemiology, describes the most important types of studies, and introduces some elementary methods of analysis. That chapter focuses largely on the following questions:

- Are the objectives of the study stated precisely and clearly?
- Is the study design appropriate for the purpose?
- Does the study population represent the target?
- Were enough subjects enrolled to meet the objectives?
- Were the measures of outcome and exposure reliable and valid?
- Were potential confounding variables assessed?
- Are the statistical models appropriate?

When answers to these questions show that the data are suitable for analysis, what statistical methods can be applied? Table 1 summarizes the main methods of analysis for epidemiologic data, organized by type of study. These statistical methods include simple stratified techniques to adjust for confounding in the analysis of rates and proportions and several types of regression analysis. The simple and stratified analyses of rates and proportions, with or without standardization, present little difficulty in concept. For outcomes measured on

Table 1. Common Statistical Methods Used to Analyze Epidemiological Studies.*

Statistical Method	Parameter to Be Estimated	Type of Data	Comments
Cohort Studies: Stratified Analyses of Incidence			
Internal or external analysis			
Directly standardized incidence or mortality ratio (also known as cumulative mortality figure (CMF))	Ratio of incidence or mortality rates in a cohort to rates in a standard population	Outcome: failure Exposure: categorical Covariates: categorical and can be time-dependent	For each of the types of analysis: Standard population can be external (e.g., population rates) or internal (e.g., a sub-cohort or total cohort) Typical adjustment variables for external analyses: age, gender, calendar year, ethnic group. Tests of linear trend and homogeneity across the levels of exposure can be obtained. Person-years must be distributed into all mutually exclusive categories of the cross-classification of covariates.
Indirectly standardized incidence or mortality ratio (also known as standardized rate) (SIR, SMR)			
Mantel-Haenszel			
Cohort Studies: Regression Analyses of Incidence			
Poisson regression	Ratio of incidence or mortality rates in a cohort to that of an external or internal population	Outcome: failure Exposure: categorical Covariates: categorical, and can be time-dependent	This method is an extension of the stratified techniques described above. The assumption is that person-years of observation are distributed into variables defined categorically, such as age and calendar year. Standard population can be external (e.g., population rates) or internal (e.g., a sub-cohort or total cohort). Tests of linear trend and homogeneity across the levels of exposure can be obtained. Person-years must be distributed into all mutually exclusive categories of the cross-classification of covariates before conducting the analyses.

Table 1. Common Statistical Methods Used to Analyze Epidemiological Studies (*continued*).[*]

Proportional-hazards (Cox)	Ratio of incidence rates in cohort to that of an internal reference population	Outcome: failure Exposure: any type Covariates: any type, and can be time-dependent	Any measured explanatory variable of any type can be used in the model (e.g., continuous, categorical). Tests of linear trend and homogeneity across the levels of exposure can be obtained. Person-years do not have to be tabulated. Survival functions are estimable from the model, and the proportional-hazards assumption can be tested.
Nested case-control	Ratio of incidence rates in cohort to that of an internal reference population	Outcome: failure Exposure: any type Covariates: any type	Used if computer processing time is a concern or if selected covariates have been measured for a subset of cases and a subset of controls. The method is based on matching non-cases to cases at time of event; the controls at one time can become cases at another time. Two types of software can be used for the analysis: conditional logistic (see below) or the Cox model. Any measured variable of any type can be used as a covariate. Tests of linear trend and homogeneity across the levels of exposure are available. The analysis is equivalent to a full proportional-hazards analysis except that estimates have more variability because only a subset of potential controls is selected.
Case-Control Studies			
Mantel-Haenszel	Odds ratio	Outcome: failure Exposure: categorical Covariates: categorical	Any categorized variable can be used. Tests of linear trend and homogeneity across the levels of exposure can be obtained. Homogeneity of the odds ratio across strata is assumed, but this can be tested using a chi-squared test.

Table 1. Common Statistical Methods Used to Analyze Epidemiological Studies (continued).*

Logistic regression	Odds ratio	Outcome: failure Exposure: any type Covariates: any type	Any measured variable can be used. Tests of linear trend and homogeneity across levels of exposure can be obtained. The model allows different functional forms, other than stratification, to be used to represent the effects of potential confounding factors as well as the exposure of interest. In addition, interactions between the exposure and the covariates can be tested explicitly.
Conditional logistic regression	Odds ratio	Outcome: failure Exposure: any type Covariates: any type	Similar to logistic regression but used for matched studies. This method can also be used in nested case-control studies (matching on time of event). Any measured variable can be used. The effects of the matching variables cannot be estimated, but effect-modification by these variables can be assessed. Tests of linear trend and homogeneity across the levels of exposure can be obtained. Homogeneity of the odds ratio across strata is assumed, and this can be tested. Effect-modification can be assessed explicitly.
Polytomous regression	Odds ratio	Outcome: mutually exclusive categorical variable Exposure: any type Covariates: any type	Similar to logistic regression but the outcome variable consists of more than two unordered categories. Any measured variable can be used. Adjustments are not just between variables but also between categories. Tests of linear trend and homogeneity across the levels of exposure can be obtained. Homogeneity of the odds ratio across strata is assumed, and this can be tested. Effect-modification can be assessed explicitly.

Table 1. Common Statistical Methods Used to Analyze Epidemiological Studies (continued).*

Method	Measure	Variable types	Assumptions
Ordinal logistic regression	Odds ratio	Outcome: ordinal categorical variable; Exposure: any type; Covariates: any type	Similar to logistic regression except that the outcome variable is rank-ordered. Two different models are available: continuation ratio and cumulative odds models. Homogeneity of the odds ratio across strata is assumed, and this can be tested. Effect-modification can be assessed explicitly.
Cross-Sectional Studies**			
Multiple linear regression	Mean	Outcome: interval variable; Exposure: any type; Covariates: any type	Main assumptions are: continuous nature of outcome variable, outcome variable distributed normally, and homogeneity of variance.
Mantel-Haenszel, logistic regression, polytomous regression, ordinal regression	Odds ratio	Outcome: prevalence binary, nominal, or ordinal variable; Exposure: dependent on method; Covariates: dependent on method	See descriptions above.
Longitudinal Cohort Studies: Regression Analyses of Studies Where Endpoints Are Recurrent**			
Multi-level linear regression	Mean	Outcome: interval variable; Exposure: any type; Covariates: any type	Main assumptions are: continuous nature of outcome variable, outcome variable distributed normally, and homogeneity of variance. Correlated nature of study needs to be accounted for explicitly in the analysis.

Table 1. Common Statistical Methods Used to Analyze Epidemiological Studies (continued).*

Multi-level logistic regression	Odds ratio	Outcome: failure Exposure: any type Covariates: any type	Any measured variable can be used. Tests of linear trend and homogeneity across the levels of exposure are available. Assumption of homogeneity of the odds ratio across strata; this can be tested and effect-modification assessed. Correlated nature of study needs to be accounted for explicitly in the analysis.

*See text for lists of assumptions in the various statistical models.

**Standard methods of analysis can be used if there is little correlation between the measurements of outcome across time. Two other procedures are available when correlations are important: hierarchical (multi-level) random-effects models[8, 54] and the Generalized Estimating Equations models (see [45, 55–57]).

interval scales, simple *t*-tests can be used in some instances. Most of the more-advanced methods involve some form of regression (introduced in Chapter 10), including multiple linear regression for interval outcome variables and logistic and Poisson-type analyses for categorical outcomes. The focus here is on what the reader should know to understand the analysis of a study and its results; appropriate application of the methods to produce those results often requires a trained statistician or epidemiologist.

After some introduction, I take up, in turn,

- Incidence cohort studies (Poisson models; Cox proportional-hazards models)
- Case-control studies (incidence; nested)
- Longitudinal cohort studies
- Cross-sectional studies
- Some general issues in regression modeling, and overall considerations

Two main objectives drive most statistical analyses of epidemiological data: 1) to identify one or more explanatory factors for the health endpoint under consideration, and/or 2) to estimate the magnitude of the risk of that health outcome according to the presence of explanatory factors. For the former objective, it is usual to include only those factors that may confound the relationship under investigation, whereas the latter may require more variables to maximize predictive power. In particular, the set of variables to be included in a model (e.g., accepted and possible risk factors that may confound associations) needs careful thought, as do questions about whether they are truly direct contributors to risk or are surrogates for other variables or for each other and whether each variable is a single entity (e.g., a single food substance) or a complex mixture (e.g., diet as a whole). Some other issues include whether the variables are intermediate between exposure and outcome, whether plausible mechanisms of action suggest composite indices of exposure based on measured components (e.g., cumulative exposure to cigarette smoke, derived from duration, frequency, and intensity), and whether important changes in levels of exposure have occurred over time. Thus, the choice of statistical models should depend on the objectives of the analysis, and different models can produce different results. More-sophisticated models tend to be increasingly efficient in teasing out information as long as the model is approximately correct; otherwise, the advantage lies with simpler models, but it is usually unclear where the boundary lies. Modeling is an art, working within biological, statistical, and epidemiological considerations that constrain the range of plausible models. To repeat an often-quoted remark of George E. P. Box, "All models are wrong, but some are useful."

In large data sets that contain many variables, the modeler faces the additional challenge of accounting for the role of chance in finding that associations are statistically significant (a version of the "problem of multiple comparisons").[1-7] In addition, analysis of epidemiological data is least complicated when the observations are statistically independent (an important assumption of the basic methods). In practice, observations often are not statistically independent, sometimes by design, and the analysis needs to account for departures from independence. Examples in which data are non-independent by design include surveys of households that enroll all family members, case-control studies of twins, and longitudinal studies investigating risk factors for exacerbation of asthma, with multiple outcomes per subject. Non-independence may also arise from inherent clustering; for example, persons in certain geographic areas may be more similar to one another than to persons in other areas. A variety of departures from statistical independence can be handled by multi-level or random-effects models, discussed in many texts (e.g., Pinehiro and Bates[8]).

Many kinds of models are available for the analysis of epidemiologic data (Table 1 shows those in common use). I focus briefly on several regression approaches, with their ranges of application, underlying assumptions, strengths, and weaknesses, and provide some examples.

For flexibly modeling and comparing rates of disease, regression methods allow for some control of confounding and for assessing interactions, and provide powerful techniques for predicting incidence.

REGRESSION MODELS

A common object of regression analysis is to reduce a large set of possible covariates and effect modifiers to a smaller set by removing those that contribute little to the model. Among the many approaches to selecting variables, the simplest two are step-up (which adds one variable at a time until further additions do not improve the model) and step-down (which starts with the full set and deletes, one by one, those contributing least, stopping when the next deletion impairs the fit to an unacceptable degree). In assessing associations between a covariate and an outcome, such stepwise regression methods may inadvertently exclude known risk factors if they do not reach a specific level of significance, and this violates a rule to *not* use significance testing to assess confounding.[9] In developing predictive models, these procedures are not stable and may not lead to reproducible results.[10] Unfortunately, most authors do not report use of stepwise procedures, even implicitly, to reach the set analyzed. The procedures can be used with any of the methods described in this chapter.

A standard strategy for reducing these problems uses validation or cross-validation. One validation procedure separates the data set into three parts (say,

50%, 25%, and 25%, respectively) and uses the first part to develop candidate models, the second part to choose a final model, and the third part to evaluate that model's performance. When the data set is not large enough to support this approach, cross-validation may still be feasible. This strategy divides the data set into a number of roughly equal parts (perhaps 20), withholds each part in turn, develops a model on the non-withheld data, evaluates the model on the withheld data, and summarizes those leave-one-out assessments. An important limitation is that these approaches sacrifice considerable statistical power, adding further uncertainty to the findings.

Another concept that often arises in regression studies, especially those with multiple explanatory variables, is a distinction between fixed and random effects. Though the distinction between these is not always sharp, a variable that takes on specific values that we care about (e.g., a study of the incidence of drug abuse in schools, targeted toward the adoption of steps to control use in those schools where incidence is high) deals with fixed effects (we care about which schools have high incidence of use). Where we have a random sample of subjects and care about the population but not the specific subjects (e.g., a random sample of schools in a study targeted toward a decision about adopting a school-district-wide drug intervention program), the effects of the subjects are regarded as random. The results of applying fixed-effects models and random-effects models to the same data tend to be similar, with somewhat narrower confidence bounds for fixed effects, but the appropriate choice of model is always important. A model that includes fixed effects for some explanatory variables and random effects for others is called a mixed model, and these are common in the medical literature. Mixed models are often used in the analysis of clustered longitudinal data (e.g., with multiple measures of health effects in each subject and a random effect for subjects). Software for mixed linear models is readily available in many statistical packages, but application and interpretation of such models require substantial training and experience.

INCIDENCE COHORT STUDIES

Incidence cohort studies are designed for an event that can occur only once (e.g., death, or the first repeat myocardial infarction (MI) in patients who are under observation following an initial MI). We usually wish to estimate a ratio of (or difference between) rates observed at different levels of some explanatory variable, after adjusting for potential confounding variables.

Where combinations of potential confounding variables can be used to define strata, stratified techniques (direct, indirect, and the Mantel-Haenszel technique—first part of Table 1) can be used to estimate a rate ratio by a weighted average of stratum-specific rate ratios. The two main regression methods for these data are Poisson regression and the Cox proportional-hazards regression model,[11] which are more flexible than the stratified methods in that they can use various functional forms for the exposure variables and covariates and goodness-of-fit can be assessed. Unlike the stratified methods, the regression model provides estimates of rate ratios for the confounding and exposure variables. The Cox proportional-hazards model has come into broad use because it is very flexible and because it seems to fit many sets of data in medicine.

The stratification procedures and the two types of regression models usually lead to similar estimates of effect.[11, 12] However, the regression models allow for continuous as well as categorical covariates; thus, variables measured on interval scales do not have to be stratified. Use of the scale in which the variable was recorded ensures that important information is not lost and eliminates misclassification that may occur with arbitrary cut-points. In addition, if an explanatory variable affects risk in a nonlinear way, its functional form can be assessed by testing various parametric representations (e.g., using more-appropriate functional forms) or using smoothing functions (e.g., natural cubic splines[13]), aiding the interpretation of the findings and reducing residual confounding from the misclassification of covariates. Other advantages of the Cox model are that it allows the control of confounding through a readily interpretable regression approach, produces estimates of rate ratios for all parameters, can incorporate time-dependent covariates, allows the estimation of interaction terms between covariates, and provides estimates of incidence rates and survival functions.

All of these failure-time procedures rely on the *independent censoring assumption*. That is, censoring is statistically independent of the outcome (failure time), though its extent may vary among exposure groups. If the censoring mechanisms are not statistically independent of outcome, a valid estimate of survival for each group is not possible. In practice, this means that the reasons for withdrawals from the study must be assessed carefully to determine whether withdrawals may have introduced selection bias. For example, a patient who is lost to follow-up may be feeling well and see no need to return—a strong link between the outcome and the reason for censoring. An equally strong link would exist if the patient did not return because she was dissatisfied with the outcome and was seeking care elsewhere, or had died.

Poisson Models

The Poisson probability distribution describes the occurrence of binary events that are uncommon (i.e., have a low probability of occurrence). It is characterized by a single parameter, the average number of occurrences, which determines the probability of each possible number of occurrences (0, 1, 2, ...). Non-medical examples include the number of particles emitted by decay of a quantity of a radioactive substance in time intervals of fixed length and the number of misprints per page in a book. A typical Poisson analysis involves some important assumptions:

- outcomes in different subjects are statistically independent;
- the outcome variable is a non-recurrent binary health state (also referred to as a "failure," though it may sometimes be a desired outcome);
- losses to follow-up and death (censoring) are statistically independent of both exposure and outcome (independent censoring assumption);
- the rate ratios do not vary by time (proportional-hazards assumption);
- the rate ratios from different factors multiply each other (multiplicative model).

Statistical techniques can deal with some kinds of departures from these assumptions, but a strong study design serves to minimize problems before any data are collected.

An important property of the Poisson distribution is that the variance of the number of events is equal to the mean number of events. (If the variance is greater than the mean [overdispersed], special methods are required.) Similarly, when an event can occur more than once to an individual (e.g., respiratory illness during a six-month period) or among a group (e.g., new cases of breast cancer in groups of women during several years of study), one common probability model for the number of occurrences is the Poisson distribution. A historical reason for using the Poisson model is that for very large data sets other regression methods, such as the Cox proportional-hazards model, required considerable computing power. With the advent of very fast personal computers, this reason no longer holds. Even studies as large as the American Cancer Society CPS-II study,[14] with about 1,500,000 subjects, can now be analyzed on a high-speed desktop computer.

Poisson regression of rates is a straightforward extension of the stratified methods. Indeed, the method requires as input person-time and the number of events, both tabulated by the pre-defined strata. The strata can be independent of time (e.g., fixed exposure at baseline) or time-dependent (for example, age, calendar year, or cumulative exposure). The model relates the stratum-specific incidence rates (on a natural logarithmic scale) to the set of covariates. Poisson models can handle many situations in which covariates either confound or modify the effects of exposure.

In some instances, however, an intermediate variable can also act as a confounding variable. The usual methods of analysis (Poisson, Cox) cannot handle these types of situations, so special techniques need to be used. For example, suppose the investigator wants to determine whether Zidovudine improves survival in AIDS.[15] Zidovudine may improve survival in AIDS, and if past CD4 counts are associated with survival and also predict future Zidovudine use, then CD4 counts would act as both a confounding and effect-modifying variable. These complex methods are not described here (see [15-19]).

Example of Poisson Regression

The Agricultural Health Study,[20] a cohort study in two U.S. states that investigates occupational exposure to pesticides and herbicides, included a sub-study of the wives of 43,475 private pesticide applicators. The investigators obtained completed questionnaires regarding exposures of these women to pesticides on the farm and their general and reproductive health (for potential confounding factors). Incident cases of breast cancer were identified through state cancer registries, and vital status was ascertained through state death registries and the National Death Index. Subjects with a diagnosis of malignant or in situ breast cancer before the beginning of follow-up (1993) were excluded. The mean duration of follow-up was about five years (146,653 person-years). Person-years of observation were partitioned between the various levels of covariates and exposure, cases were assigned to the cells in which the events occurred, and Poisson regression was used to estimate the rate ratios. (This process entails a categorization of the variables, so standard stratified analyses could also have been used.) The known risk factors for breast cancer included age (5 categories), race (2), state (2), body mass index (4), age at menarche (2), parity (2), age at first birth (3), menopausal status (2), age at menopause (4), family history of breast cancer (2), smoking (3), and education (3). A full cross-classification on these risk factors would have had to assign person-years and cases to a total of 138,240 cells. With exposure categorized into five categories (e.g., years of pesticide application), the full analysis would have had 691,200 cells. The authors indicated that most of these factors did not have an influence on the association with exposure to pesticides, although it is unclear from the paper what modeling strategy was actually used to select variables. Table 2 shows the results for an analysis of all potential risk factors as well as exposure to pesticides and shows that the usual risk factors for breast cancer (adjusted for one another) were identified in the data. There was little evidence for an association between breast cancer and exposure to pesticides.

Cox Proportional-Hazards Model

As indicated above, another popular method for analyzing rates of failure is the Cox proportional-hazards model,[12] discussed in Chapter 11. The model assumes that each subject has a probability of failure, and a hazard rate (the probability

Table 2. Selected Results of Poisson Regression Analysis for the Incidence of Malignant Breast Cancer among Wives of Pesticide Applicators in the Agricultural Health Study.[20]

Characteristic	Cases (n = 309) No.	%	Noncases (n = 30,145) No.	%	Adjusted RR[‡,†]	95% CI
Age (years)						
18–39	29	9.4	9494	31.5	1[§]	
40–49	69	22.3	8653	28.7	2.7	1.7–4.1
50–59	120	38.8	7085	23.5	4.6	3.0–6.9
60–69	70	22.7	3964	13.2	4.5	2.9–7.1
70–96	21	6.8	949	3.2	7.0*	3.9–12.4
Race						
White	303	98.1	29,626	98.3	1[§]	
Other	6	1.9	519	1.7	1.5	0.6–3.4
State of residence						
Iowa	207	67.0	20,592	68.3	1[§]	
North Carolina	102	33.0	9553	31.7	0.7	0.6–1.0
Highest educational level[¶]						
Less than high school	16	5.7	1453	5.4	1[§]	
High school	129	46.1	10,866	40.4	1.1	0.6–1.9
More than high school	135	48.2	14,611	54.3	1.2	0.7–2.1
Smoking						
Never smoker	222	73.0	21,612	72.6	1[§]	
Former smoker	53	17.4	5085	17.1	1.0	0.8–1.4
Current smoker	29	9.5	3057	10.3	1.1	0.8–1.7
First-degree family history of breast cancer	74	24.7	3360	11.4	2.1	1.6–2.8

Table 2. Selected Results of Poisson Regression Analysis for the Incidence of Malignant Breast Cancer among Wives of Pesticide Applicators in the Agricultural Health Study (continued).[20]

Characteristic	Cases (n = 309) No.	%	Noncases (n = 30,145) No.	%	Adjusted RR[‡,†]	95% CI
Body mass index[§,#,]**						
<22.0	44	17.8	4792	22.6	1[§]	
22.0–24.9	71	28.7	5843	27.6	1.3	0.7–2.3
25.0–29.9	78	31.6	6670	31.5	1.4	0.8–2.4
≥30.0	54	21.9	3882	18.3	1.9*	1.1–3.4
Age (years) at menarche						
<12	125	43.9	10,730	44.6	1[§]	
≥12	160	56.1	13,310	55.4	1.1	0.8–1.4
Parous[§]	273	96.1	22,630	94.5	1.0	0.6–1.5
Age (years) at first birth[††]						
<20	53	19.6	3934	17.6	1[§]	
20–29	189	70.0	16,781	75.0	0.8	0.6–1.2
≥30	28	10.4	1668	7.5	1.3	0.8–2.2
Postmenopausal[§]	192	68.8	10,736	45.1	1.6	0.8–3.1
Age (years) at menopause**						
<40	30	13.2	2631	20.8	1[§]	
40–44	33	14.5	1891	14.9	1.4	0.8–2.5
45–49	58	25.6	3133	24.7	1.5	0.9–2.4
50–54	84	37.0	3890	30.7	1.6	1.0–2.6
≥55	22	9.7	1125	8.9	1.3	0.7–2.5

Table 2. Selected Results of Poisson Regression Analysis for the Incidence of Malignant Breast Cancer among Wives of Pesticide Applicators in the Agricultural Health Study (*continued*).[20]

Characteristic	Cases (n = 309) No.	%	Noncases (n = 30,145) No.	%	Adjusted RR[‡,†]	95% CI
Years of pesticide application						
0	152	57.6	13,297	51.4	1[‡]	
1–5	37	14.0	4608	17.8	1.0	0.7–1.4
6–10	22	8.3	2444	9.5	1.1	0.7–1.7
11–20	20	7.6	2918	11.3	0.7	0.4–1.1
≥21	33	12.5	2592	10.0	0.8	0.6–1.2

*p for trend < 0.05.

†RR, rate ratio; CI, confidence interval.

‡All factors were adjusted for the other factors in the table, except where indicated.

§Reference category.

‖Missing data (including those for questions for which the participant answered "Do not know") exceeded 10% for highest educational level (9.4% of cases and 10.7% of noncases among all study subjects; 8.5% of cases and 8.1% of noncases who never used pesticides), body mass index (20.1% of cases and 29.7% of noncases among all study subjects; 21.7% of cases and 32.6% of noncases who never used pesticides), age at menarche (7.8% of cases and 20.3% of noncases among all study subjects; 7.2% of cases and 21.6% of noncases who never used pesticides), parity (8.1% of cases and 20.6% of noncases among all study subjects; 7.2% of cases and 21.9% of noncases who never used pesticides), and menopausal status (9.7% of cases and 21.0% of noncases among all study subjects; 8.6% of cases and 22.0% of noncases who never used pesticides).

#Weight (kg)/height (m)².

**Restricted to postmenopausal women.

††Restricted to parous women.

Engel LS, Hill DA, Hoppin JA, et al., Pesticide use and breast cancer risk among farmers' wives in the Agricultural Health Study. American Journal of Epidemiology 2005, 161(2):121–35, by permission of Oxford University Press.

of failure, conditional on not having failed up to a specific time) at each time during follow-up. It then assumes that the relationship betwen these hazard rates does not vary by time; for example, suppose that the cohort can be divided into an unexposed group and an exposed group. If the rate ratio in the exposed is 3.2, for example, then the interpretation is that the rate is 3.2 times higher than in the unexposed group and that this ratio is constant across the follow-up period. As with the Poisson model, strata may be defined by a combination of explanatory variables, multiple exposure categories can be defined, and multiple confounding factors can be included. The Cox proportional-hazards model does not require that the outcome data follow a Poisson distribution.

Figure 1 shows graphically how the Cox model works. This example involves three failures. The *risk set* comprises the subject who has had the event and all

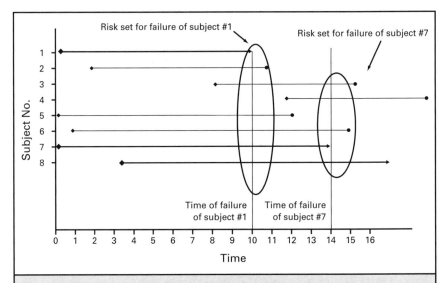

Figure 1. Incidence density sampling and the Cox proportional-hazards model.

A line ending in an arrow represents a subject who had an event, and a line ending in a small circle represents a subject who was censored (i.e., lost to follow-up, died of other causes, end of study). The risk period for the entire study is defined as the period of time from start to end of follow-up. The actual risk period for a particular subject is defined as the period of time between entering and leaving the cohort. The exposure period can occur during the risk period, but it can also be defined as occurring before entry into the cohort. Subjects who are censored are still at risk until the time they are censored; thus, in counting incidence time, one must include the person-time experience of these subjects. In this example, the first failure was subject 1, who had an event at time = 10. Subjects 2, 3, and 5–8 would serve as comparison subjects in the Cox model for this failure; subject 4 would not because she entered the study after the failure. Subjects 7 and 8 must be included even though they failed later on. To see this, consider that the incidence rate up to time = 10 would be 1 failure / (sum of the person-time of all subjects who are still under observation, including future cases).

those subjects who, at the time of the event, are still under observation and are still at risk of developing the event. All subjects who are in view when the first case (subject 1) becomes a case are selected as "controls" and the exposure profiles of the case and these "control" subjects are compared. A subject who becomes a case subsequently (subjects 7 and 8) is not excluded from this first risk set. For the second failure (subject 7), the risk set excludes the first case as well as those subjects who are lost to follow-up before the second failure time (subjects 2 and 5). Exposures can be defined at any time before the event occurred (including before the start of the study) or at the beginning of follow-up or reassessed at each failure time (time-dependent exposures). This sampling scheme is referred to as *incidence density sampling*, and in this example all potential controls are taken (100% sampling fraction).

The Cox model uses this sampling and then takes an "average" of the rate ratios across all risk sets; this is where the proportional-hazards assumptions comes in, as it is assumed that the rate ratios do not vary by time across the risk sets.

Examples of Cox Proportional-Hazards Model

The American Cancer Society's Cancer Prevention Study II (CPS-II), a population-based, prospective cohort study, included an investigation of whether obesity was associated with increased rates of death from cancer.[14] In 1982, volunteers enrolled almost 1.2 million study subjects from across the contiguous United States. Enrollment focused on persons who were considered unlikely to move, and comprised mostly relatives and friends of the volunteers, so the cohort does not necessarily reflect the general population of the United States. A self-administered questionnaire elicited information on a variety of personal characteristics and exposures (e.g., smoking, alcohol, body mass index). Among roughly 900,000 subjects who were cancer-free at enrollment, over 57,000 died from cancer during 16 years of follow-up.

A proportional-hazards analysis used age at time of entry (in single years) to define strata, and the relative risks associated with categories of body mass index (BMI) were adjusted for education, smoking status and (for smokers) the average number of cigarettes, physical activity, alcohol use, marital status, race, aspirin use, fat consumption, and vegetable consumption. A score (1, 2, 3, 4, 5) for the categories of BMI was used to assess whether the response function was compatible with linearity.

Directly standardized rates (i.e., adjusted only for age) were computed using the age distribution of the entire male or female study population, and rate ratios (cumulative mortality figure, Chapter 7) were obtained by dividing the rate in each category of BMI by the rate in the lowest group (18.5 to 24.9 kg/m^2). Analyses

Table 3. Rate Ratios among Men for Categories of Body Mass Index from the American Cancer Society's Cancer Prevention Study II, for All Cancers Combined, Adjusted for Selected Covariates.[14]

	Body mass index (kg/m^2)				
	18.5–24.9	25.0–29.9	30.0–34.9	35.0–39.9	≥40.0
Number of cancer deaths	13,855	15,372	2683	350	43
Directly standardized death rates per 100,000 person-years*	578.30	546.21	636.30	738.69	841.62
Relative risk from comparing directly standardized rates	1 (reference)	0.94	1.10	1.28	1.46
Relative risk from Cox model**	1 (reference)	0.97	1.09	1.20	1.52
95% CI		0.94–0.99	1.05–1.14	1.08–1.34	1.13–2.05

Source: Adapted from Table 1 of Calle et al.[14]

*Standardized by age using as a standard the entire sub-cohort of men.

**The Cox proportional-hazards model adjusted for age, education, smoking status and number of cigarettes smoked, physical activity, alcohol use, marital status, race, aspirin use, fat consumption, and vegetable consumption.

using the Cox model, adjusted for a number of factors including age, were also computed. From either analysis for men (Table 3), the risk of dying from cancer increased with body mass index. The test for linear trend in the Cox model ($p = 0.001$) supports this conclusion, though the pattern of increase in the relative risk is not exactly linear. The 95% confidence intervals show that the rate ratios for the three highest categories of BMI were statistically greater than the null value (rate ratio of 1), corresponding to the cancer mortality rate in the reference category. Categorization of a continuous variable is not optimal (misclassification across arbitrary cutpoints, assumption that the relative risks are constant within each subgroup); and other methods that make full use of the original, uncategorized data should be used to investigate nonlinearity with flexible functions such as natural cubic splines.[13]

Several applications of the Cox model come from a three-year follow-up study of chronic renal failure among patients who had transplants of non-renal organs.[21] The investigators used a variety of clinical transplant databases to assemble a cohort of 69,321 individuals in the United States who received a heart, lung, heart-lung, liver, or intestine transplant between 1990 and 2000 and were followed until 2001. The primary outcome variable was chronic renal failure or onset of end-stage renal disease (ESRD). The authors used one Cox regression model to investigate the relation between chronic renal failure and a number of baseline variables and a separate time-dependent Cox model to study the long-term effect of chronic renal failure on mortality. Patients who developed ESRD received renal-replacement therapy, either a kidney transplant or dialysis (while on a waiting list for a transplant). A time-dependent Cox regression model was used to estimate the effect of a kidney transplant on mortality among those who had ESRD and were on a waiting list, adjusting for the duration of ESRD before placement on a waiting list. Mortality after kidney transplantation, as compared to patients on dialysis, was higher for about the first five months, and transplanted subjects then had lower mortality rates (Figure 2). These results, showing non-proportionality of the relative risks through time, are of great importance for understanding the effects of the treatments.

MATCHING IN COHORT STUDIES TO CONTROL FOR CONFOUNDING

One method of controlling for confounding in the design stage is matching. In cohort studies, this is used rarely (but see [22-28]), but one example is a study in Sweden that was used to determine whether appendectomy decreased the risk of developing ulcerative colitis.[22] Patients who had an appendectomy before the

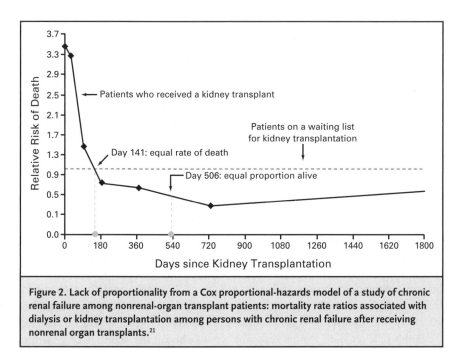

Figure 2. Lack of proportionality from a Cox proportional-hazards model of a study of chronic renal failure among nonrenal-organ transplant patients: mortality rate ratios associated with dialysis or kidney transplantation among persons with chronic renal failure after receiving nonrenal organ transplants.[21]

age of 50 years, identified from the central Inpatient Register (1964–1993), were matched individually on age, sex, and residence to subjects who did not have the procedure. After all exclusions, there were 212,963 individuals in the cohort of persons with appendectomies and the same number in the comparison cohort. An issue with individual matching is that subjects may be excluded if a match cannot be found or if a comparison subject had to be excluded (80 died and were excluded in this study). Both groups were then followed, and the incidence rate of ulcerative colitis was assessed and compared using the Cox proportional-hazards model. It is incorrect to use an ordinary (non-matched) analysis for a matched study; a matched analysis will increase statistical precision. For example, the crude rate ratio for perforated appendicitis was 0.59 (95% CI: 0.34 to 0.99), whereas the adjusted estimate was about the same but with a smaller range (0.58, 95% CI: 0.38 to 0.87). In addition, although matching at the beginning of the study may guarantee balance, this balance may be upset through follow-up time because of deaths and censoring, so that adjustments are usually still needed. Thus, matched cohort studies may have lower statistical precision than unmatched designs.[19, 29] In general, matching is seldom advantageous for cohorts, but it is in case-control studies (see below).

NESTED CASE-CONTROL STUDIES

A variation of incidence cohort studies is the nested case-control study. This design is useful when individual outcomes are known, but potential confounders and modifiers are not known, and there are high costs to obtaining person-specific information after the cohort was defined (for example, a cancer registry may include all known cases in a defined population, with little or no other information about either cases or the population that does not have cancer). This approach allows for the collection of individual data for all known cases but for only a random sample of the much larger group of potential control subjects (i.e., those subjects who have not had the outcome and are still "in view"). The data from this reduced sample of controls are equivalent to the data that would be obtained from study of the whole population except that variances are larger. One has two choices for the types of software that can be used for the analysis, and they are equivalent: a Cox model or a conditional logistic model (discussed in Chapter 12).

Figure 1 can be used to describe the process used in the nested case-control study. The risk set for the first failure (subject 1 at time = 10) comprises the case and potential controls (subjects 2, 3, 5, 6, 7, and 8), and the Cox model would include all of these subjects in the analysis. In the nested case-control study, at each failure, a random number of control subjects would be selected from the risk set, and the investigator would choose the number of controls.

(The more controls, the greater the statistical precision of the analysis, but the cost of obtaining extra information would increase.) For example, if the investigator chose two controls per case, then she would develop a process to select these subjects randomly; for example, subjects 2 and 7 could be chosen, and the remaining controls would be ignored in the analysis. However, all possible controls still in view would be available for selection at the next failure (this is called sampling with replacement), so subjects 3, 4, 6, and 8 could be selected for the second failure (subject 7 at time = 14). Thus, eligibility of a subject as a control at the time of each failure in a proportional-hazards study can be thought of in terms of the calculation of person-time and incidence rates. This implies that 1) all subjects who were censored or failed before the case became a case would be ineligible and 2) all subjects who had not yet become a case or censored would still be eligible for selection. Excluding this latter group of subjects as controls may lead to serious biases.[30] If additional matching criteria were used in selecting controls (e.g., gender, age), the set of eligible controls would be those who fit the criteria. This matching is equivalent to defining strata in the Cox model. The process of the nested case-control study is just the Cox analysis except that the sampling fraction is no longer 100%, and this explains why Cox or conditional logistic software could be used for the analysis.

As suggested above, although nested case-control studies provide unbiased estimates of rate ratios, those estimates will be more variable than estimates from the full-cohort analysis because only a sample of control subjects is studied.[31, 32] However, improvements in statistical precision are small after the first few controls for each case. For example, using 11 cases per control rather than 3, a 3-fold increase in total number of subjects, decreases the variance of case-control differences by only 18%. The number of control subjects in the sample must be large enough so that sampling variations will not mask what would have been found had the full cohort been analyzed. It is often assumed that three controls for each case suffice, but the optimal number of controls will depend on the prevalence of exposure and the expected rate ratios. Thus, as in any study, due consideration must be given in advance to estimating sample size.[11, 31]

Two examples show the use of this design. In a study of HMG-CoA reductase inhibitors (statins) and the risk of fractures within the U.K. General Practice Research Database, up to six control subjects were matched (by age, gender, general practice attended, calendar time, and years of prior history in the database) to each of the 3940 cases having a first fracture.[33] This database comprised more than 3 million subjects, so that the full-cohort analysis would have taken an inordinate amount of computer resources with little further reduction in the variance of comparisons between cases and controls. The results of the analysis are shown in Table 4. Current use of statins decreased the risk of having

Table 4. Rate Ratios for Statin Use and Fractures from a Nested Case-Control Study Conducted within the U.K. General Practice Research Database.

	No Statin Use	Past Statin Use	Current Statin Use			
				Number of Prescriptions for Statins		
			Total	1–4	5–19	≥20
Number of cases (3940)*	3235	58	112	23	55	34
Number of controls (23,379)*	19223	321	918	213	404	301
Odds ratio**	1	0.87	0.55	0.51	0.62	0.52
95% CI		0.65–1.18	0.44–0.69	0.33–0.81	0.45–0.85	0.36–0.76

Adapted from Table 2 of Meier et al.[33]

*The total numbers of cases and controls in the first column include subjects with other drug use, so the sum of subjects who used statins does not correspond to the total.

**The odds ratios are interpreted as direct estimates of the rate ratios for statin use to no statin use, adjusted for body mass index, smoking, number of general practitioner visits, and steroid or estrogen use.

a fracture, although there was no indication of decreasing risks by number of computer-recorded prescriptions prior to the index date.

This next example illustrates the use of the design when costly information that was not available at the time the cohort was defined is required. In a study of cervical cancer in Scandinavia, stored serum samples were analyzed for IgG antibodies to *Chlamydia trachomatis* and *C. pneumoniae* for 181 women with cervical cancer and for three controls matched to each case.[34] Such an analysis on the complete cohort would have been extremely expensive and also would have depleted the biological samples that could be used for further analyses.

LONGITUDINAL COHORT STUDIES

Longitudinal studies are cohort studies in which outcomes may be reversible, may recur, and may for each subject be measured more than once during the follow-up period. As explained in Chapter 7, health states can be defined on nominal, ordinal, or continuous scales. An example of a binary, recurrent outcome is relapse of moderate symptoms of multiple sclerosis, and an example of a continuous scale is blood pressure. Incidence (and prevalence) rates are not defined for outcomes measured on continuous scales. At the cost of losing important information, incidence can be estimated by transforming the outcome to a binary scale and by including the dimension of time (e.g., first time that lung function was less than 80% of predicted). As in any cohort study, exposures can be measured before or during the period of observation.

The advantage of a longitudinal study over a standard cohort study is its ability to assess changes in health states over time. For health outcomes that may recur, the basic methods of regression analysis are modified to account for within-subject correlation between observations. Thus, the statistical methods become more complicated: Because each subject contributes more than one observation, one cannot assume statistical independence of the observations. One consequence is that the effective sample size will generally be less than the number of observations (though greater than for a single observation per subject) and, thus, estimates of population-wide variances will be greater. In addition, there may be important questions related to change of outcomes through time and how covariates affect this change. Repeated measures can give much more precise estimates of change, which is usually the object of most interest, though they give less precise estimates of population-wide levels.

Depending on the study design and the nature of the data, many types of outcomes can be assessed, even in one study, and these evaluations can be carried out in various ways. Of course, standard analyses of incidence can be undertaken for variables that are non-recurring. Cross-sectional analyses can also be conducted using categorical or continuous measures (e.g., lung function, prevalence of asthma), and mean values or proportions between groups, such as exposure groups, can be estimated. In these instances, a range of models is available (multiple linear regression, logistic regression, polytomous regression,[35] ordinal regression[36]). The accumulated person-time experience of the cohort is disregarded, so the validity and interpretation of the findings depend strongly on whether those subjects who were excluded from analysis because of censoring (from death or loss to follow-up) or because of missing data differ importantly from those who were part of the analysis (selection bias).

The British Doctors Study,[37] which made assessments of cigarette smoking throughout the study period, is not considered a longitudinal study because the outcome was defined exclusively as a failure (namely, cause-specific mortality). The Framingham study,[38] which administered examinations and questionnaires periodically throughout the follow-up period, can be considered a failure-time study for outcomes that do not recur (e.g., a first breast cancer),[39] but a longitudinal study for outcomes such as changes in lung function.[40]

Examples of Longitudinal Cohort Studies

A study of intellectual impairment in children and blood levels of lead[41] illustrates many of the issues. The original cohort comprised 276 children born between July 1994 and January 1995 who were enrolled at birth in a study of the efficacy of control of household dust and were enrolled in the present study when they were between 24 and 30 months of age. One hundred ninety-eight children (71.7%) were tested for intelligence at 3 and 5 years of age, and 172 had fairly complete data (about 150 children at each assessment). Blood lead levels were measured at 6, 12, 18, 24, 36, 48, and 60 months of age, and lifetime averages were estimated by the area under the blood-lead concentration curve from 6 to 36 months and from 6 to 60 months. The intelligence tests used the Stanford-Binet Intelligence Scale, which is designed to produce an age-standardized score relative to a baseline value of 100 and a standard deviation of 16.1 in the population at large. Use of age-standardized IQ scores allows for fair comparisons among subjects who had different concentrations of lead across time.

Consider first an analysis of this study using only the first assessment of intelligence. Because each subject contributed one observation, the analysis was a multiple linear regression (with a random effect for each child), in which intelligence scores were regressed on exposure to lead. (It is unclear why a random effect was needed, as the analysis did not involve repeated measures.) Specifically, after adjusting for maternal IQ, race, level of education, use of tobacco during pregnancy, household income, and the score on the Home Observation for Measurement of Environment Inventory (an index that reflects the quality and quantity of emotional and cognitive stimulation in the home environment), and the child's sex, birth weight, and iron status, the mean IQ measured at age three years decreased by 0.35 points for each increase of 1 µg per deciliter of lifetime exposure to lead (95% CI: −0.69 to −0.00). A similar analysis at age five years showed a stronger effect (−0.57 points; 95% CI: −0.93 to −0.20). Because these analyses were conducted separately, there was no need to account for multiple observations per subject. However, the two results are not statistically independent of each other because in any one subject the IQ score at age five can be roughly predicted from that at age three (Pearson correlation coefficient, $r = 0.67$).

The slightly stronger effect at age five may suggest that continued exposure to lead is associated with decreases in IQ. The investigators reported a crude test of equality (a t-test of the regression coefficients) that assumed statistical independence. This test is too liberal because the observations are correlated, but more-complex regression models that accounted for the correlations led to the same conclusion. Thus, because the estimates at the two ages were similar, the mean value of the assessments at ages three and five years is a reasonable representation across these ages: the reduction in mean IQ averaged over these ages was −0.46 points per µg/dL, and, with more data contributing to the combined estimate, confidence bounds were somewhat narrower (95% CI: −0.76 to −0.15). The extensive adjustments for covariates increase the likelihood that this relationship is one of cause-and-effect.

Had there been important differences in the effect of lead between these two ages, the interaction effect between lead and age would have been statistically significant. This interaction effect would be interpreted as representing how age affects the relationship between lead and mean IQ. A simple way of thinking about this is to plot on one graph, for each subject separately, the adjusted IQ scores against age. If the rate of change of IQ (the slope) for each subject is similar (i.e., the lines are approximately parallel), then the interaction term described above would be equal to the slope averaged across subjects.

Use of change scores in longitudinal studies is described in more depth in Chapters 4 and 9, on randomized clinical trials. The message is that adjusting for baseline (regression of the final on the initial value, the difference of values on the initial, or the difference of values on the mean) is non-optimal and should be avoided. Rather, models that can handle different starting values of the dependent variable by including a random-effects component on the intercept should be used. Thus, the intercepts or starting values for each subject are that person's actual initial observation. In addition, these random-effects models allow for the slopes to vary among subjects; in this case, an average slope and the range across subjects (the random-effects component) are estimated.

The analyses described above assume that the relationship between IQ and lead exposure is linear. Simple ways to avoid this assumption, as discussed above, are to use polynomial functions or nonparametric or semi-parametric smoothers. Indeed, the authors used both methods: Figure 3, based on a model that included a penalized spline (a complicated type of flexible smoother), shows a nonlinear relationship between IQ and lifetime average blood lead concentration.

An important methodological point in longitudinal studies is that subjects who do not participate in a scheduled evaluation are generally omitted from that part of the analysis, as they were in this study of lead and IQ. If the reasons for not participating are related to outcome (IQ) and exposure (lead), such exclusions may introduce a selection bias. Authors often present a table comparing participants to non-participants to show whether these groups are similar in baseline characteristics, as was done in the present study. Because of the short interval between IQ assessments and because there were few missing observations, it is unlikely that missing follow-up data are a serious problem here, but this may not be true in other studies.

Another issue is related to tailoring the methods used in the statistical analysis to account closely for the design of the study. A cohort study on inhaled glucocorticoids and changes in bone density in premenopausal women[42] used the data to their fullest extent. This cohort study followed 109 asthmatic women for three years. Subjects were classified into one of three groups: those not taking inhaled glucocorticoids ($n = 28$); those taking four to eight puffs per day

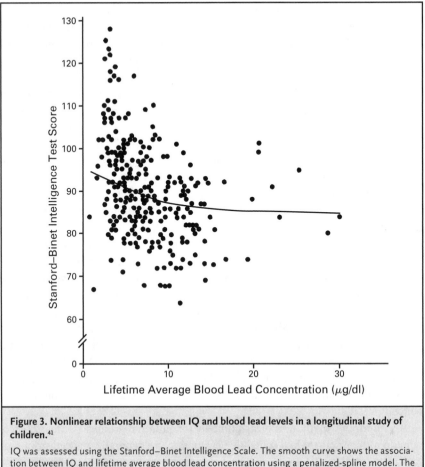

Figure 3. Nonlinear relationship between IQ and blood lead levels in a longitudinal study of children.[41]

IQ was assessed using the Stanford–Binet Intelligence Scale. The smooth curve shows the association between IQ and lifetime average blood lead concentration using a penalized-spline model. The individual data points represent unadjusted lifetime mean concentrations of blood and IQ values.

of inhaled glucocorticoids ($n = 39$); and those taking more than eight puffs per day ($n = 42$). Women who were taking glucocorticoids other than triamcinolone acetonide were switched to triamcinolone acetonide. Annualized changes in bone density were regressed against average number of puffs taken per day, adjusting for a priori confounding variables and covariates that were found to be associated with the dose of inhaled glucocorticoids, and a mixed regression model was used to account for correlations in bone density measurements over time. The authors found that each additional puff was associated with a decrease of 0.00044 g/cm^2 in bone density of the total hip.

A study designed to identify factors that influence reductions in microalbuminuria among persons with Type 1 diabetes[43] illustrates how data in longitudinal studies are often analyzed as failure-time data despite possible losses in information. In a cohort of 386 patients, urinary albumin excretion was measured approximately every eight months over an eight-year period. Rather than analyze the rate of change of albumin excretion over time, the investigators divided the total period of observation into four two-year intervals. At the end of each two-year period a subject was classified as having microalbuminuria if the median of all measurements of albumin excretion rate in the period was in the range of 30 to 299 µg/minute. A favorable change was defined as a reduction of at least 50% from the median in the preceding two-year period. The authors then used a failure-time analysis where time to event was defined in each two-year interval. Shortcomings with this method of analysis include categorizing, in an essentially arbitrary manner, an interval variable (albumin excretion) and loss of valuable information on the time intervals between measurements. Mixed models could have been used to estimate changes in albumin excretion through time, and the influence of explanatory variables (e.g., cholesterol levels, systolic blood pressure) on rate of change could have been assessed.

A longitudinal study of a birth cohort of New Zealand children illustrates how arbitrary definitions of health states can constrain the analysis and interpretation of a study. The study was designed to investigate health and behavior through time, and the specific objective was to identify risk factors for persistence and relapse of wheeze.[44] The cohort comprised children who were born in 1972–1973 and who were followed until age 26 years. Figure 4 shows the time points at which relevant factors were measured, as well as the percentage of subjects participating at each time. Asthma was characterized by wheezing, and its occurrence through time is marked by exacerbations and relapses. In order to capture the various aspects of the temporal patterns of asthma, the outcome measure was a 7-level variable based on a classification of reported symptoms (Figure 5): no wheezing ever; transient wheezing; intermittent wheezing; remission; relapse; persistent wheezing from onset; and persistent wheezing from nine years of age. The analytic strategy was driven by this definition: it required data from subjects who completed all assessments, so only 613 of the base cohort of 1037 (59.1%) were included in the analysis of persistence, remission, and relapse of wheezing. Concern about this high exclusion rate is reinforced by concerns that lost patients may be atypical and hence this exclusion may bias results. The authors addressed this in a table comparing selected baseline characteristics of the 613 subjects to those who were not seen at all assessments and used hypothesis tests to determine whether there were differences. Differences were found in some variables (current asthma and wheezing at age nine

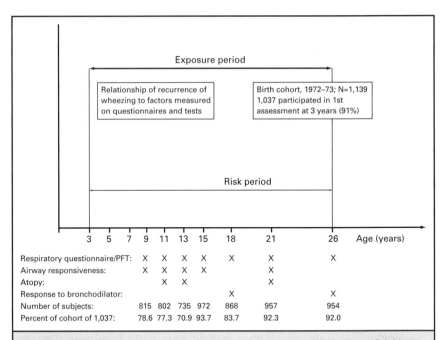

Figure 4. Layout of the longitudinal follow-up study of wheezing in a birth cohort of children living in New Zealand.[44]

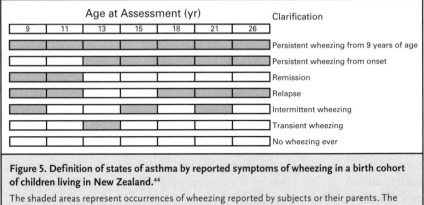

Figure 5. Definition of states of asthma by reported symptoms of wheezing in a birth cohort of children living in New Zealand.[44]

The shaded areas represent occurrences of wheezing reported by subjects or their parents. The categories of time are illustrative and are not part of the definitions.

years, atopy at 13 years, dust mite allergies at 13 and 21 years), but the authors concluded that the analyzed sample was representative of the base cohort.

The proportions of characteristics were compared among the outcome categories from persistent from onset to never wheezed using a chi-squared test for linear trend. For example, the proportion of subjects with a positive skin test for house dust mite allergens increased with increasing levels of wheezing (p-value for linear trend <0.001; Table 5). However, the "distances" among these categories are not defined: for example, is the increase in severity from transient to intermittent wheezing the same size as the increase from relapse to persistent? (Analysis of data in such ordered categories is discussed in Chapter 13.) It seems unlikely that adjacent categories are even approximately equidistant in any meaningful clinical sense; thus, linear regression is not appropriate. Instead, the authors used logistic regression, excluding subjects without wheeze, comparing subjects with persistent wheeze to all other subjects, and comparing subjects with relapses to all other subjects except those who had persistent wheeze. For example, for a positive skin test for house dust mite allergens at 13 years, the odds ratio of persistence compared to all other categories except never wheezed was 3.38 (95% CI: 2.12 to 5.37), and that for relapse compared to all other categories except persistence and never was 4.17 (95% CI: 2.49 to 7.01).

This analytic procedure is not optimal for ordinal outcomes. The comparisons are arbitrary, the exclusion of subjects without wheeze is not explained, and the differences in odds ratios between categories might be chance events. A

Table 5. Proportion of Subjects with a Positive Skin Test for House Dust Mite Allergens at 13 Years by Pattern of Wheezing and Odds Ratios from the Proportional-Odds Ordinal Model.[44]

	Wheezing pattern					
	Persistent	Relapse	Remission	Intermittent	Transient	Never
Number of subjects with data	88	71	87	56	129	166
Proportion of subjects with a positive skin test (%)*	55.7	54.9	35.6	30.4	23.3	12.7
Number with positive skin test	49	39	31	17	30	21
Number without positive skin test	39	32	56	39	99	145
Reanalysis of these data using an unadjusted proportional-odds ordinal regression model						
Odds ratio (95% CI) for proportions with a positive skin test, comparing each category of wheezing to all other categories**	3.4 (2.1–5.4)	4.2 (2.9–6.2)	3.9 (2.7–5.6)	3.9 (2.7–5.7)	4.3 (2.6–7.1)	1

*The p-value for linear trend across the categories of wheezing was <0.001.

**The odds ratios represent comparing persistent wheezing versus all other categories, relapse versus all other categories, etc. The summary estimate from the proportional-odds model was 4.0 (95% CI: 2.9 to 5.5), with $p = 0.72$ for the test of homogeneity across the categories.

more appropriate analysis is through ordinal regression. I conducted a reanalysis of these data, although it was not possible to adjust for other factors. The odds ratio of each category compared to all others is presented in the last row of Table 5, and the findings are close to those obtained by the authors. These simple logistic models are based on the same categorizations used in the proportional-odds ordinal regression model. However, the proportional-odds model produces a summary estimate across the ordinal categories; specifically the odds ratio was 4.0 (95% CI 2.9 to 5.5). As well, a test of homogeneity across the categories can be obtained ($p = 0.72$), and this is interpreted as meaning that it does not matter how the ordinal categories are combined, and the best estimate of the effect of positive skin test on severity of wheezing was statistically independent of the categorization of wheezing. This conclusion is in contrast to the interpretation of the test of linear trend ($p < 0.001$).

In addition to analyzing wheeze, the authors used a generalized estimating equations (GEE) framework[45] for analysis of pulmonary function tests using the interval variable FEV_1:FVC ratio. (To handle correlated data, this regression method makes simplifying assumptions about the structure of the within-subject correlations between observations.) The investigators compared average differences in FEV_1:FVC between the wheezing groups across all time points. This index of pulmonary function was modeled using multiple regression, but accounting for the fact that multiple measurements on each subject were taken and were correlated. The analysis is similar to a repeated-measures analysis with each observation being used as the unit of analysis, but taking into account within-subject correlations. The regression coefficients represent the average mean change in FEV_1:FVC, after accounting for the correlations in the data. Figure 6 shows the patterns by age according to the wheezing categories. A conclusion of this analysis was that men with persistent wheezing had a 6.8% lower mean FEV_1:FVC ratio than men without wheezing ($p < 0.001$). An alternative and likely more powerful analysis (including all subjects) would have made use of the binary time-dependent outcome variable suggested above for wheezing and then tested specifically the interaction between wheezing and age on FEV_1:FVC.

INCIDENCE CASE-CONTROL STUDIES

As with cohort studies, stratified procedures (such as Mantel-Haenszel) can be used to analyze case-control studies (see Chapter 7). Regression methods have been developed to handle binary outcome data, and these are now used routinely by researchers. For unmatched data, the appropriate model is logistic regression (discussed in Chapter 12); for matched designs, it is conditional logistic regression.

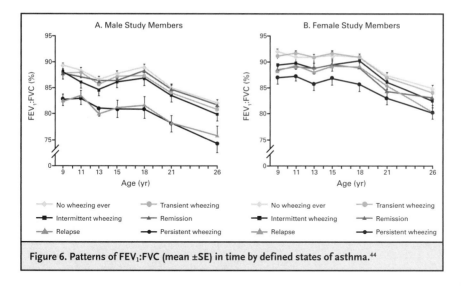

Figure 6. Patterns of FEV₁:FVC (mean ±SE) in time by defined states of asthma.[44]

Generally, well-designed case-control studies can be thought of as nested case-control studies, except that the cohort is not defined explicitly. A usual assumption is that the target population is stationary (steady state), namely that the distributions of key variables (e.g., age, gender) and their effects remain approximately constant in time during the study period. The parameter estimated in the logistic model can be interpreted as odds on the natural logarithmic scale, and odds ratios comparing values of covariates can be computed from the regression coefficients. Thus, the interpretation of a logistic model is similar to that of a simple 2×2 table, but the odds ratio for any one covariate is adjusted for all other covariates in the model. The conditional logistic model extends this model to data that have been matched in the design stage. For example, if one has matched three controls to each case based on year of birth, then a conditional logistic model would be appropriate.

Examples of Case-Control Studies

A study of the association of a mother's own birth weight and gestational diabetes during her first pregnancy[46] illustrates important lessons about analyzing case-control data. Table 6 shows the principal results for the mother's own birth weight. The results in the first row treat birth weight as a continuous variable, and show a protective effect. The units of birth weight for this odds ratio were not stated, but it can be inferred from the categorical analysis that it corresponds to an approximately 500 g increase in maternal birth weight. (The odds ratio for a continuous variable in a logistic model is based on a

Table 6. Selected Results from a Case-Control Study of Mother's Birth Weight and Subsequent Development of Gestational Diabetes.*

Birth weight (g)	No. of cases	No. of controls	OR (95% CI) adjusted for gestational age	p-value**	OR (95% CI) adjusted for gestational age and other factors	p-value**
Continuous variable	N/A	N/A	0.84 (0.75–0.94)	0.002	0.73 (0.62–0.86)	<0.001
Categorical variable						
<2000	10	328	2.16 (1.04–4.50)		4.23 (1.55–11.51)	
2000–2499	34	1291	1.57 (1.03–2.40)		2.58 (1.44–4.60)	
2500–2999	111	5024	1.35 (1.02–1.80)	0.002	1.93 (1.25–2.99)	<0.001
3000–3499	156	9226	1.05 (0.80–1.36)		1.42 (1.00–2.01)	
3500–3999	91	5548	1		1	
≥4000	35	1460	1.53 (1.03–2.27)		0.92 (0.54–1.57)	

*Adapted from Table 3 of Innes et al.[46]

**p-values on the first row (continuous variable) are derived from a Wald test for linear trend. p-values for the categorical variable are based on an unspecified test for trend. In the analysis that adjusted only for gestational age, the test for trend included only birth weights less than 4000g.

Adapted with permission from JAMA. Innes KE, Byers TE, Marshall JA, et al. Association of a woman's own birth weight with subsequent risk for gestational diabetes. Table 3. JAMA 2002; 287(19):2534–41. Copyright © 2002 American Medical Association. All rights reserved.

particular amount of change in the variable; hence that change, the units, must be reported.) The p-value associated with this odds ratio ($p = 0.002$) comes from a test of linear trend. The categorical analysis, presented below the continuous one, is based on arbitrarily cutting the birth weight distribution into six mutually exclusive categories, using the category 3500–3999 g as reference (OR = 1). In the analysis adjusted for gestational age, risks decreased until 3999 g and then increased (a "J-shaped" pattern). Thus, the odds ratio using birth weight as a continuous variable may be misleading, because it does not show the J-shape produced by the increment in risk in the last category.

On the other hand, the odds ratio for ≥4000 g may be an artifact of the specific cut points used. A more appropriate analysis[47] could use a larger number of narrower categories or a polynomial (e.g., a linear-quadratic) model or splines to determine whether there is indeed some upward trend at the high end of the birth weight scale. The fitted function can also be plotted with the residuals. Use of flexible functions would lessen residual confounding arising from not capturing the correct functional form of the covariates.[48, 49]

In the categorical analysis, the p-values of 0.002 and <0.001 are labeled as coming from a test for trend. Categorical variables do not lead to a formal test for trend. The authors apparently assigned scores to the categories.

This example also shows how confounding can affect the results. The odds ratios in the right-hand column are adjusted for several potentially confounding factors. The J-shaped pattern has now vanished, and instead the odds ratios show a monotonically decreasing trend, confirmed by the much lower p-value ($p < 0.001$). More importantly, the confidence intervals have increased in length; for example, the interval for the birth weight category <2000 g has increased nearly 3-fold in length from 3.46 to 9.96. This increase is most likely due to adjusting for factors that are collinear with birth weight (i.e., so highly correlated that variables are measuring nearly the same trait). In summary, the initial J-shaped pattern may have been an artifact of arbitrarily assigning cut points to a continuous variable, and the fully adjusted analysis may be incorrect because of collinearity, although one may have some confidence that the overall trend is a decrease in risk as birth weight increases. (As a general rule in statistics, whenever small changes in the data or methods cause large and unexpected changes in standard errors, it may be useful to look for collinearity.)

CROSS-SECTIONAL STUDIES

In cross-sectional studies of health, in which the sampling of subjects is independent of health or exposure (i.e., many surveys), the health outcome is commonly a health state, defined by a continuous, nominal, or ordinal variable. The type of outcome variable determines the choice of regression technique. When the health outcome is a non-recurrent failure-type event, prevalence is estimated, and the appropriate analysis is a Mantel-Haenszel stratified analysis or logistic regression. (Incidence rate ratios may be estimable from prevalence ratios when the duration of disease is statistically independent of risk factors.) For nominal outcomes, prevalence can also be estimated using polytomous or ordinal regression methods.

For health outcomes that are measured on continuous or interval scales, simple linear regression can be used. The main statistical assumptions are statistical independence of the outcome among subjects (no clustering by design), the outcome is distributed normally, and the population variance does not differ among subjects.

Examples of Cross-Sectional Studies

A cross-sectional study of children and adolescents, part of the Child and Adolescent Trial for Cardiovascular Health, examined individual-level variables and homocysteine levels measured at the time of the eighth-grade risk factor screening survey (1997). In a cross-sectional analysis a mixed linear regression model accounted for the nested design of the original study, namely school nested within field site. The analysis of serum homocysteine and its correlates[50] (Table 7) showed that homocysteine levels were higher in boys (5.44 µmol/L) than in girls (5.05; $p < 0.001$). The adjusted means were based on a linear regression model in which the slightly skewed values of homocysteine levels were first transformed to a natural logarithm scale and then regressed on individual covariates as well as variables related to the original study design (CATCH field site [and original CATCH intervention condition fixed effects] and school within field site and intervention condition [random effect]).

Chapter 7 introduced a study[51] that used logistic regression to identify variables associated with the prevalence of advanced colonic neoplasia. Table 8 shows the results of a multivariable logistic analysis comparing, at the time of the survey, subjects with advanced colonic neoplasia (prevalence) with those not having any colonic polyps. The prevalence odds ratio for these selected factors was estimated after adjusting for age and total energy intake (from dietary assessments conducted at the time of the survey) and the other factors in the table. Some of the significant odds ratios on continuous variables may seem very small because of scaling. For example, the odds ratio for vitamin D (OR = 0.94; 95%CI: 0.90 to 0.99) is based on an increase of 100 IU; perhaps a more easily interpretable increase would be change per 1000 IU or a change across the interquartile range (from the 25th to the 75th percentile). However, an important issue with this study is the interpretation of these factors as "risk factors." The term "risk factor" is meant to convey that it may be related causally to the development of new cancers (incidence), whereas prevalence odds ratios reflect the effects of both incidence and duration of disease (survival). For example, although vitamin D was found to be protective, this effect may be related to changes of diet because of illness or to the possibility that consumption of vitamin D is also related to survival after the cancer was present.

Table 7. Distribution of Serum Homocysteine Levels (µmol/L) by Gender in a Cross-Sectional Study of Cardiovascular Risk Factors in Children and Adolescents.[*]

	Mean (SD)	Adjusted Geometric Mean (95% CI)[**]	Percentile 25th	Percentile 50th	Percentile 75th
Boys	5.48 (1.90)	5.44 (5.21–5.68)	4.3	5.1	6.2
Girls	5.09 (1.78)	5.05 (4.84–5.27)	4.0	4.8	5.8

[*]Adapted from Tables 2 and 3 of Osganian et al.[50]

[**]The p-value was <0.001 for the difference in means from a mixed model that adjusted for age, original CATCH intervention condition, site, school, sex, race, multivitamin use, smoking, family history of cardiovascular disease, body mass index, serum total and high-density lipoprotein cholesterol, and systolic blood pressure among 3151 girls and boys with complete data.

Table 8. Multivariable Logistic Analysis of Factors Associated with the Prevalence of Advanced Neoplasia.

Factor	Adjusted Prevalence Odds Ratio*	95% Confidence Interval
Family history of colon cancer	1.66	1.16–2.35
Current smoking	1.85	1.33–2.58
Current moderate to heavy alcohol consumption, per serving per week	1.02	1.01–1.03
Physical activity index, per 5 units	0.94	0.86–1.02
Daily nonsteroidal anti-inflammatory drug use	0.66	0.48–0.91
Body mass index, per 5 units	1.06	0.94–1.20
Cereal fiber, per 1 g	0.95	0.91–0.99
Beef, pork, or lamb as main dish	1.06	0.98–1.15
Vitamin D, per 100 IU	0.94	0.90–0.99

Adapted from Table 4 of Lieberman et al.[51]

*The logistic model included age and total energy intake as well as the factors listed in the table. Fat derived from beef, pork, or lamb was expressed as a percentage of total energy intake.

Adapted with permission from JAMA. Lieberman DA, Prindiville S, Weiss DG, Willett W. Risk factors for advanced colonic neoplasia and hyperplastic polyps in asymptomatic individuals. Table 4. JAMA 2003; 290(22):2959–67. Copyright © 2003 American Medical Association. All rights reserved.

SOME GENERAL ISSUES IN REGRESSION MODELING

Incorrect use of statistical adjustment procedures may introduce bias. In a study of upper gastrointestinal bleeding, both population-based and hospital controls were frequency-matched by gender and age in five-year age groups.[52] The investigators used a stepwise procedure to select variables for a logistic regression model. Although gender and age were included as potential covariates in the stepwise procedure, the matching would have led to large p-values, so these variables would not have been retained in the model. Because the distributions of age and sex were almost identical between cases and controls (successful frequency-matching), excluding these variables from the model would probably not have introduced an important bias, although it might have inflated standard errors. This may not be true in all studies where the matching was not as close, and the general rule is to force into the model these matching variables as well as, usually, all accepted risk factors.

A study of Factor XI and deep venous thrombosis illustrates a loss of information through the categorization of a continuous covariate.[53] The distributions in cases and controls are shown in boxplots (Figure 7). The median in the cases is larger than in the controls. This would imply that the odds ratio comparing cases to controls is greater than unity. The analysis was based on comparing

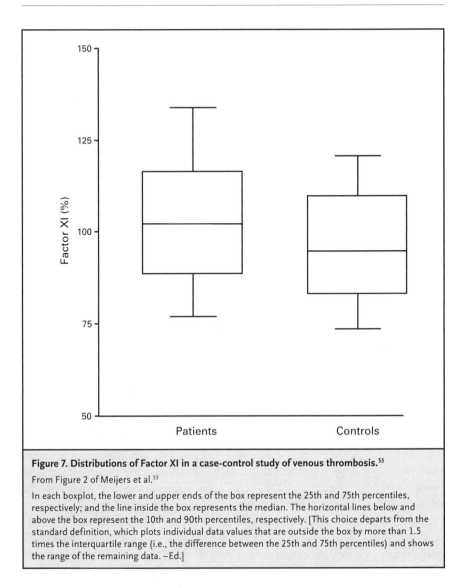

Figure 7. Distributions of Factor XI in a case-control study of venous thrombosis.[53]

From Figure 2 of Meijers et al.[53]

In each boxplot, the lower and upper ends of the box represent the 25th and 75th percentiles, respectively; and the line inside the box represents the median. The horizontal lines below and above the box represent the 10th and 90th percentiles, respectively. [This choice departs from the standard definition, which plots individual data values that are outside the box by more than 1.5 times the interquartile range (i.e., the difference between the 25th and 75th percentiles) and shows the range of the remaining data. –Ed.]

subjects above the 90th (and 95th) percentiles of Factor XI to those below it (odds ratios of 2.2 [95%CI: 1.5 to 3.2] and 2.3 [95%CI: 1.4 to 3.9], respectively). The form of the exposure response curve cannot be estimated using such crude methods and, again, use of natural splines or other functional forms might have been more informative.

OVERALL CONSIDERATIONS

The above descriptions of methods and examples illustrate some broad issues in statistical analysis. In particular, the design of the study as well as the health outcome variable (dependent variable in a regression model) will dictate the general type of statistical analysis. Simpler, more-intuitive analysis may be carried out so that the researcher is assured that the findings from more-complex models are appropriate, but when the design is complicated, these simpler methods may actually lead to incorrect conclusions. Before a complex design is chosen, the investigator should ensure that appropriate analytical methods are available and that sufficient expertise will be available to apply them correctly.

Missing data, especially in longitudinal studies, and the biases they may cause are very important but are not discussed in depth in this chapter. Imputation of missing data is beyond the scope of this chapter but is becoming more important as research designs become more complex.

All models require some assumptions; when the assumptions for a specific model are close to correct, that model will be more powerful (in a statistical sense) than alternatives; but if they are not adequately fulfilled, the model may be a lot worse than a model that is less demanding. Thus, the investigator should know what assumptions are behind each model, and how closely the data must agree with the assumptions to support reliable results. Only then can the best model be selected. Moreover, the investigator needs to verify that the assumptions inherent in the models were met; regression diagnostics (generally explained in the documentation for statistical software that offers them) should be employed routinely in all analyses.

REFERENCES

1. Greenland S. A semi-Bayes approach to the analysis of correlated multiple associations, with an application to an occupational cancer-mortality study. Stat Med 1992; 11(2):219–30.

2. Greenland S. Methods for epidemiologic analyses of multiple exposures: a review and comparative study of maximum-likelihood, preliminary-testing, and empirical-Bayes regression. Stat Med 1993; 12(8):717–36.

3. Greenland S. Hierarchical regression for epidemiologic analyses of multiple exposures. Environ Health Perspect 1994; 102(Suppl 8):33–9.

4. Greenland S. When should epidemiologic regressions use random coefficients? Biometrics 2000; 56(3):915–21.

5. Witte JS, Greenland S. Simulation study of hierarchical regression. Stat Med 1996; 15(11):1161–70.

6. Steenland K, Bray I, Greenland S, Boffetta P. Empirical Bayes adjustments for multiple results in hypothesis-generating or surveillance studies. Cancer Epidemiol Biomarkers Prev 2000; 9(9):895–903.

7. Wacholder S, Chanock S, Garcia-Closas M, et al. Assessing the probability that a positive report is false: an approach for molecular epidemiology studies. J Natl Cancer Inst 2004; 96(6):434–42.

8. Pinehiro JC, Bates DM. Mixed-effects models in S and S-PLUS. 1st ed. New York, NY: Springer-Verlag; 2000.

9. Dales LG, Ury HK. An improper use of statistical significance testing in studying covariables. Int J Epidemiol 1978; 7:373–5.

10. Austin PJ, Tu JV. Automated variable selection methods for logistic regression produced unstable models for predicting acute myocardial infarction mortality. J Clin Epidemiol 2004; 57:1138–46.

11. Breslow NE, Day NE. Statistical methods in cancer research. Volume II—The design and analysis of cohort studies. Lyon, France: International Agency for Cancer; 1987.

12. Hosmer DW, Lemeshow S, May S. Applied survival analysis: regression modeling of time-to-event data. 2nd ed. Hoboken, NJ: John Wiley; 2008.

13. Cao J, Valois MF, Goldberg MS. An S-Plus function to calculate relative risks and adjusted means for regression models using natural splines. Comput Methods Programs Biomed 2006; 84(1):58–62.

14. Calle EE, Rodriguez C, Walker-Thurmond K, Thun MJ. Overweight, obesity, and mortality from cancer in a prospectively studied cohort of U.S. adults. N Engl J Med 2003; 348(17):1625–38.

15. Hernan MA, Brumback B, Robins JM. Marginal structural models to estimate the causal effect of zidovudine on the survival of HIV-positive men. Epidemiology 2000; 11(5):561–70.

16. Robins JM. A graphical approach to the identification and estimation of causal parameters in mortality studies with sustained exposure periods. J Chron Dis 1987; 40(Suppl 2):139S–61S.

17. Robins JM. A new approach to causal inference in mortality studies with a sustained exposure period-application to control of the healthy worker survivor effect. Math Modeling 1986; 7:1393–512.

18. Arrighi HM, Hertz-Picciotto I. Controlling for time-since-hire in occupational studies using internal comparisons and cumulative exposure. Epidemiology 1995; 6(4):415–8.

19. Rothman KJ, Greenland S, Lash TL. Modern epidemiology. 3rd ed. Philadelphia, PA: Lippincott Williams & Wilkins; 2008.

20. Engel LS, Hill DA, Hoppin JA, et al. Pesticide use and breast cancer risk among farmers' wives in the Agricultural Health Study. Am J Epidemiol 2005; 161(2):121–35.

21. Ojo AO, Held PJ, Port FK, et al. Chronic renal failure after transplantation of a nonrenal organ. N Engl J Med 2003; 349(10):931–40.

22. Andersson RE, Olaison G, Tysk C, Ekbom A. Appendectomy and protection against ulcerative colitis. N Engl J Med 2001; 344(11):808–14.

23. Cecchi F, Olivotto I, Gistri R, et al. Coronary microvascular dysfunction and prognosis in hypertrophic cardiomyopathy. N Engl J Med 2003; 349(11):1027–35.

24. Wilson BJ, Watson MS, Prescott GJ, et al. Hypertensive diseases of pregnancy and risk of hypertension and stroke in later life: results from cohort study. BMJ 2003; 326(7394):845.

25. Helms M, Vastrup P, Gerner-Smidt P, Molbak K. Short and long term mortality associated with foodborne bacterial gastrointestinal infections: registry based study. BMJ 2003; 326(7385):357.

26. Ray WA, Stein CM, Hall K, et al. Non–steroidal anti–inflammatory drugs and risk of serious coronary heart disease: an observational cohort study. Lancet 2002; 359(9301):118–23.

27. Mollerup CL, Vestergaard P, Frokjaer VG, et al. Risk of renal stone events in primary hyper-parathyroidism before and after parathyroid surgery: controlled retrospective follow up study. BMJ 2002; 325(7368):807.

28. Stelfox HT, Bates DW, Redelmeier DA. Safety of patients isolated for infection control. JAMA 2003; 290(14):1899–905.

29. Greenland S, Morgenstern H. Matching and efficiency in cohort studies. Am J Epidemiol 1990; 131:151–9.

30. Lubin JH, Gail MH. Biased selection of controls for case-control analyses of cohort studies. Biometrics 1984; 40:63–75.

31. Breslow NE, Lubin JH, Marek P, Langholz B. Multiplicative models and cohort analysis. J Am Stat Assoc 1983; 78:1–12.

32. Langholz B, Thomas DC. Efficiency of cohort sampling designs: some surprising results. Biometrics 1991; 47(4):1563–71.

33. Meier CR, Schlienger RG, Kraenzlin ME, et al. HMG-CoA reductase inhibitors and the risk of fractures. JAMA 2000; 283(24):3205–10.

34. Anttila T, Saikku P, Koskela P, et al. Serotypes of *Chlamydia trachomatis* and risk for develop-ment of cervical squamous cell carcinoma. JAMA 2001; 285(1):47–51.

35. Thomas DC, Goldberg M, Dewar R, Siemiatycki J. Statistical methods for relating several exposure factors to several diseases in case-heterogeneity studies. Stat Med 1986; 5:49–60.

36. Scott SC, Goldberg MS, Mayo NE. Statistical assessment of ordinal outcomes in comparative studies. J Clin Epidemiol 1997; 50(1):45–55.

37. Doll R, Peto R. Mortality in relation to smoking: 20 years' observations on male British doc-tors. BMJ 1976; 2:1525–36.

38. Gillman MW, Cupples LA, Gagnon D, et al. Margarine intake and subsequent coronary heart disease in men. Epidemiology 1997; 8(2):144–9.

39. Longnecker MP. The Framingham results on alcohol and breast cancer. Am J Epidemiol 1999; 149(2):102–4.

40. Gottlieb DJ, Wilk JB, Harmon M, et al. Heritability of longitudinal change in lung function: the Framingham study. Am J Respir Crit Care Med 2001; 164(9):1655–9.

41. Canfield RL, Henderson CR Jr, Cory-Slechta DA, et al. Intellectual impairment in children with blood lead concentrations below 10 μg per deciliter. N Engl J Med 2003; 348(16):1517–26.

42. Israel E, Banerjee TR, Fitzmaurice GM, et al. Effects of inhaled glucocorticoids on bone density in premenopausal women. N Engl J Med 2001; 345(13):941–7.

43. Perkins BA, Ficociello LH, Silva KH, et al. Regression of microalbuminuria in type 1 diabe-tes. N Engl J Med 2003; 348(23):2285–93.

44. Sears MR, Greene JM, Willan AR, et al. A longitudinal, population-based, cohort study of childhood asthma followed to adulthood. N Engl J Med 2003; 349(15):1414–22.

45. Liang KY, Zeger S. Regression analysis for correlated data. Annu Rev Public Health 1993; 14:43–68.

46. Innes KE, Byers TE, Marshall JA, et al. Association of a woman's own birth weight with subsequent risk for gestational diabetes. JAMA 2002; 287(19):2534–41.

47. Greenland S, Longnecker MP. Methods for trend estimation from summarized dose–response data, with applications to meta-analysis. Am J Epidemiol 1992; 135(11):1301–9.

48. Brenner H. A potential pitfall in control of covariates in epidemiologic studies. Epidemiology 1998; 9(1):68–71.

49. Brenner H, Blettner M. Controlling for continuous confounders in epidemiologic research. Epidemiology 1997; 8(4):429–34.

50. Osganian SK, Stampfer MJ, Spiegelman D, et al. Distribution of and factors associated with serum homocysteine levels in children: Child and Adolescent Trial for Cardiovascular Health. JAMA 1999; 281(13):1189–96.

51. Lieberman DA, Prindiville S, Weiss DG, Willett W. Risk factors for advanced colonic neoplasia and hyperplastic polyps in asymptomatic individuals. JAMA 2003; 290(22):2959–67.

52. Lanas A, Bajador E, Serrano P, et al. Nitrovasodilators, low-dose aspirin, other nonsteroidal antiinflammatory drugs, and the risk of upper gastrointestinal bleeding. N Engl J Med 2000; 343(12):834–9.

53. Meijers JC, Tekelenburg WL, Bouma BN, et al. High levels of coagulation factor XI as a risk factor for venous thrombosis. N Engl J Med 2000; 342(10):696–701.

54. Singer JD. Using SAS PROC MIXED to fit multilevel models, hierarchical models, and individual growth models. J Educ Behav Stat 1998; 24(4):323–55.

55. Liang KY, Zeger S. Longitudinal data analysis using generalized linear models. Biometrika 1986; 73:13–22.

56. Zeger S, Liang KY. Longitudinal data analysis for discrete and continuous outcomes. Biometrics 1986; 42:121–30.

57. Zeger S, Liang KY. An overview of methods for the analysis of longitudinal data. Stat Med 1992; 11:1825–39.

CHAPTER 19

ঙ্গ

Genetic Inference

DAN L. NICOLAE, PH.D., THORSTEN KURZ, PH.D.,
AND CAROLE OBER, PH.D.

ABSTRACT   The mathematical properties of inheritance described over 50 years ago serve as the theoretical framework for testing genetic hypotheses. In this chapter we discuss methodological approaches for estimating the genetic component of a trait and for localizing genes on chromosomes.

The field of statistical genetics can be traced back to the early 1900s, following the rediscovery of Mendel's classic experiments demonstrating the principles of heredity (now referred to as Mendelian genetics) and beginning with the seminal work of R.A. Fisher, Sewall Wright, and J.B.S. Haldane. The mathematical properties of inheritance worked out over the next half century still serve as the theoretical framework for testing genetic hypotheses.

Genetic inference addresses three central questions: 1) What is the genetic (or hereditary) component of a trait? 2) What is the location on a chromosome of the locus that influences it? 3) What is the specific gene (or variation within a gene)? This chapter discusses the methods used to address the first two questions, particularly as they relate to genetic studies of human disease. Chapter 20 discusses the methods used to address the third question. Genetic terms used in both chapters are defined in a Definition Box.

ESTIMATING GENETIC CONTRIBUTIONS

TO DISEASE

Though the genetic contributions to simple Mendelian (or monogenic) traits may be obvious and easy to measure, the relative contributions of genetic and environmental factors to the expression of complex traits are less so. Complex traits are those that "cluster in families" but do not follow patterns of inheritance that are predicted for monogenic traits (autosomal recessive, autosomal dominant, X-linked, Y-linked, or mitochondrial). Complex traits include nearly

Term	Definition
Additive	A trait in which the phenotype of the heterozygote is intermediate between the two homozygotes
Allele	An alternative form of a gene at a given location (locus)
Autosome	Any chromosome other than the sex chromosomes
Cross-over	The exchange of DNA segments between two homologous chromosomes during meiosis; cross-overs result in recombination
Dominant	A trait that is expressed in the individuals with one (heterozygote) or two (homozygote) copies of a mutation
Epistasis	The expression of one gene depends on the expression of another gene
Exon	The part of a gene that is retained in the mature mRNA
Genetic Marker	A segment of DNA with a known location on a chromosome that varies among individuals (is polymorphic)
Genetic Map	A "map" of the location of the genes and markers relative to each other, and the recombination rates between them. The units used in genetic maps are recombination fractions and/or Morgans and centi-Morgans (cM). A cM is equivalent to 1% recombination in meiosis between two loci
Genotype	The genetic composition of an individual. Also refers to the pair of alleles inherited at a given locus
Haplotype	The alleles present at linked loci on an individual chromosome
Hardy-Weinberg Equilibrium	A population's genotype and allele frequencies will remain unchanged over successive generations in a randomly breeding population where there is no selection, migration, or mutation. Under Hardy-Weinberg equilibrium, genotype frequencies can be calculated directly from allele frequencies
Heterozygote	The presence of two different alleles at a given locus; can also refer to an individual with two different alleles at a locus
Homozygote	The presence of two identical alleles at a given locus; can also refer to an individual who has identical alleles at a given locus
Interference	The interaction between cross-overs (recombination events) such that the occurrence of one cross-over reduces the likelihood of another in its neighborhood
Intron	The non-coding DNA sequence of a gene between exons
Locus	The position on the chromosome of a particular gene or DNA sequence
Microsatellite DNA	Repetitive segments of DNA. Some have variable numbers of repeat units between chromosomes and are often used in linkage analysis (also referred to as short tandem repeat polymorphisms, or STRPs)

Definition Box

Mitochondrial DNA	A circular chromosome contained within the cytoplasm of cells; mitochondrial DNA is maternally inherited, and mutations in mitochondrial DNA are maternally transmitted
Penetrance	The probability of individuals with a particular genotype expressing the phenotype
Phenotype	The observable characteristics of an individual with a particular genotype
Polymorphism	The presence of two or more DNA sequences (alleles) at a given location (locus) for which the minor allele occurs at 1% frequency or greater in the population
Promoter	DNA sequences, usually upstream of the first exon, that bind transcription factors and RNA polymerase and initiate transcription
Recessive	A trait that is expressed only in individuals with two copies of the mutation (homozygotes)
Recombination	The formation of new combinations of linked genes in gametes by crossing over
Recombination Fraction (θ)	The proportion of meioses that lead to recombination between two given loci
Single Nucleotide Polymorphism (SNP)	A variant DNA sequence in which a single nucleotide has been replaced by another nucleotide
X-linked	Traits caused by mutations in genes on the X chromosome

Definition Box (continued)

all the common human diseases, such as most cancers, heart disease, hypertension, diabetes mellitus, asthma and allergy, autoimmune diseases, psychiatric and neurological disorders, and common birth defects, as well as quantitative phenotypes that are often associated with common diseases, such as systolic and diastolic blood pressure, blood levels of various cholesterols or antibodies, and measures of body size or composition.

The expression of complex traits in any individual reflects both genetic and environmental factors. Further, because the phenotypic effects of genotypes at any particular locus are variable, and often influenced by environmental exposures, the penetrance of genotypes at loci influencing common diseases is always less than 100%. *Penetrance* is defined as the proportion of individuals with the susceptibility genotype that manifest the phenotype. For genes that influence multiple phenotypes, penetrance can refer to the expression of any of the phenotypes, or it can be phenotype-specific. Though penetrance can be less than 100% for monogenic traits, it is generally high and around 90 to 100%, reflecting the modifying effects of other genes and environmental factors on some Mendelian traits. However, locus-specific penetrances are generally much less than 10% for common diseases, because most genes that influence common diseases have relatively small effects. For example, the HLA-DR3 and DR4 alleles are well-established independent risk factors for type 1 diabetes; 95% of Caucasian type 1 diabetes cases carry one or both of these alleles. Yet only approximately 1 in 200 individuals in the population with one or both of these alleles will develop type 1 diabetes.[1] Thus, the penetrance of this major susceptibility locus for type 1 diabetes is only 0.5%.

Estimating the Heritability of Traits

A first step in any genetic study is to estimate the contribution of genes to the trait under investigation. The value of twins in genetic studies was first pointed out by Galton in 1865,[2] and twins remain important in genetic studies today. Because monozygotic (MZ) twins share 100% of their genes and dizygotic (DZ) twins share only 50% of their genes (similar to any sibling pair), and because twin pairs raised together are assumed to share much more similar "environments" than other sibling pairs, comparing the concordance of qualitative traits or the correlations of quantitative (or measured) traits, such as height, between MZ and DZ twins provides an estimate of the genetic contribution to that trait. Although twin studies provide more-robust estimates of genetic contributions, heritability can be estimated using sibling pairs, parent-offspring pairs, or any other pairs of relatives.

Heritability is the proportion of total phenotypic variance (V_P) that is due to genetic variance (V_G), and can range between 0 and 1. It is assumed that the remainder of the inter-individual variation in susceptibility is due to non-genetic factors (i.e., environment). The total genetic variance (V_G) is composed of additive and non-additive genes. The term narrow heritability, denoted by h^2, refers to the proportion of total phenotypic variance due to additive genetic variance (V_A/V_P), and the term broad heritability, denoted by H^2, is the proportion of total phenotypic variance due to all genetic variance (additive, dominant, recessive, epistastic, etc.) (V_G/V_P). The ability to estimate h^2 or H^2 largely depends on the sampling strategy. For example, estimates of H^2 require studying extended pedigrees because in siblings it is impossible to separate non-additive genetic effects from shared environment effects. As a result, estimates of heritabilities from siblings are inflated. Further, because the variance in environmental risk factors differs among populations, estimates of heritability can also differ among populations. That is, estimates of h^2 and H^2 are properties of the population under investigation and are not intrinsic properties of a phenotype. In general, samples drawn from more-homogeneous environments will provide higher estimates of heritability because the proportion of V_P due to variance in environmental (or non-genetic) factors (V_E) is lower (for a more-detailed discussion and examples, see Abney et al.[3]).

A twin study to determine the heritability of breast tissue density, modeled as a continuous variable measured from mammograms,[4] serves as an example. Because menopausal status, weight, and parity account for 20 to 30% of the age-adjusted variation in tissue density, the authors adjusted for these variables in their analysis to estimate the proportion of the residual variance that is due to additive genetic factors (h^2) in 353 MZ twin pairs and 246 DZ twin pairs from Australia and in 218 MZ twin pairs and 134 DZ twin pairs from Canada and the United States. The results of this study are shown in Table 1. In both samples the correlation in the adjusted percentage of dense tissue was approximately two times greater among MZ than among DZ twin pairs ($p < 0.001$). Further, the best-fitting model included only components for additive genetic factors and person-specific environmental factors; the estimated contribution of environmental factors that are common to twins was not significant in any model. A model including just additive genetic and person-specific environmental components of variance yielded estimates of $h^2 = 0.60$ in the Australian sample and 0.67 in the North American sample, after adjustment for age and other covariates. The similarity of these estimates may reflect the fact that both were drawn from predominantly European populations living in "Western" environments. However, it is possible that in other populations common environmental factors may contribute more significantly to the variation in breast density and that estimates of heritability may differ from these. These global estimates of heritability reflect the effect of all contributing loci.

Measuring Familial Clustering of Traits

Another measure related to heritability, lambda (λ), measures the familial clustering of a trait. It is calculated as the prevalence of disease among specific relatives of an affected individual divided by the prevalence of that disease in the population. The most common estimate, the risk to siblings, λ_s, is calculated by determining the prevalence of disease among siblings of affected individuals in a particular population, divided by the prevalence of the disease in the same population. Because the denominator of λ is the population prevalence,

Table 1. Correlations (±1SE) between Twin Pairs and Estimates of Heritability in MZ and DZ Twin Pairs of Dense Breast Tissue Adjusted for Covariates. Modified from Boyd et al. 2002.[4]

Variable	Australia	North America	Combined Samples
Correlation Coefficient for MZ twins	0.61 ± 0.03	0.67 ± 0.03	0.63 ± 0.02
Correlation Coefficient for DZ twins	0.25 ± 0.06	0.27 ± 0.08	0.27 ± 0.05
Heritability (h^2)	0.60 ± 0.03	0.67 ± 0.04	0.64 ± 0.02

a property of λ is that it tends to be higher for diseases with low population prevalences, as illustrated in Table 2.

Estimates of heritability and λ both have the limitation that the likelihood of identifying specific genetic loci that contribute to disease risk through genetic linkage or association studies relies on the locus-specific heritability or λ_S and not on the global values, such as those shown in Table 2. Thus, it may be more difficult to map genes' underlying traits with high heritabilities that are influenced by the small cumulative effects of many genes, than to map traits with lower heritabilities that are largely due to the greater effects of a smaller number of genes (for examples, see Ober et al.[5]). Unfortunately, it is not possible to determine *a priori* whether the genetic component of a trait consists of many genes with small effects or fewer genes with larger effects, so estimates of heritability and λ_S should be interpreted cautiously when designing genetic mapping studies.

Estimating Effect Size

Once a gene is identified as contributing to the risk for disease, the locus-specific effects and the *population attributable risk*, or etiologic fraction, can be estimated. Whereas odds ratios and relative risks estimate the risk of disease among individuals with a specific genotype, the population attributable risk provides related information from a national or public health perspective.[6] The population attributable risk is the proportion of all cases in the target population attributed to an allele or genotype. If we denote with K the prevalence of the disease in the population and with K^W the prevalence of the disease in the subpopulation having the non-risk genotype for the risk marker, the population attributable risk for that marker is given by $(K - K^W) / K = 1 - (K^W / K)$. These prevalences are simple functions of penetrances of the marker genotypes that

Table 2. Population Prevalences and Estimates of λ_S for Some Common Diseases.

Disease	Population	Prevalence (%)		λ_S	Reference
		Among Sibs	In Population		
Sarcoidosis	United Kingdom	1.46	0.02–0.4	3.6–73	McGrath et al.[18]
Autism	United States	4.5	0.1–0.2	22.5–45	Veenstra-VanderWeele and Cook[19]
Autoimmune Thyroid Disease	United States	13.5	0.8	16.9	Villanueva [20]

can be calculated from retrospective studies using Bayes's Rule. For example, if we denote with D the disease subjects and with W the non-risk genotype, K^W / $K = P(D|W) / P(D) = P(W|D) / P(W)$, and these can be obtained from the genotype counts in cases and controls. To illustrate, the *CARD15* gene was identified as a susceptibility locus for Crohn's disease (reviewed in Cho[7]). Three common polymorphisms in a leucine-rich region of the *CARD15* gene independently contribute to risk. The incidence of Crohn's disease in a European cohort was 1.5- to 4-fold higher in heterozygous carriers of any allele and 15- to 40-fold higher in homozygotes for the risk alleles, compared with non-carriers of any risk alleles. However, among carriers of two risk alleles (homozygotes or compound heterozygotes) fewer than 10% develop Crohn's disease. The population attributable risk for each of the three risk alleles ranges from 6.4% to 8.3%, with the total locus accounting for 21.7% of Crohn's disease patients in the United States. Similar to λ, the population attributable risk varies from population to population because it is a function of the allele frequencies in each population.

LOCALIZING DISEASE GENES THROUGH
LINKAGE STUDIES

Linkage refers to the co-inheritance of alleles at two loci because they are located on the same chromosome and close to each other. Genetic linkage studies are often the first step in localizing and identifying a disease gene. These studies aim to locate regions on the genome that are very likely to contain disease-susceptibility genes. The basic principle of linkage analysis is derived from the mechanism of storage and transmission of hereditary information. During the formation of gametes each pair of homologous chromosomes will break and recombine at one or more locations in each parent, so the resulting egg or sperm contains chromosomes that are a mixture of the two grandparental chromosomes. This reshuffling allows specific DNA variants in genes on chromosomes to be mapped, as DNA pieces that lie close together on the same chromosome tend to have the same grandparental origin. The data used in linkage studies consist of disease (phenotype) information for family members, and genotype data on markers distributed throughout the genome (i.e., spaced across the chromosomes) for the same family members.

Genome-wide linkage studies require adequate coverage of the genome with polymorphic markers. This can be accomplished by genotyping family members with a minimal set of 300–400 highly polymorphic microsatellite (or short tandem repeat [STR]) markers or with 1500–3000 bi-allelic SNPs evenly spaced across the genome.[8]

Parametric Linkage

Classical linkage analyses estimate the recombination fraction (an estimate of distance) between a fixed position on the genome (i.e., at a marker locus) and a putative disease gene, and test whether these two loci are linked (referred to as two-point analysis) or whether a distribution of markers with known locations is linked to a disease-susceptibility gene (multipoint analysis). Two-point linkage analyses are less powerful than multipoint analyses, but have the advantage of not requiring that the order and inter-marker distances are known. In general, for any two loci, the proportion of recombinant and non-recombinant gametes can be used to predict the distance between them; the more recombinants, the farther apart the loci are. The simplest way of deciding whether a gamete is recombinant or non-recombinant uses family data (Figure 1). In some situations genotypes allow deterministic counting of recombination and non-recombination

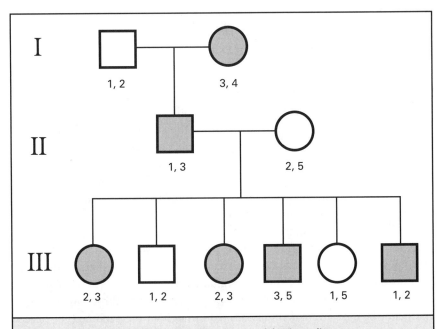

Figure 1. A 3-generation family segregating an autosomal dominant disease.

Genotypes at a marker locus are shown under each symbol, and affected individuals are shown as shaded symbols. The "3" allele at the marker locus is co-segregating with the disease in this family. The last child in generation III has the disease but inherited the "1" allele from the affected father in generation II, representing a recombination between the disease locus and the marker locus in the father's gamete. Therefore, a recombination occurred in one out of six paternal meioses, yielding an estimated recombination frequency, θ, of 16.7% between the marker and disease loci.

events within pedigrees, as in Figure 1, but usually a statistical assessment of the strength of the evidence in favor of or against linkage is required.

Parametric linkage analysis tests for linkage between a marker (or markers) and the trait and requires specifying a genetic model, including the mode of inheritance (e.g., dominant, recessive), the disease allele frequency, and the penetrances of genotypes at the disease locus. The penetrance specifies the probability that an unaffected individual is in fact a non-penetrant (i.e., unaffected) carrier of the susceptibility allele or genotype. The parameter of interest is the location of the susceptibility gene relative to the markers that provide the data, denoted by the recombination fraction, θ, between a marker and the susceptibility locus. The test for linkage is usually based on a likelihood-ratio statistic. The likelihood calculation can be computationally challenging, and it requires specialized software. Linkage can be tested using a *logarithm of the odds* (lod) score,

$$\text{lod} = \log_{10} \frac{L(\theta)}{L(\theta = 1/2)}$$

in which the denominator shows the likelihood of observing the pedigree and marker data under the null hypothesis of no linkage, or free recombination (θ = 0.5).

A useful feature of the lod score is that it can be summed over families. In practice, this means that additional families are studied until the lod score reaches a threshold for significance (discussed below), or becomes sufficiently negative (i.e., the data show that non-linkage is more likely than tight linkage) to exclude the location as one harboring a disease gene. In parametric linkage analysis, however, misspecification of the genetic model (mode of inheritance, allele frequency, penetrances, phenocopy rates) can lead to incorrect conclusions about linkage.

In a study using multipoint parametric linkage analysis, Gunel et al.[9] concentrated on a part of chromosome 7 that was thought to harbor a gene causing cerebral cavernous malformation, based on a prior linkage analysis. They genotyped members of 14 pedigrees for 20 markers across this region. The linkage analysis used an autosomal dominant trait model and assumed a disease allele frequency of 0.001 and 80% penetrance. The results of the analyses, summarized in the lod scores, are shown in Figure 2. The lod score peaked at marker D7S657 and allowed the investigators to narrow the region harboring the disease gene to a 7 centiMorgan (cM; roughly equivalent to 7% recombination) interval, which represents a 95% confidence interval for the location of the susceptibility locus. In linkage analysis all of the locations that reside within 1 of the maximum lod score form a 95% confidence interval. For example, the maximum lod score is 10.6 in Figure 2. At lod = 9.6 (= 10.6 − 1) the lod curve spans 7 cM between D7S492 and D7S479, defining a 95% confidence interval.

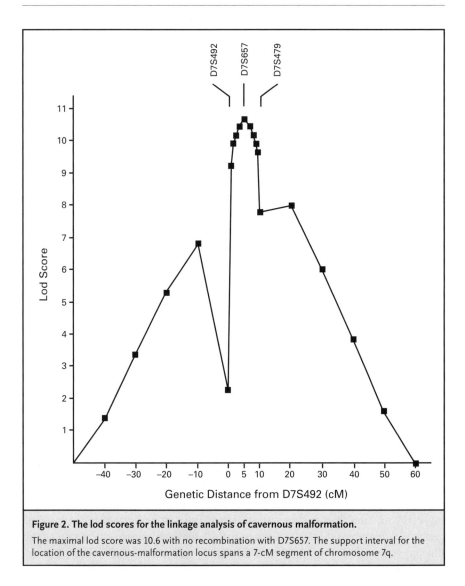

Figure 2. The lod scores for the linkage analysis of cavernous malformation.
The maximal lod score was 10.6 with no recombination with D7S657. The support interval for the location of the cavernous-malformation locus spans a 7-cM segment of chromosome 7q.

Model-Free Linkage

Allele-sharing methods were introduced as a nonparametric approach of investigating the data and, compared with the classical parametric methods, have the advantage of not employing a specific mode of inheritance. As a result these approaches are more appropriate for studies of common, complex diseases in which the true genetic models are unknown. Most of these methods focus on affected individuals, but unaffected relatives can be used to reconstruct the paths of inheritance. The idea behind allele-sharing methods is simple: if a gene is contributing to disease in all the affected persons in a family, then the genetic material at and around the disease locus should be more similar among those affected than expected by chance. For a given location on the genome, the evidence for a disease-susceptibility locus linked to it is given by the sharing of alleles *identical by descent* (IBD) among affected relatives in excess of what is expected under no linkage. Alleles are IBD if they are inherited from the same common ancestor. The statistical methods capture the deviations (excess in sharing) from the null identical-by-descent distribution H_0.

As an example, consider an affected sib pair, the pedigree structure for which data are often collected. Figure 3 shows a family with two affected brothers in which the parental genotype at a locus is denoted by "1,2" for the father and "3,4" for the mother. Each parent transmits one allele to each offspring. The siblings in Figure 3 have one allele IBD that they inherited from their father (allele "2"), and different alleles inherited from their mother. In general, siblings share either two, one, or no alleles IBD. In pedigrees unselected with respect to disease status, the maternal allele is shared IBD in 50% of the meioses, and the paternal allele is independently shared IBD in 50% of meioses. This implies that the expected proportion of alleles that are IBD is 0.5. Conditioned on the status of the sibs, an increase in the proportion of alleles IBD among affected sib pairs from different families is expected in the neighborhood of a

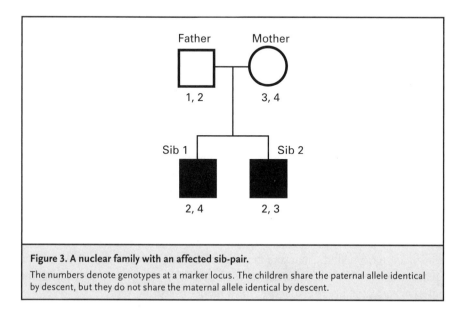

Figure 3. A nuclear family with an affected sib-pair.

The numbers denote genotypes at a marker locus. The children share the paternal allele identical by descent, but they do not share the maternal allele identical by descent.

disease gene. Statistical testing methods can measure the strength of the deviation from the expected proportion of alleles IBD, which can provide evidence for linkage. The significance of the excess in IBD sharing can be assessed using large-sample approximations to the distribution of the statistic measuring the mean proportion of alleles IBD.

In a study using sib-pairs to identify a genetic location for bronchial hyper-responsiveness (BHR), Postma and colleagues[10] studied 303 children and grandchildren of 84 probands with asthma selected from a homogeneous population in the Netherlands. Clinical measurements included BHR to histamine, ventilatory function, and total serum IgE. BHR is a component of the asthma phenotype in which the amount of a stimulus required to induce a given degree of airway narrowing is measured. Patients with asthma require less stimulus to achieve the same obstructive response as a normal subject. The goal of this study was to test for linkage between BHR and 10 genetic markers on chromosome 5q31-q33, a region that had previously been shown to be linked to a genetic locus regulating serum total IgE levels. The mean proportion of alleles IBD in siblings who were concordant for BHR varied between 0.53 and 0.64, and the most significant results were obtained with the marker D5S436 ($p = 0.009$). More-detailed analysis revealed that, when both siblings were negative for BHR (the study contained 173 such pairs), there was also greater sharing of marker alleles (mean proportion of alleles IBD = 0.55, $p = 0.02$), whereas in discordant pairs in which one member was positive for BHR and one member was negative (114 such pairs), the pair tended not to share parental alleles (mean = 0.39, $p < 0.001$). These results are consistent with a disease locus linked to D5S436, where we would expect excess of sharing among concordant siblings (both affected or both unaffected) and a deficiency of sharing among discordant siblings (one affected and one unaffected).

In practice, data are not as simple as in the above example. Pedigree structures can contain more-complicated relations than sib pairs and more than two affected individuals. Another complication is that the IBD status cannot always be determined with certainty. Suppose that, in the sib pair example in Figure 3, the father has two copies of allele "2." The sibs have one allele that has the same state (*identical by state* or IBS), but it is unknown whether this allele was inherited from the same paternal chromosome. It can be inferred that the siblings have zero or one alleles IBD and, without further information, the probabilities of sharing zero or one allele IBD are equal to one-half, under the null hypothesis. In general, a probability distribution for the IBD sharing is calculated from genotype data. Multipoint IBD calculations are used to extract efficiently the information from all the markers in a region, or on a chromosome. The inferred distribution for the IBD sharing is used in constructing an extension to the inference process described above[11] or a model-based lod score.[12]

Quantitative Traits

Statistical methods for mapping quantitative traits were first proposed by Penrose[13]; his test used sib pairs from different families (i.e., independent pairs). More recently, Haseman and Elston proposed a test based on the regression of the trait differences in sib pairs on the estimated number of alleles shared IBD.[14] Several extensions to the original Haseman-Elston method are applicable to pedigrees of arbitrary structure and to pedigrees selected on the basis of trait value.[15] These methods are suitable for traits that are normally distributed.

An alternative approach to regression-based methods has been developed from classical variance-components analysis.[16] This approach models the phenotypic covariance between a pair of related individuals as a function of the average IBD sharing (over the genome) between the two individuals and their specific IBD sharing at a given chromosomal location. It allows covariate effects along with variance components. The variance is decomposed into a major genetic component that is linked to a marker, a component due to genes unlinked to the genetic marker, and non-genetic sources of variability. The variance-component approach allows the joint analysis of all familial information, and also can be easily modified for multivariate phenotypes.

Assessment of Significance

Genome-wide linkage scans are usually performed using hundreds of markers, and linkage tests can be performed at each location on the genome. It is therefore important to develop testing methods that take into account the large number of statistical comparisons. The *nominal significance* level is the probability of observing a statistically significant deviation at a given locus by chance (most often set at 5%); the *genome-wide significance* level is the probability of observing a deviation somewhere in the whole genome scan. The test at the nominal level is based on the properties of the statistic; for lod scores, large-sample approximations to the null distribution of a likelihood-ratio statistic are often used. Genome-wide levels are usually calculated from simulations. For single-gene, Mendelian traits, a lod score of 3 (odds 1,000 to 1 in favor of linkage) is considered significant. However, for studies of complex traits, which are likely to examine many susceptibility loci in the genome and generally involve genotyping many more markers, a lod score of 3 is no longer sufficiently stringent to establish significance. Lander and Kruglyak[17] formulated a set of criteria for reporting the significance of a linkage result for complex traits. They suggested "lod threshold values" for different study designs that could be used for strong control of type I error, to ensure a low rate of reporting false-positive signals. A "significant linkage" (usually a lod score larger than 3.6) refers to signals expected to occur 0.05 times in a genome scan. They also provided criteria for "suggestive linkage" (usually a lod score greater than 2), which are signals that would be expected to occur once at random in a genome scan. These threshold values are useful as guidelines, but they are stringent because they assume that allele sharing among relatives is known at all locations in the genome. In practice, this never occurs.

Computer simulations are a general approach for obtaining threshold values that are adjusted for multiple comparisons. With this approach, simulated genome scans are analyzed to build empirical estimates of null distributions. Although they do not apply to all situations because of the nature of the ascertainment schemes and patterns of missing data, this is the preferred method for assessing significance, whenever possible.

CONCLUSIONS

Well-established methods provide estimates of the genetic contributions to quantitative phenotypes and diseases, and of the effect size of a given genotype. Interpretation of these estimates should consider population-specific attributes, such as allele frequencies, pedigree structure, and environmental variation. Localizing disease genes on chromosomes by linkage analysis can utilize parametric or model-free approaches, depending on the disease and pedigree under consideration. Genome-wide assessments of significance require appropriate correction for multiple testing, either by pre-specified thresholds or by computer simulation, using any of the many available statistical packages.

ACKNOWLEDGMENTS

The authors were supported in part by NIH grants HD21244, HL56399, HL66533, HL70831, HL72414, and DK55889.

REFERENCES

1. Raffel LJ, Rotter JI. Type 1 diabetes mellitus. In: King RA, Rotter JI, Motulsky AG, eds. The genetic basis of common diseases. 2nd ed. New York: Oxford University Press; 2002:431–56.

2. Galton F. Hereditary talent and character. Macmillan Mag 1865; 12:157.

3. Abney M, McPeek MS, Ober C. Estimation of variance components of quantitative traits in inbred populations. Am J Hum Genet 2000; 66:629–50.

4. Boyd NF, Dite GS, Stone J, et al. Heritability of mammographic density, a risk factor for breast cancer. N Engl J Med 2002; 347(12):886–94.

5. Ober C, Abney M, McPeek MS. The genetic dissection of complex traits in a founder population. Am J Hum Genet 2001; 69(5):1068–79.

6. Schlesselman JJ. Case-control studies. Oxford: Oxford University Press; 1982.

7. Cho JH. Significant role of genetics in IBD: the NOD2 gene. Rev Gastroenterol Disord 2003; 3(Suppl 1):S18–22.

8. Kruglyak L. The use of a genetic map of biallelic markers in linkage studies. Nat Genet 1997; 17(1):21–4.

9. Gunel M, Awad IA, Finberg K, et al. A founder mutation as a cause of cerebral cavernous malformation in Hispanic Americans. N Engl J Med 1996; 334(15):946–51.

10. Postma DS, Bleecker ER, Amelung PJ, et al. Genetic susceptibility to asthma—bronchial hyperresponsiveness coinherited with a major gene for atopy. N Engl J Med 1995; 333(14):894–900.

11. Kruglyak L, Daly MJ, Reeve-Daly MP, Lander ES. Parametric and nonparametric linkage analysis: a unified multipoint approach. Am J Hum Genet 1996; 58(6):1347–63.

12. Kong A, Cox NJ. Allele-sharing models: LOD scores and accurate linkage tests. Am J Hum Genet 1997; 61(5):1179–88.

13. Penrose LS. Genetic linkage in graded human characters. Ann Eugen 1938; 8:233–7.

14. Haseman JK, Elston RC. The investigation of linkage between a quantitative trait and a marker locus. Behav Genet 1972; 2(1):3–19.

15. Sham PC, Purcell S, Cherny SS, Abecasis GR. Powerful regression-based quantitative-trait linkage analysis of general pedigrees. Am J Hum Genet 2002; 71(2):238–53.

16. Goldgar DE. Multipoint analysis of human quantitative genetic variation. Am J Hum Genet 1990; 47(6):957–67.

17. Lander E, Kruglyak L. Genetic dissection of complex traits: guidelines for interpreting and reporting linkage results. Nat Genet 1995; 11(3):241–7.

18. McGrath DS, Daniil Z, Foley P, et al. Epidemiology of familial sarcoidosis in the UK. Thorax 2000; 55(9):751–4.

19. Veenstra-VanderWeele J, Cook EH. Molecular genetics of autism spectrum disorder. Mol Psychiatry 2004; 9(9):819–32.

20. Villanueva R, Greenberg DA, Davies TF, Tomer Y. Sibling recurrence risk in autoimmune thyroid disease. Thyroid 2003; 13(8):761–4.

CHAPTER 20

Identifying Disease Genes in Association Studies

DAN L. NICOLAE, PH.D., THORSTEN KURZ, PH.D.,

AND CAROLE OBER, PH.D.

ABSTRACT This chapter reviews approaches for identifying specific genes that contribute to disease risk by genetic association studies. We summarize applications to candidate gene studies, positional candidate gene studies, and genome-wide association studies and discuss the limitations and interpretations of these studies.

In Chapter 19 we posed three central questions that are addressed by genetic inference: First, what is the heritability of a trait? Second, where does the disease locus reside on a chromosome? Third, what is the specific gene (or variation within a gene)? In this chapter we address the third question and describe methods for identifying the specific gene (or variation within a gene) that influences disease susceptibility. As discussed in Chapter 19, genome-wide linkage approaches to gene discovery have the potential to identify novel genes and pathways involved in disease susceptibility. Association studies generally focus on genes selected on the basis of either their function (*functional candidate genes*) or their position near a linkage signal (*positional candidate genes*). Because the methods for assessing the potential role of functional or positional candidates are similar, this chapter discusses them together. Furthermore, although genome-wide association studies were not feasible in the past because of the density of markers required for such studies (400,000 to >1 million single nucleotide polymorphisms [SNPs], depending on the population) (see Definition Box in Chapter 19), technological advances in genotyping now make these studies possible. The methods and issues discussed below are also relevant to genome-wide association studies.

CASE-CONTROL ASSOCIATION STUDIES

Traditionally, association studies were conducted in unrelated samples of cases (affected individuals) and controls (unaffected individuals). Controls are typically matched to the cases on race or ethnicity and variables that may affect penetrance, such as age, sex, and socioeconomic status, which vary from study to study. This approach has the advantage that it is usually much easier and less expensive to study large numbers of unrelated cases and controls than to study families. The main disadvantage is that poor matching of cases and controls on variables that are associated with genotype frequencies can increase type I errors. Type I error can arise from ethnic heterogeneity between the case and control groups, despite attempts to match the groups for ethnicity, and is referred to as *population stratification* or *substructure*. In such cases allele frequency differences that are unrelated to the presence or absence of the disease, but due to subtle differences in the ethnic composition of the two groups, can result in spurious associations. This limitation of the case-control design led to the development of family-based association tests (discussed below). However, methods have been developed that directly test for population stratification and correct for any imbalances.[1, 2] These methods require genotyping the case and control samples for 30 or more informative loci (i.e., loci that discriminate between pairs of racial or ethnic groups[2]). In the case of genome-wide association studies, the large number of genotyped SNPs provides sufficient information for inferring structure.

    With the case-control design, investigators test the hypothesis that a particular allele or genotype at a specific locus is significantly more common in the cases than in the controls. Standard statistical methods, such as chi-squared tests, logistic regression, and trend tests, can be used to test the hypothesis. Although studies are usually designed to detect alleles or genotypes that confer susceptibility to the disease, these approaches will also detect alleles or genotypes that are protective. In that situation the associated allele or genotype will be significantly less frequent in the cases than in the controls.

FAMILY-BASED ASSOCIATION STUDIES

Family-based association tests overcome the potential confounding of population stratification. The most commonly used family-based test is the transmission disequilibrium test (TDT),[3] which examines trios consisting of an affected child and his/her parents. Extensions of the TDT allow for missing parents, additional relatives, multi-locus analyses, and quantitative traits (reviewed in Schulze and McMahon[4]). The basis of this approach is that each allele in a heterozygous parent has equal (50%) probability of being transmitted to an offspring. However, if an allele is associated with a disease, it will be overtransmitted (>50%) to affected children and undertransmitted to children without the disease. The non-transmitted alleles from the same heterozygous parents serve as the "controls," and a chi-squared test determines whether a particular allele is transmitted to affected children significantly more often than expected by chance alone. This approach has the advantage of avoiding spurious associations from population stratification because the "control" alleles are drawn from the same persons as the "case" alleles. A disadvantage is that it requires DNA (for genotyping) from both parents, which is often difficult to obtain, particularly for late-onset disorders. Furthermore, because only transmissions from heterozygous parents are included, many parents do not contribute to the analyses. For example, at a SNP with maximum informativeness (i.e., alleles at equal frequency), only half of the parents are expected to be heterozygotes. As a result, this method has considerably lower power than the case-control design in samples of equivalent size.[5]

For example, Infante-Rivard et al. examined the relationship between four polymorphisms previously associated with thrombophilias and intrauterine growth restriction (IUGR).[6] They used a hospital-based case-control design as well as a family-based study. They first compared genotype frequencies at each of the four loci between cases (493 IUGR neonates and mothers) and controls (472 normal weight neonates and mothers). Only the 677TT genotype at the methylenetetrahydrofolate (*MTHFR*) locus differed between case and control neonates (odds ratio after adjusting for mother's genotype and other confounders, 0.52; 95% confidence interval, 0.29 to 0.94). Genotypes for 258 case fathers were available. Therefore, to ensure that the results of the case-control study were not due to population stratification, they tested for association in the case trios. The TDT with the *MTHFR* C677T polymorphism was not statistically significant (TDT = 0.51, $p = 0.47$). This result may reflect the lower power of the TDT, as discussed above, but it leaves open the possibility that the result of the case-control study was a type I error. The facts that their initial finding was only modestly significant and that they did not take into account multiple comparisons (discussed below) make this a likely interpretation of their study.

LINKAGE DISEQUILIBRIUM, HAPLOTYPE BLOCKS, AND MULTILOCUS METHODS

The concept of *linkage disequilibrium* (LD) is basic to interpreting the results of association studies. LD is the nonrandom association of alleles at linked loci. Mendel's law of independent assortment predicts that alleles at different loci assort independently into gametes. Recombination during meiosis ensures that this is approximately true even for most genes on the same chromosome.

However, because the probability that a recombination will occur between two loci increases with the distance between them (discussed in Chapter 19), alleles at loci that are very close to each other on a chromosome may show nonrandom patterns of association if there has not been sufficient opportunity for recombination to "break" the association that occurs when a mutation arises on a chromosome background (Figure 1). In the human genome LD extends on average 60 kilobases (kb), but the range is from <10 to >100 kb, depending on local recombination rates and the evolutionary history of the particular chromosomal segment.[7, 8] As a result, when a disease is associated with an allele in the population (case-control studies) or in families (TDT studies), it will also be associated with all alleles that are in strong LD with it. Because human genes are on average 40 kb in size, LD can extend across entire genes and sometimes across more than one gene. It remains one of the greatest challenges in human

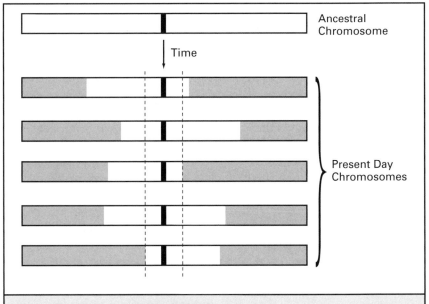

Figure 1. Illustration of linkage disequilibrium.

A mutation (black bar) arises on an ancestral chromosome (shown in white). Over time, recombination with other chromosomes (shown in gray) will narrow the length of the ancestral chromosome that flanks the mutation. In this example all present-day chromosomes that carry the disease mutation retain the ancestral segment between the dashed lines, referred to as a shared segment. As a result, the mutation will show strong association in the population with all other alleles on this shared segment, and more modest associations with alleles of genes that are located in ancestral segments retained on most (but not all) disease chromosomes. The older the mutation, the smaller the ancestral segment containing the disease locus, and the smaller the shared segment among individuals with the disease.

genetics today to determine which allele among a group of alleles that are in strong LD is actually the risk allele. Ultimately, this task requires replication (discussed below) and studies demonstrating that the variant under consideration affects the function of the gene or protein and is involved in disease pathogenesis.

LD patterns in the human genome create "blocks" of polymorphisms that are in relatively high LD, separated from each other by small regions that do not show LD with adjacent blocks. This is likely due to adjacent stretches of regions with lower and then higher recombination rates ("cold" and "hot" spots, respectively). In regions of low recombination LD will be more extensive, whereas in regions of high recombination LD will be less so. This "patchlike" characteristic of LD has been referred to as *haplotype blocks*,[9, 10] where haplotype refers to the alleles present on an individual chromosome. A useful measure of LD in association studies is r^2, the correlation between alleles at two loci. When two alleles occur at identical frequency and are on the same haplotypes, $r^2 = 1$. When $r^2 \geq 0.8$, the two alleles are in sufficient LD that they can substitute for each other in association studies. Haplotype blocks are defined using prespecified sets of rules based on LD measures, such as r^2. Within a block a small fraction of SNPs, called haplotype tag (ht) SNPs, is sufficient to capture most of the haplotype structure. This feature of LD blocks greatly reduces the number of SNPs to be tested and allows for a relatively comprehensive survey of an entire gene or region. The NIH-funded HapMap project has as one of its goals to identify all htSNPs in the genome of the major racial groups (http://www.hapmap.org/index.html.en).

Furthermore, unless we select the causal SNP for genotyping, association studies are really aimed at detecting association with SNPs that are in LD with the causal SNP (or SNPs). In these situations methods that analyze haplotypes (composed of two or more SNPs) may provide more information than analysis of individual SNPs.

Two general approaches to association mapping use haplotypes. The first is similar to those discussed above for single loci, but it analyzes the frequencies or transmissions of haplotypes instead of individual alleles. This approach may identify SNPs that interact to confer susceptibility or haplotypes that include the causal SNP (or SNPs). The second is based on the assumption that affected individuals will share a longer haplotype that is IBD as compared with unaffected control individuals, such as in the haplotype sharing analysis (HSA)[11] and the decay of haplotype-sharing (DHS)[12] methods. However, these methods are computationally intensive and are usually used to study regions that have high probabilities of containing disease genes, based on prior linkage or association studies.

AN ASSOCIATION STUDY OF DRUG RESISTANCE

Siddiqui et al.[13] used several of the approaches discussed above to examine an association between a polymorphism in the drug-transporter gene *ABCB1* and response to antiepileptic-drug treatment. A prior study had shown that the C3435T SNP, a silent SNP in exon 12 of the *ABCB1* gene, was associated with expression levels and function;[14] the investigators hypothesized that this SNP influences the response to antiepileptic-drug treatment. They genotyped 200 drug-resistant epileptic individuals, 115 drug-responsive epileptic individuals, and 200 individuals without epilepsy (controls). Using a chi-squared test, they found that the CC genotype was significantly more common in the drug-resistant group (27.5%) than in the drug-responsive group (15.7%) or the controls (18.5%) (p = 0.006 and 0.01, respectively; odds ratio compared to controls 2.58, 95% CI 1.25–5.36). Because the subjects were largely White but included some Asians, they re-analyzed the data of the White subjects only, with similar results.

To further ensure that the differences between groups were not because of population admixture, they genotyped their samples for nine SNPs that were unlinked to the *ABCB1* locus. Two SNPs, for which genotype frequencies deviated from Hardy-Weinberg expectations (see discussion below), were discarded due to high genotyping errors. The genotype frequencies of the remaining seven SNPs did not differ between the two epileptic groups (p > 0.15 for each comparison). Further, they divided the observed chi-squared by the maximal chi-squared across the unlinked markers, and the *ABCB1* 3435C allele remained significantly overrepresented among patients with drug-resistant epilepsy as compared with drug-responsive epilepsy (p < 0.05). Pritchard and Rosenberg recommended that case-control studies should include 15–20 unlinked microsatellite markers or at least 30 SNPs to detect stratification,[2] so it is possible that undetected stratification existed in their study.

Next, to determine the LD pattern in this gene, Siddiqui et al. genotyped five SNPs in the *ABCB1* gene in 32 Centre d'Etude du Polymorphisme Humain (CEPH) trios (mother, father, child). The family information allowed them to determine haplotypes in 52 unrelated parents, who were used in the analysis. The C1236T SNP was in significant LD with a SNP in exon 21 (r^2 = 0.61, p < 0.001) and a SNP in exon 26 (r^2 = 0.20, p < 0.001). The associated 3435C allele occurred on three haplotypes (A, C, and D in Table 1). Similar to other human genes in which relatively few haplotypes account for most of the observed haplotypes, three common haplotypes (A, B, and C) at the *ABCB1* locus accounted for 73.1% of parental chromosomes. They concluded that, because of the LD within this gene, it is not possible to identify the SNP (or SNPs) that determine responsiveness to epileptic drugs but that the 3435C allele is in LD with the causal SNP. Moreover, because the pattern of LD can differ among populations, this SNP may not predict drug-responsiveness in other populations.

Table 1. Haplotype Structure of the *ABCB1* Gene in 52 CEPH Parents; 1 Corresponds to the More Common Allele and 0 the Minor Allele at Each SNP (modified from Siddiqui et al.[13]).

Haplotype	Intron 2 SNP (rs2888599)	Exon 12 (C1236T)	Exon 12 (C+44T)	Exon 21 (G2647A)	Exon 26 (C3435T)	Frequency (%) in Parents
A	1	0	1	0	1	34.6
B	1	1	1	1	0	23.1
C	1	1	1	1	1	15.4
D	1	1	1	0	1	7.7
E	1	1	0	1	0	7.7
F	1	0	1	1	0	5.8
G	1	0	1	0	0	3.8
H	0	1	1	1	0	1.9

TYPE I ERRORS IN ASSOCIATION STUDIES

The interpretation of association studies is not always straightforward because a statistically significant association between a genetic variant and a disease phenotype can have three possible explanations. First, the variant may affect gene function by altering the amino-acid sequence or by modifying splicing, transcriptional properties, or mRNA stability, and thereby directly affect disease risk. We refer to this as the "causal" SNP. Second, the marker allele may merely be in LD with the causal variant, as discussed above in the context of the study of an *ABCB1* association with drug-resistant epilepsy. In that study, the investigators correctly concluded that they could not identify the causal variant, but possibly only a marker for the drug-resistance allele. Third, the association could be a false-positive result (type I error). Using a *p*-value of 0.05 as the threshold for significance corresponds to a 5% type I error rate. However, genetic studies are often small, and *p*-values are usually calculated using large-sample approximations to the distributions of the test statistics. As a result, the probability of type I errors for many of these approximations is higher than the nominal *p*-value. Furthermore, a large number of negative association studies are never reported, and reported *p*-values are rarely adjusted for the total number of tests performed (both reported and unreported). The result is, again, that the type I error rate in reported studies is actually higher than the nominal level of 5%.

False-positive results are especially likely to occur if multiple comparisons are made, either with multiple polymorphisms in the same gene, with polymorphisms in multiple genes, or with multiple phenotypes. In these situations the 5% false-positive rate expected under the null hypothesis (of no association) no longer applies because each individual comparison (for example, with polymorphisms in different genes) has a 5% error rate. A common correction for multiple comparisons (known as the Bonferroni correction) divides the threshold by the number of comparisons and compares the individual p-values to the adjusted threshold. Therefore, in a study of a single variant in each of 20 genes, one would need to obtain an individual p-value of 0.0025 to have a 5% "simultaneous" type I error rate (i.e., the chance of one or more type I errors among the 20 comparisons is only 5%). However, the Bonferroni correction is overly conservative if the multiple tests correspond to correlated variables. For example, phenotypes considered in single studies are often correlated (e.g., systolic and diastolic blood pressures, asthma and IgE levels), as are the genotypes of SNPs that are in LD. Thus, these comparisons do not represent independent tests, and the Bonferroni correction can be extreme in these circumstances. In fact, the Bonferroni correction can be conservative even for independent tests.[15]

Because no simple correction handles multiple correlated comparisons, alternative methods are used. One such approach randomly permutes either genotypes or phenotypes among the study subjects to obtain empirical null distributions of the test statistics. Permutation tests are useful because they preserve the correlation structure of the data and provide accurate p-values. They can be used to control the probability of committing any type I error and thus produce stringent thresholds in studies with a large number of candidate genes. An alternative approach is to control the False Discovery Rate (FDR),[16] which is the proportion of false positives in the set of rejected hypotheses. FDR is a more liberal (but often more useful) rate to control, and it generally yields higher statistical power. When a large number of tests are performed, controlling the FDR will generally lead to a larger number of discoveries than the Bonferroni correction, although tests on correlated variables may require a modification in the FDR-controlling procedure.[16] For example, in a genome-wide association study with 1 million SNPs, the expected number of false discoveries at the $p = 10^{-5}$ significance level is approximately 10 (1 million $\times$ 10^{-5}). If the observed number of SNPs with $p < 10^{-5}$ is 30, then the FDR is estimated to be 10/30, or 33%.

Type I errors can also result from genotyping errors, particularly from systematic errors such as overcalling one genotype over another in the cases or in the controls (but not in both). In studies in families Mendelian error checks and estimates of allele sharing among relatives identify some genotyping errors. However, comparable tests are not possible for samples of unrelated individuals, such as those used in case-control studies. One way to minimize genotyping error is to make sure that the genotypes in the cases and controls are in *Hardy-Weinberg* proportions (see Definition Box in Chapter 19). Systematic errors in genotyping often yield genotype frequencies that are not in Hardy-Weinberg proportions. Indeed, a surprisingly large number of published associations either did not check for Hardy-Weinberg equilibrium or presented data that were not in Hardy-Weinberg proportions.[17] When published association studies were re-examined, 12% of the 133 SNPs reported were not in Hardy-Weinberg equilibrium in the controls, suggesting genotyping error. Moreover, the deviation from equilibrium was higher among the SNPs for which a positive association was reported. Some of these markers were not identified by the authors as showing deviations from equilibrium.

One explanation could be that authors used incorrect tests of significance, which may not be uncommon (e.g., Ozaki et al.,[18] Brody et al.[19]). In particular, the significance test for Hardy-Weinberg equilibrium for a SNP with three genotypes is a 1-degree-of-freedom test. Incorrectly assuming 2 degrees of freedom will undercall deviations from Hardy-Weinberg equilibrium. On the other hand, markers showing departure from Hardy-Weinberg equilibrium should not be automatically discarded, because many genetic models predict such deviations in cases for variants close to a susceptibility locus.[20, 21] Regardless, markers showing deviations from expectations should be closely scrutinized and retyped to ensure that they are genotyped correctly. Lastly, type I errors can result from population substructure, which can be addressed either by correcting for imbalances[1, 2] or by conducting family-based association studies,[3] as discussed above.

AN ASSOCIATION STUDY OF MYOCARDIAL INFARCTION

As an example of a study that conducted a large number of statistical tests using a case-control design, Yamada et al.[22] wanted to identify genetic risk factors for myocardial infarction (MI). They first selected 71 genes that had been previously characterized and were considered to be good functional candidate genes for MI, and then selected 112 known polymorphisms in these genes. Most of the polymorphisms were in regions of the gene that could influence expression or function (i.e., the promoter regions, exons, or intron-exon boundaries). Their sample included 2819 unrelated Japanese patients with MI (2003 men and 816 women) and 2242 unrelated Japanese controls (1306 men and 936 women). They used a two-step approach to address the difficulty in interpreting the results of multiple comparisons (112 polymorphisms and three genetic models analyzed separately in men and in women). They first examined the 112 polymorphisms in 909 randomly selected subjects (219 male and 226 female cases; 232 male and 232 female controls). Using a liberal cut-off of $p < 0.10$ and three genetic models (dominant, recessive, additive) in multivariate logistic regression analyses to adjust for non-genetic risk factors, they identified 19 polymorphisms in the men and 18 in the women for further studies. Only four polymorphisms overlapped in men and women.

In the second step, they genotyped these 33 polymorphisms in the remaining 2858 men and 1294 women. Statistical analysis in this step was limited to these polymorphisms and a single model for each, which greatly reduced the number of tests. For these analyses they used multivariate logistic regression analysis with adjustment for age, body-mass index, and the prevalence of smoking, hypertension, diabetes mellitus, hypercholesterolemia, and hyperuricemia and a stringent significance level ($p < 0.001$) to identify associated alleles. If they had utilized a Bonferroni correction for the number of tests, the threshold for significance (allowing for a 5% false-positive rate) would have been 0.0028 (= 0.05/18) in females and 0.0026 (= 0.05/19) in males. Because some of the polymorphisms that they examined were in the same gene, and therefore not independent, this would have been a conservative threshold, as discussed above. Moreover, because they had identified these polymorphisms in the first stage of their analysis, albeit at a liberal threshold of $p < 0.10$, requiring a p-value < 0.001 in the follow-up study was conservative.

The investigators identified one polymorphism in men (connexin 37) and two in women (plasminogen-activator inhibitor type 1 and stromelysin-1) for increased risk for MI that met this level of significance. Although these results are robust because of the two-step approach and the very large sample size, it is still possible that they represent false-positive results (type I errors) because of the very large number of tests performed. As discussed above, replication in a second population that was independently ascertained would substantially strengthen the evidence that these are true associations. Ultimately, however, identifying the causal variant or variants and demonstrating its functional consequences may provide proof that these are indeed genetic risk factors for MI.

REPLICATION OF ASSOCIATION STUDIES

Because of the potential for type I errors in genetic-association studies, especially when sample sizes are small and/or many tests are performed, replication with different subjects (often from different populations) is a standard for publication in many journals. Although replication in a second population significantly increases the likelihood that a gene identified in the first study is a true association, failure to replicate may not mean that the first result was a false positive. An association may not be replicated because of different patterns of LD in different populations, which can be caused by differences in allele frequencies and/or the presence of more than one causal variant. In such instances haplotype analysis can be helpful. Because a shared haplotype that contains the disease variant will be more common in cases than in controls, even when the disease-causing variant itself is not studied, examining haplotypes instead of single SNPs is often useful and could help to identify the true susceptibility variant, as discussed above.

Lastly, positive associations may not be replicated because the true model of genetic susceptibility for common diseases is complex. In these diseases, susceptibility variants may have relatively minor effects on the phenotype, and the magnitude of the effect may be influenced by genes at other loci (gene-gene interactions) and by environmental factors (gene-environment interactions). In fact, some variants may only confer susceptibility in combination with other genes (epistasis) or in certain environments. Because background genes and environmental exposures differ among populations, it should not be surprising that associations are not replicated in all subsequent studies.

ACKNOWLEDGMENTS

The authors were supported in part by NIH grants HD21244, HL56399, HL66533, HL70831, HL72414, and DK55889.

REFERENCES

1.   Devlin B, Roeder K. Genomic control for association studies. Biometrics 1999; 55(4):997–1004.

2.   Pritchard JK, Rosenberg NA. Use of unlinked genetic markers to detect population stratification in association studies. Am J Hum Genet 1999; 65(1):220–8.

3.   Spielman RS, Ewens WJ. The TDT and other family-based tests for linkage disequilibrium and association. Am J Hum Genet 1996; 59(5):983–9.

4.   Schulze TG, McMahon FJ. Genetic association mapping at the crossroads: which test and why? Overview and practical guidelines. Am J Med Genet 2002; 114(1):1–11.

5.   Teng J, Risch N. The relative power of family-based and case-control designs for linkage disequilibrium studies of complex human diseases. II. Individual genotyping. Genome Res 1999; 9(3):234–41.

6.   Infante-Rivard C, Rivard GE, Yotov WV, et al. Absence of association of thrombophilia polymorphisms with intrauterine growth restriction. N Engl J Med 2002; 347(1):19–25.

7.   Ardlie KG, Kruglyak L, Seielstad M. Patterns of linkage disequilibrium in the human genome. Nat Rev Genet 2002; 3(4):299–309.

8.   Wall JD, Pritchard JK. Haplotype blocks and linkage disequilibrium in the human genome. Nat Rev Genet 2003; 4(8):587–97.

9.   Gabriel SB, Schaffner SF, Nguyen H, et al. The structure of haplotype blocks in the human genome. Science 2002; 296(5576):2225–9.

10. Cardon LR, Abecasis GR. Using haplotype blocks to map human complex trait loci. Trends Genet 2003; 19(3):135–40.

11. Van der Meulen MA, te Meerman GJ. Haplotype sharing analysis in affected individuals from nuclear families with at least one affected offspring. Genet Epidemiol 1997; 14(6):915–20.

12. McPeek MS, Strahs A. Assessment of linkage disequilibrium by the decay of haplotype sharing, with application to fine-scale genetic mapping. Am J Hum Genet 1999; 65(3):858–75.

13. Siddiqui A, Kerb R, Weale ME, et al. Association of multidrug resistance in epilepsy with a polymorphism in the drug-transporter gene ABCB1. N Engl J Med 2003; 348(15):1442–8.

14. Hoffmeyer S, Burk O, von Richter O, et al. Functional polymorphisms of the human multidrug-resistance gene: multiple sequence variations and correlation of one allele with P-glycoprotein expression and activity in vivo. Proc Natl Acad Sci USA 2000; 97(7):3473–8.

15. Schwager SJ. Bonferroni sometimes loses. Am Statistician 1984; 38:192–7.

16. Benjamini Y, Yekutieli D. The control of the false discovery rate in multiple testing under dependency. Ann Stat 2001; 29(4):1165–88.

17. Xu J, Turner A, Little J, et al. Positive results in association studies are associated with departure from Hardy-Weinberg equilibrium: hint for genotyping error? Hum Genet 2002; 111(6):573–4.

18. Ozaki K, Ohnishi Y, Iida A, et al. Functional SNPs in the lymphotoxin-alpha gene that are associated with susceptibility to myocardial infarction. Nat Genet 2002; 32(4):650–4.

19. Brody LC, Conley M, Cox C, et al. A polymorphism, R653Q, in the trifunctional enzyme methylenetetrahydrofolate dehydrogenase/methenyltetrahydrofolate cyclohydrolase/formyltetrahydrofolate synthetase is a maternal genetic risk factor for neural tube defects: report of the Birth Defects Research Group. Am J Hum Genet 2002; 71(5):1207–15.

20. Nielsen DM, Ehm MG, Weir BS. Detecting marker-disease association by testing for Hardy-Weinberg disequilibrium at a marker locus. Am J Hum Genet 1998; 63(5):1531–40.

21. Lee WC. Searching for disease-susceptibility loci by testing for Hardy-Weinberg disequilibrium in a gene bank of affected individuals. Am J Epidemiol 2003; 158(5):397–400.

22. Yamada Y, Izawa H, Ichihara S, et al. Prediction of the risk of myocardial infarction from polymorphisms in candidate genes. N Engl J Med 2002; 347(24):1916–23.

CHAPTER 21

Risk Assessment

A. JOHN BAILER, PH.D., AND JOHN C. BAILAR III, M.D., PH.D.

ABSTRACT   *Risk assessment* describes 1) the process for considering the evidence for the association between some hazard and an adverse outcome, coupled with 2) examination of the magnitude of exposure to this hazard and the frequency or severity of the adverse outcome. Historically, steps in a risk assessment have been hazard identification, dose-response modeling, exposure assessment, and risk characterization. Recent additions to this process include problem formulation and a scoping of the problem, so that the risk assessment can better inform risk management decisions. This chapter introduces the vocabulary of risk assessment, describes statistical concepts important for risk assessment (e.g., uncertainty, variability, conditional probability, and regression models), and discusses how medical and healthcare professionals may be involved in this process.

E very day, people weigh the benefits of decisions against the likelihood of adverse outcomes. This process might be something as trivial as comparing different routes for driving home during rush hour, or as important as deciding whether to use a medical intervention with potentially serious side effects.

A medical professional is on the proverbial "front lines" of the risk assessment process. Any decision process that balances a predicted risk of adverse health outcomes (e.g., coronary heart disease (CHD) or cancer) with the risk of treatments (e.g., surgery risks or drug side effects) reflects a comparative risk assessment. Similarly, balancing injury against benefits unrelated to health requires risk assessment, at least implicitly. We argue that implicit risk assessment is not good enough: important factors affecting major decisions should be explicit. A medical professional may be advising an individual, such as a patient with high cholesterol, or may be involved in balancing risks when making decisions at national levels, as in a consideration of food guidelines that encourage consumption of fish while recognizing that some fish may have levels of mercury or other contaminants too great to ignore.

A colleague of ours likes to quote the wisdom of a folk singer as it applies to risk assessment: "nothing is certain, and that's for sure" (from the song "One Man's Trash" by John McCutcheon © 1988, from the album "What It's Like" © 1990). It is critical to recognize the uncertainties that affect the process of risk assessment. Starting with a statistical modeling perspective, the relation of risk to dose or exposure is generally unknown, and often controversial. Should linear terms be required in the model? Should threshold parameters be included? Should one use point estimates of regression-based potency endpoints, or lower confidence limits, which incorporate sampling variability? Though these questions may seem esoteric, different answers often lead to dramatically different conclusions about the size and nature of the risk, and hence to different strategies for managing the risk. This is especially true in the prediction of responses to very low exposures.

An educated citizenry should understand that there is a reason for federally recommended exposure limits, that risk is not the only important factor considered in the regulation of hazards, that risk assessment is inherently uncertain (even when human data are available), and that our understanding of specific risks is likely to change only slowly with the accumulation of sound research studies, each adding a bit to the evidence for or against the existence of a hazard and our ability to quantify it accurately. Finally, and perhaps most importantly for physicians in clinical practice, understanding what risk estimates mean to individuals can also help physicians communicate risks to their patients.

This chapter provides an introduction to risk assessment concepts relevant to medical practice and other aspects of healthcare. Sections include a basic introduction to the vocabulary of risk and hazards, relevant risk-related statistical concepts, and how medical and healthcare professionals might be involved in the risk assessment process. The format for a portion of this chapter was first published in 2001.[1] We illustrate the process and concepts of risk assessment by using a clinical example along with examples of environmental and occupational hazards to health. Before we begin, it is important to recognize a potential source of terminological confusion when discussing "risk." In clinical settings, "risk" factors describe variables that are thought to be prognostic variables (not necessarily cause and effect) for some adverse health outcome or disease. In general "risk assessment" parlance, "risk" describes the likelihood and magnitude that some exposure (in a very broad sense) will cause some adverse response. Finally, this chapter targets two audiences: the practicing physician who is seeing patients and the research physician who is studying disease etiology. It is particularly important for physicians to know enough about risk and risk assessment to communicate important information to their patients. For example, a natural question from the cholesterol study that permeates this chapter would be: Could the patient control CHD risk by changes in lifestyle (e.g., diet, exercise)? A patient would need to be informed about how any intervention affects the risk. If diet and exercise could reduce cholesterol levels to low-risk levels, say < 200 mg/dL, then no other intervention would be necessary. If these lifestyle changes (assuming patient compliance was complete) still would not reduce cholesterol to a level associated with low CHD risk, then other interventions would be required. To facilitate an informed decision, a physician would need to be able to present this comparative risk exercise in a manner accessible to the patient.

A CLINICAL EXAMPLE WITH RISK-MOTIVATED INTERVENTION

We begin with a short, motivating example that examines the probability of adverse response for an individual with a certain profile of risk factors (here, we use "risk factor" in its clinical, prognostic sense). Suppose a 45-year-old male patient presents with the following test results: cholesterol of 311 mg/dL, high-density lipoprotein (HDL) of 32 mg/dL, and systolic blood pressure (SBP) of 110 mmHg. The patient is not currently treated for hypertension and is not a smoker. A risk calculator based on the Framingham Heart Study (http://hp2010.nhlbihin.net/atpiii/riskcalc.htm, accessed 21 April 2009) yields a 10-year risk of coronary heart disease (CHD) of 9% (here "risk" is a probability of a CHD event such as a myocardial infarction). This risk calculation is based on the Third Report of the Expert Panel on Detection, Evaluation, and Treatment of High Blood Cholesterol in Adults (Adult Treatment Panel or ATP III). A quick desk reference to these guidelines is available on the web at http://www.nhlbi.nih.gov/guidelines/cholesterol/dskref.htm (accessed 15 November 2008). This reference also provides a categorical prediction of risk where categories of risk factors are assigned scores (e.g., age category 20–34 is assigned a score of "–7", age category 35–49 is assigned a score of "–3", total cholesterol 240–279 mg/dL or age category 50–59 is assigned a score of "5", etc.), and the sum of these scores is then linked to a 10-year risk of CHD (e.g., point total = 9 has a risk of 1%, point total = 20 has a risk of 11%). The clinical intervention in this case may be clear—drug therapy (e.g., statins) to reduce cholesterol levels, plus certain lifestyle changes (e.g., diet, exercise)—but a question remains: what does it mean to say a 10-year risk of CHD is 9%? Does it mean that 9 of 100 individuals with these characteristics (age, cholesterol, HDL, SBP, smoking status, etc.) will experience CHD within 10 years? Or does it mean that the risk of CHD is 9 percentage points higher in an individual with these characteristics than in an individual with normal values for the risk factors? Both of these interpretations correspond to an absolute risk definition. This "9 percentage points higher" risk could be rephrased to mean that we expect 9 additional CHD cases per 100

45-year-old male non-smokers with cholesterol = 311, HDL = 32, and SBP = 110, over and above the CHD cases in 45-year-old male non-smokers with low cholesterol (say, < 160), desirable HDL (say, > 60), and SBP = 110 (a risk-difference definition). Finally, this "9%" risk value may correspond to a risk ratio or an odds ratio, relative risk definitions. A risk ratio corresponds to the probability of disease in an "exposed" individual relative to an unexposed individual, whereas the odds ratio corresponds to the odds of disease in an exposed individual relative to the odds in an unexposed individual. Here, "exposed" means a 45-year-old, non-hypertensive, male non-smoker with cholesterol = 311 and HDL = 32; and "unexposed" corresponds to a 45-year-old, non-hypertensive, male non-smoker with cholesterol < 160 and HDL > 60. If an odds ratio of 1.09 were reported, it would suggest that the odds of CHD in a group of exposed individuals was 9% higher than the odds of CHD in a group of unexposed individuals. In this instance the 9% actually reports absolute risk. The development and application of the model for CHD risk estimation have been studied in a series of articles (a subset[2-4] provides a starting point for further investigation). Ideas from this example serve to illustrate the various risk concepts that we introduce in later sections.

The example above focuses on risks to an individual. Other risk assessments are better conceptualized as population-oriented—e.g., post-market surveillance of drugs or devices (the "active, systematic, scientifically valid collection, analysis, and interpretation of data or other information about a marketed device. The data can reveal unforeseen adverse events, the actual rate of anticipated adverse events, or other information necessary to protect the public health." [http://www.fda.gov/cdrh/devadvice/352.html, accessed 15 November 2008]). These concepts also apply to food additives, potentially hazardous consumer products, and many other possible hazards.

RISKS, HAZARDS, AND HEALTH CARE

Risk corresponds to the probability of some adverse outcome. In risk assessment, the questions of greatest interest are generally the size of the risk caused by a specific exposure to some *hazard* and how the risks are likely to change after some intervention. Disease is an adverse outcome commonly studied in medicine, and CHD is the outcome highlighted in our motivating example. In this instance risks are related to both the incidence of disease and possible treatments (see Chapter 7). These include the risk of unwanted side effects of treatment as well as the expected probabilities of CHD or death associated with various treatment regimes. For example, if statins were used to treat the high-cholesterol case described above, joint pain is a possible side effect of the treatment.

Direct medical care often requires interactions (not in a statistical sense) that might result in injury or illness of patients or staff members. For example, injuries with contaminated needles are a potential source of transmission of disease (see, e.g., Ridzon et al.[5]). To assess the risk that a healthcare worker will become ill from a blood-borne pathogen, the probability of a needle-stick injury coupled with the probability of disease given exposure via a needle-stick injury must be determined. In this example the hazard is infected blood. Another example is the hazard of musculoskeletal injury to staff members who move patients or residents of nursing homes. The adverse response in this example may be back injury or other musculoskeletal injury. For example, workers in nursing and residential care facilities had an injury rate of 8.8 total recordable cases per 100 full-time workers per year in 2007, compared to 5.4 injuries per 100 full-time construction workers per year (http://www.bls.gov/news.release/osh.t01.htm, accessed 21 April 2009).

COMPONENTS OF A RISK ASSESSMENT

The most familiar paradigm for risk assessment was published by the National Research Council[6] and has been elaborated upon in many later NRC reports. In the NRC model risk assessment has four components: hazard identification, exposure assessment, dose-response modeling, and risk characterization.

Hazard identification uses scientific data developed by physicians, epidemiologists, biologists, chemists, and others to determine whether some agent is a hazard. For example, epidemiologists evaluate the strength of human studies to determine whether the association between exposure and an adverse response is one of cause and effect. In the cholesterol example above, a host of studies have examined the etiology of CHD. This work has suggested that elevated levels of cholesterol and low levels of HDL are risk factors or hazards for CHD.

A hazard may be first identified by observing a series of unusual cases. Parmet and Von Essen[7] reported that several employees at a microwave popcorn processing plant exhibited severe pulmonary symptoms. Kreiss et al.[8] described a survey of these plants to identify potential causes of respiratory disease. They concluded that workplace exposure to diacetyl, an airborne ketone in the artificial butter flavoring, was associated with the adverse pulmonary response.

The National Toxicology Program (NTP) uses a more-structured approach to identifying potential carcinogenic hazards. In the framework employed by the Report on Carcinogens committee of the NTP, criteria are provided for listing an "agent, substance, mixture, or exposure" as "known to be a human carcinogen" or "reasonably anticipated to be a human carcinogen." These are carefully defined in operational terms. (See http://ntp.niehs.nih.gov/go/15209, accessed 15 November 2008.)

Though the 12th Report of Carcinogens is currently in process [early in 2009], previous reports addressed a broad range of exposures ranging from alcoholic beverage consumption to saccharin and tamoxifen. Alcoholic beverage consumption and tamoxifen were both categorized as known human carcinogens, but saccharin was removed from its earlier categorization as "reasonably anticipated to be a human carcinogen." Epidemiological evidence was sufficient for alcoholic beverages and tamoxifen; for saccharin, even though carcinogenic responses were observed in male rats, a mechanistic explanation for the higher sensitivity of male rats coupled with the absence of human evidence led to the delisting.

Exposure assessment often requires many kinds of expertise, including nutrition, industrial hygiene (for occupational exposures), engineering, hydrology (for waterborne hazards), meteorology (for airborne hazards), and analytical chemistry. For our hypothetical cholesterol study, laboratory blood work is required to measure cholesterol in an individual. In addition, if lifestyle changes are recommended for individuals (e.g., dietary changes), then an assessment (or measurement) of the contribution of various diets to blood cholesterol levels is required in order to evaluate the likely contribution of dietary cholesterol to the adverse outcome (in this case high blood cholesterol). Simply put, is it possible to evaluate the contribution of a patient's current diet to the patient's current blood cholesterol level? A related, critical issue is how much the target population will in fact change its diet. For the popcorn example, an industrial hygienist could be involved in measuring the levels of diacetyl in various work areas. This assessment might be used in a future dose-response analysis. Special challenges arise in the evaluation of risks of infectious disease, in which exposure assessment must include modeling of the contact with infected individuals along with modeling the probability of disease given such contact.

Dose-response modeling or exposure-response modeling requires the input of statisticians, epidemiologists, and modelers in order to develop models that predict adverse response as a function of dose or exposure. Some disciplines distinguish between "dose" and "exposure"; exposure may refer to a level of a hazard encountered in the environment, whereas dose may refer to the amount of a hazard that is delivered to some target organ or tissue. An important question involves the measurement of exposure. For some hazards, the amount of exposure accumulated over a lifetime, so-called *cumulative exposure*, might be of interest. This is appropriate for substances that accumulate in the body over time, such as many pesticides and heavy metals. Other exposures, such as to some light organic compounds and radiation, may act very quickly (though covertly) and disappear long before their effects are manifest.

The identification of the appropriate response for modeling might involve the contribution of pathologists, toxicologists (especially important for understanding mechanisms of toxicity and the relevance of animal data for human exposures), or bacteriologists (say, to elucidate the spread of an infectious disease). In the cholesterol example, we reported a predicted risk derived from a regression model. In this example a dichotomous response (presence/absence of CHD) was predicted as a function of the risk factors of primary interest (e.g., cholesterol, HDL) and other factors (e.g., age, SBP, smoking status). In the microwave pop-corn example, FEV_1 (forced expiratory volume in 1 second), a measure of the flow of air in large airways of the lungs, decreased with increasing cumulative exposure to diacetyl.[8] This analysis examined response relative to quartiles of cumulative exposure.

Risk characterization involves all of the disciplines described above and many others. It integrates the first three components of risk assessment into a full picture of what is known about the effects of exposure, of a specific kind and intensity, on specific populations or persons.

The risks associated with exposure to a hazard may be expressed by a variety of summary statistics that include individual lifetime risk, annual population risk, the percentage or proportion of increase in risk, and loss of life expec-tancy.[9] For cholesterol exposure, individual risk might be of primary interest, whereas years of potential life lost might be a relevant means of characterizing the risk of hazards that are often experienced by younger individuals (e.g., fatal occupational injuries). As noted above, the CHD risk calculations reflect an absolute risk, the change in probability of developing CHD over a 10-year period.[2] Figure 1 displays the estimated absolute risk of CHD as a function of cholesterol for a 45-year-old male non-smoker with normal SBP (here, SBP = 110 mm Hg). The top (dashed) curve corresponds to the relation of CHD risk to cholesterol level for HDL = 32 mg/dL, and the bottom (solid) curve corresponds to this relationship for HDL = 50 mg/dL. The values plotted in this figure were extracted from the risk calculator mentioned previously (http://hp2010.nhlbihin .net/atpiii/riskcalc.htm).

The risk difference, P(CHD *GIVEN* exposure to a risk factor) − P(CHD *GIVEN* no exposure to risk factor), is also commonly reported in risk assessment. In a different quantification the additional risk of disease is estimated in the group of individuals who would have been disease-free in the absence of risk factor exposure: the extra risk is

$$ER = \frac{P(\text{CHD } \textit{GIVEN} \text{ exposed}) - P(\text{CHD } \textit{GIVEN} \text{ not exposed})}{P(\text{CHD } \textit{GIVEN} \text{ not exposed})}$$

although in a clinical context, often absence of exposure might equate to pos-sessing normal values of particular risk factors such as cholesterol, blood pres-sure, etc. Other descriptions such as risk ratios or odds ratios are common in epidemiological studies, but less common in risk assessment.

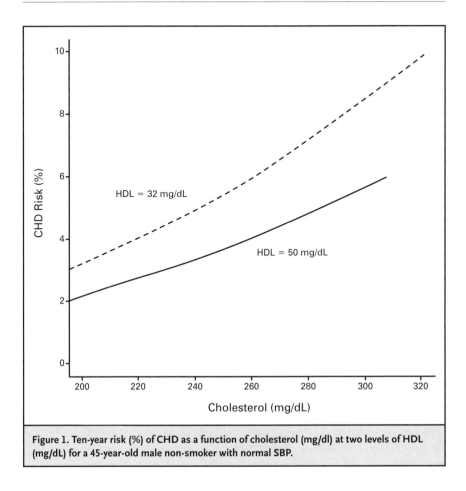

Figure 1. Ten-year risk (%) of CHD as a function of cholesterol (mg/dl) at two levels of HDL (mg/dL) for a 45-year-old male non-smoker with normal SBP.

REFLECTIONS ON RISK

First, risk prediction is probabilistic; not every individual with a particular profile of risk factors/hazard exposure will have an adverse response. Not all 45-year-old males will experience CHD in 10 years, whatever their blood pressure, cholesterol level, or smoking history. In addition, almost every adverse response may occur with no exposure. CHD is observed in individuals with low cholesterol and high HDL. Many long-term cigarette smokers may not develop lung cancer, and non-smokers sometimes get the disease. However, persons who smoke still have a 10- to 15-fold higher probability of developing lung cancer than non-smokers. Some responses, such as asbestosis, are clearly and uniquely linked to exposure to a particular hazard, but this tends to be the exception rather than the rule.

Second, the frequency of a dichotomous response (e.g., CHD) or the magnitude of a continuous response (e.g., lung function) generally depends on the degree and extent of exposure to a hazard (e.g., blood cholesterol level or diacetyl concentration). Some responses may have a threshold below which no risk is apparent or real. For example, nearly all drugs have small risks when used as approved, but a much greater risk of serious consequences at doses well above the approved dosage.

Third, persons vary in their responses to the same level of dose or exposure. As we saw from the CHD example, the risk for any individual may depend on a variety of intrinsic factors such as age, sex, prior or concurrent exposures to other hazards (e.g., smoking status, hypertension), and the level of detoxifying enzymes. Beyond individual differences, certain subpopulations may be at unusually high or low risk of adverse response. For example, infants, the elderly, and those with impaired immune systems may be at unusually high risk of contracting an infectious disease, and such diseases often hit these subpopulations particularly hard. The reasons for special sensitivity to other exposures are often poorly characterized or unknown.

Fourth, scientifically sound data for direct measurement of human risk are often absent or seriously inadequate. Thus, the carcinogenic potential for humans of a modest intake of saccharin is thought to be low because the primary evidence of carcinogenicity comes from animal studies, where doses were very high and where the mechanisms of carcinogenesis may not operate at low exposures in humans.[10]

Fifth, the acceptability of exposure to some hazard and the attendant risk depends on many, sometimes surprising, factors, including the number of persons exposed, whether exposure is voluntary, the social value of the risky exposure, mechanisms of compensation for harm or death, and familiarity with the risk.[11]

Finally, decisions must be made about the best way to balance risks and benefits in order to establish acceptable exposure limits for a hazard. This balancing moves into the fields of cost-benefit analysis, cost effectiveness, and medical decision analysis, which are beyond the scope of this chapter.

STATISTICAL CONCEPTS IMPORTANT FOR RISK

A few basic statistical concepts are critical when considering risk. First, *natural variation* in both exposures and responses exists in the population. For example, we are not surprised that there is a distribution of exposures in an occupational setting or that patients weighing 70 kg do not all have the same proportion of body fat. Thus, variability in responses (or probabilities of yes-no responses, e.g., CHD present / no CHD) may be linked to some intrinsic trait in a natural population. This is important for several risk assessment activities. For example, when studying the risk of exposure to a lipophilic chemical such as dioxin, adiposity will be an important factor because it is a predictor of the total amount of dioxin absorbed by an individual. Thus, a risk assessment of such a chemical should consider the variability of a measure of fat, such as the body mass index, in a population at risk.

Uncertainty plays an important role in risk assessment. Whereas variability is a characteristic of a trait in the population, uncertainty reflects our ignorance. We might say that BMI varies in a population; but uncertainty encompasses our ignorance about the form of the distribution of BMI in the population and the parameters that describe the distribution (e.g., mean, variance). Some researchers have described variability as a property of a system and uncertainty as a property of a researcher. So, how can data help to clarify these concepts? Additional data may allow for more precision when estimating population traits (i.e., less uncertainty), but it will not reduce variability (although variability may be better characterized with more data).

Understanding *conditional probability* is important when thinking about risk. Recall that probability can be conceptualized as a long-term relative frequency of occurrence of some event, and conditional probability can be thought of as the long-term relative frequency of the event in a subpopulation. For example, some populations may be at increased risk of adverse response, given exposure to some hazard—e.g., women with the BRCA1 gene are at higher risk of breast cancer than women without this gene. Another concern in risk assessment is that some specific exposure (say, to a pesticide) may be more likely to induce an adverse response (say, neurotoxicity) in children than in adults. This can be expressed by saying that the probability of a neurotoxic response in pesticide-exposed children is greater than the probability of a neurotoxic response in pesticide-exposed adults. As a final risk-related illustration, some xenobiotic may be innocuous but have a metabolite that is toxic. Individuals may vary in their ability to metabolize a chemical, so the risk of adverse response varies with metabolic capacity.

One more statistical concept important for risk is the problem of *unobservable outcomes.* "Censoring" is common in medical and risk research. The follow-up period of any study is often fixed, and frequently events of interests are not observed for some individuals before the study ends. For example, a worker exposed to asbestos may die from unrelated heart disease before an asbestos-related illness appears, or, a worker exposed 8 years ago may not have accumulated enough follow-up time to display an effect with an average 10-year lag between exposure and outcome. In addition, dropouts and other kinds of nonresponse are common in studies of human populations. Special statistical methods deal with some types of censoring (see Chapter 11). Nonresponse and other kinds of missing data, however, are always a statistical challenge, although newer, more-special-ized methods are being developed to address such problems. A related issue in research on risk is that the event of interest may not be observed because of some competing risk. For example, in an animal carcinogenicity study, an increase in incidence of tumors may not be observed because the animals die early from treatment-related toxicity. Finally, studies often include levels of clinically relevant exposure that lie below an instrument's limit of detection.

QUANTITATIVE RISK ESTIMATION ISSUES
(EXPOSURE-RESPONSE RELATIONSHIPS REVISITED)

Two strategies are commonly employed in quantitative risk assessment. For systemic or developmental toxins, a "margin of safety" approach historically was considered, whereas for carcinogens (for which even the smallest exposure was considered to cause a proportionately small risk, so that no safe level could exist—see Chapter 2), a regression-modeling approach was typically employed. The "margin of safety" approach involves identification of the highest dose that produced no observed effect in animal or human studies, defined as the no-observed-adverse-effect level (NOAEL), or sometimes the lowest dose that did produce adverse effects (LOAEL). A set of "uncertainty factors" is then applied, such as 10-fold reduction representing the uncertainty that the animal species may be less sensitive than humans, another 10-fold for the possibility that unexpected harm will arise later or in ways that have not been assessed, and still another 10-fold reflecting other issues such as severity of the response, ade-quacy of the database, or study length. These three factors multiplied together would lead to a human exposure limit of 1/1000 of the highest dose not found to cause problems in animals. The probability or size of risk at that point is not evaluated, but is generally assumed to be virtually zero. A problem with this approach is that increases in knowledge about harmful effects can only drive the NOAEL (and allowable exposures) downward. Criticism of the NOAEL has led to the development of a benchmark dose (BMD) method.[12] This method esti-mates the dose associated with some specified level of impact, say 5–10% above the response observed in a control group (the benchmark response). Because this added response level is not too small, this estimate should be similar for any of a number of plausible dose-response models. This helps address the fact that a variety of statistical models can be used to describe the dose-response relationship in the absence of some a priori (mechanistic, other) reason to select a particular model. A lower confidence limit on this dose, the BMDL, is calculated and substituted for the NOAEL in the margin of safety calculations. It is thought that exposures below this reference level convey negligible risk, although this is not proven.

Regression-based approaches fit a model to the data and then use it to estimate the dose associated with a specified level of response. These models assume a particular distribution for the response (e.g., a binomial for the number of people with CHD within a population of people with a particular risk-factor profile) and a specified structural form for how the response is related to the hazard of interest and other confounders (e.g., the logit of the response is related to a linear function of the factors). For example, in an animal tumorigencity experiment, the proportions of animals with liver cancer at several doses (including controls, at zero dose) may be used to estimate the risk added to background incidence by intermediate exposures. Public health interest often centers on exposures close to zero, and far below any of the exposures in the animal study, so that major assumptions are needed in order to extrapolate from the animal data to the human exposures of interest. In a validation study of risk scores for CHD, logistic regression was used to develop a CHD risk prediction from one cohort that was then applied to different cohort.[13] Brindle et al.[14] applied CHD risk scores from the Framingham cohort to British men.

UNCERTAINTY

Accurate estimation of most risks is not possible. One example is the carcinogenicity of saccharin in the human diet. Very high doses of saccharin cause bladder cancer in animals, but the biologic mechanisms may have little relevance for humans, and data from human studies are limited, imprecise, and uncertain because almost all saccharin users have also used other artificial sweeteners, which may have their own adverse effects. Another difficult situation occurs in the estimation of risks (such as from a chemical that is carcinogenic at high doses over a lifetime in small rodents) where humans are exposed intermittently to much lower levels of the hazard, and these individuals have been followed for a relatively short fraction of the usual human life span. Finally, exposure to other agents may modify effects associated with the hazard of concern. An example is the synergistic effect of smoking on those who consume alcoholic beverages as it relates to oral cavity cancers.[15] In such situations, understanding the combined impact of two risk factors may reduce uncertainty in risk estimation.

Other issues have become prominent as a result of genetic research (Chapters 19 and 20). As an example, suppose that some xenobiotic is not hazardous in its initial form, but is metabolized to a compound that is hazardous. (An example is vinyl chloride.) Further, suppose the population is polymorphic (some individuals are fast metabolizers, and others are slow metabolizers), and a high-throughput screening technology can identify the types. This relates to the challenge of how risk should be summarized. Can a single number be reported that will best characterize the risk to a population? If it is clear that the population is a mixture of highly susceptible individuals and non-susceptible individuals, then a single overall risk estimate may be nonsense because it does not apply to either group. Some other summary value, such as a percentile of the risk distribution or even stratum-specific risk estimates, may be more meaningful in this context.

NEXT STEPS

This short introduction aims to give a flavor of ideas encountered in risk assessment, including risks in a clinical setting. For more background on risk assessment, interested readers are encouraged to investigate specific books on risk assessment,[16] along with a number of National Research Council reports and government reports related to risk assessment, including exposure assessment, cancer risk assessment methods, probabilistic risk methods, and reproductive toxicity. For example, the web site of the U.S. Environmental Protection Agency's National Center for Environmental Assessment includes a page describing the agency's research in risk assessment, which has links to guidelines, a risk glossary, laws and regulations, and more (http://cfpub.epa.gov/ncea/cfm/nceariskassess.cfm?ActType=RiskAssess, accessed 02 January 2009).

The practice of risk assessment continues to evolve. New biological discoveries (e.g., the "omics" revolution—genomics, metabonomics, etc.) may inform risk assessment by providing insights into hazard exposures, earlier onset of disease, and the definition of different responses for use in risk assessment. In addition, the realization that hazards are rarely encountered in isolation of other stressors has led to calls for aggregative assessments and cumulative risk assessments that simultaneously consider multiple stressors (for both chemical stressors and non-chemical stressors, such as socioeconomic status).

A recent NRC report[17] reviews the history of risk assessment and considers how to improve the utility of risk assessments. This report provides a nice definition of risk assessment as an "important public policy tool for informing regulatory and technologic decisions, setting priorities among research needs, and developing approaches for considering costs and benefits of regulatory policies" (p. 3). The report also emphasizes the design of risk assessment to include a *problem formulation and scoping phase* prior to the four steps historically encountered. This phase would allow risk management options for potentially addressing a hazard to be considered early, so that the risk assessment will support "risk-based decision-making."

HOW MIGHT MEDICAL PROFESSIONALS BE INVOLVED IN THE RISK ASSESSMENT PROCESS?

There is a need for scientists with a broad understanding of the risk assessment process. In the United States, these individuals may support risk assessment activities in organizations that include the National Research Council or federal agencies such as the Environmental Protection Agency, the National Institute of Environmental Health Sciences, the Food and Drug Administration, the Consumer Product Safety Commission, the Occupational Safety and Health Administration, and the National Institute for Occupational Safety and Health. The process of establishing exposure limits involves scientific inquiry and policy and can trigger an extended and contentious debate (see, e.g., Stayner[18] and Monforton[19] for a discussion of issues associated with diesel exposure rulemaking).

Physicians and other medical professionals can and should contribute to the risk assessment process as clinicians (identifying problems, participating in clinical solutions) and as research investigators (estimating individual and population risks as well as conducting research studies needed for risk assessment).

ACKNOWLEDGMENTS

The authors thank Drs. William Halperin and Christine Sofge for their comments and suggestions on an earlier draft of this chapter.

REFERENCES

1. Bailar JC, Bailer AJ. Environment and health: 9. The science of risk assessment. CMAJ 2001; 164(4):503–6.

2. Grundy SM, Pasternak R, Greenland P, et al. Assessment of cardiovascular risk by use of multiple-risk-factor assessment equations: a statement for healthcare professionals from the American Heart Association and the American College of Cardiology. J Am Coll Cardiol 1999; 34:1348–59.

3. Sullivan LM, Massaro JM, D'Agostino RB. Presentation of multivariate data for clinical use: The Framingham Study risk score functions. Stat Med 2004; 23:1631–60.

4. D'Agostino RB Sr, Grundy S, Sullivan LM, Wilson P. Validation of the Framingham coronary heart disease prediction scores: results of a multiple ethnic groups investigation. JAMA 2001; 286:180–7.

5. Ridzon R, Gallagher K, Ciesielski C, et al. Simultaneous transmission of human immunodeficiency virus and hepatitis C virus from a needle-stick injury. N Engl J Med 1997; 336:919–22.

6. National Research Council. Committee on the Institutional Means for Assessment of Risks to Public Health. Risk assessment in the federal government: managing the process. Washington, DC: National Academy Press, 1983.

7. Parmet AJ, Von Essen S. Rapidly progressive, fixed airway obstructive disease in popcorn workers: a new occupational pulmonary illness? J Occup Environ Med 2002; 44:216–8.

8. Kreiss K, Gomaa A, Kullman G, et al. Clinical bronchiolitis obliterans in workers at a microwave-popcorn plant. N Engl J Med 2002; 347:330–8.

9. Cohrssen JJ, Covello VT. Risk analysis: a guide to principles and methods for analyzing health and environmental risks. Springfield, VA: National Technical Information Service, 1989.

10. Ellwein L, Cohen S. The health risks of saccharin revisited. Crit Rev Toxicol 1990; 20:311–26.

11. Slovic P. Perception of risk. Science 1987; 236(4799):280–5.

12. Crump K. A new method for determining allowable daily intakes. Fundam Appl Toxicol 1984; 4:854–71.

13. Thomsen TF, McGee D, Davidsen M, Jorgensen T. A cross-validation of risk-scores for coronary heart disease mortality based on data from the Glostrup population studies and Framingham Heart Study. Int J Epidemiol 2002; 31:817–22.

14. Brindle P, Emberson J, Lampe F, et al. Predictive accuracy of the Framingham coronary risk score in British men: prospective cohort study. Br Med J 2003; 327:1267–72.

15. Choi SY, Kahyo H. Effect of cigarette smoking and alcohol consumption in the aetiology of cancer of the oral cavity, pharynx and larynx. Int J Epidemiol 1991; 20:878–85.

16. Rodricks J. Calculated risks: the toxicity and human health risks of chemicals in our environment. 2nd ed. Cambridge, UK: Cambridge University Press, 2007.

17. National Research Council. Committee on Improving Risk Analysis Approaches Used by the U.S. Environmental Protection Agency. Science and decisions: advancing risk assessment. Washington, DC: National Academy Press, 2009.

18. Stayner LT. Protecting public health in the face of uncertain risks: the example of diesel exhaust. Am J Public Health 1999; 89:991–3.

19. Monforton C. Weight of the evidence or wait for the evidence? Protecting underground miners from diesel particulate matter. Am J Public Health 2006; 96:271–6.

Index